Case Studies in Global School Health Promotion

Cheryl Vince Whitman • Carmen E. Aldinger

Editors

Case Studies in Global School Health Promotion

From Research to Practice

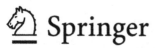 Springer

Editors

Ms. Cheryl Vince Whitman
Education Development Center, Inc
Health and Human Development
  Programs
55 Chapel St.
Newton MA 02458
USA
cvincewhitman@edc.org

Dr. Carmen E. Aldinger
Education Development Center, Inc
Health and Human Development
  Programs
55 Chapel St.
Newton MA 02458
USA
caldinger@edc.org

ISBN   978-1-4419-2827-6   e-ISBN   978-0-387-92269-0
DOI: 10.1007/978-0-387-92269-0

Printed on acid-free paper

Springer is part of Springer Science+Business Media (www.springer.com)

This book is dedicated to Mr. Jack T. Jones – inspiring mentor and colleague, and devoted public servant. Mr. Jones dedicated his professional efforts to advance health promotion through schools, to improve the lives of students, teachers, and families around the world.

In 1991, Mr. Jones, a Public Health Adviser at U.S. Centers for Disease Control and Prevention (CDC), was seconded by CDC's Division of Adolescent and School Health to the World Health Organization, where he served to promote the implementation and improvement of school health programs until his retirement in 2005. Under his leadership, the Global School Health Initiative was launched in 1995. Prior to his secondment, he was responsible for designing and developing new nationwide public health programs in collaboration with national, state, and local agencies. Today, Mr. Jones and his wife spend their days meandering the byways of France and the United States, searching for goodness and sharing it with friends.

Acknowledgments

Throughout the past decade, key people at the World Health Organization (WHO) and other agencies provided the leadership and advocacy to promote health through school settings. We thank Dr. Ilona Kickbusch, Dr. Desmond O'Byrne, Dr. Pekka Puska, and Mr. Jack Jones from WHO; Dr. Maria Teresa Cerqueira from the Pan-American Health Organization; Dr. Lloyd Kolbe, Mr. Charles Gollmar, and Dr. Laura Kahn from the U.S. Centers for Disease Control and Prevention; and our FRESH partners Ms. Anna Maria Hoffmann, Dr. Amaya Gillespie, Dr. Donald Bundy, and Dr. Lesley Drake.

We acknowledge Dr. Kwok-Cho Tang for taking the initiative, under the leadership of Dr. Robert Beaglehole, to organize the WHO Technical Meeting, "Building School Partnerships for Health, Education Achievements and Development," in Vancouver, Canada, 5–8 June 2007, for which we collected and analyzed an initial set of school health case studies, which we expanded upon in this book.

We sincerely thank all of the case study authors for contributing their time to write and revise the cases and share with us their experiences and lessons learned. And we genuinely thank the leadership of the thousands of schools reported about in all of the cases, their students, parents, and communities, for taking active part in the school health programs around the world.

Last, but not least, we want to thank those who helped us analyzing the cases and editing the book manuscript: Elizabeth Magner, Ian McManus, Matthew Biewener, and Nanni Feurzeig.

Contents

Europe

Eastern Mediterranean

Contributors

Sean B.A. Abrahams
Kleinskool Community School, Port Elizabeth, South Africa

Carmen Aldinger
Health and Human Development Programs, Education Development Center, Newton, MA, USA

Mariam Al Mulla Al Harmas Al Hajeri
Ministry of Health, Manama, Bahrain

Mariam Al Matroushi
Ministry of Health, Abu Dhabi, United Arab Emirates

Lulwa Abd Al Aziz Al Thukair
Ministry of Health, Manama, Bahrain

Laurie Bechhofer
Coordinated School Health and Safety Programs Unit, Grants Coordination and School Support, Michigan Department of Education, Lansing, MI, USA

Sheila R. Bonito
University of the Philippines Open University, Los Baños, Laguna, Philippines

Gourdas Choudhuri
Sanjay Gandhi Postgraduate Institute of Medical Sciences, Lucknow, India

Odete Moises Cossa
World Health Organization, African Region, Harare, Zimbabwe

Bruce P. Damons
Sapphire Road Primary School, Port Elizabeth, South Africa

Carlos da Silva
Rio de Janeiro Municipal Health Secretariat, Rio de Janeiro, Brazil

Elton D'Souza
La Martiniere College, Lucknow, India

Le Thi Kim Dung
Ministry of Training and Education, Hanoi, Vietnam

Barbara Flis
Parent Action for Healthy Kids, Farmington Hills, MI, USA

Ly Foung
Department of Secondary Education, Ministry of Education, Vientiane Capital,
Lao PDR

Debi Futter
Ministry of Education, Rarotonga, Cook Islands

Uday Chand Ghoshal
Sanjay Gandhi Postgraduate Institute of Medical Sciences, Lucknow, India

Kyle Guerrant
Coordinated School Health & Safety Programs Unit, Grants Coordination & School
Support, Michigan Department of Education, Lansing, MI, USA

Sahar Abdou Helmi
Ministry of Health, Muscat, Oman

Le Thi Thu Hien
Department of Preventive Medicine, Ministry of Health, Hanoi, Vietnam

Bjarne Bruun Jensen
Danish School of Education, University of Aarhus, Copenhagen, Denmark

Kimberly Kovalchick
Coordinated School Health and Safety Programs Unit, Grants Coordination and
School Support, Department of Education, Lansing, MI, USA

Yvette Laforêt-Fliesser
Family Health Services, Middlesex-London Health Unit, and School of Nursing,
University of Western Ontario, London, ON, Canada

Daniel Lang'o
Center for Research and Strategic Development, Nairobi, Kenya

Albert Lee
Department of Community & Family Medicine, Division of Health Improvement,
School of Public Health, The Chinese University of Hong Kong (CUHK), Shatin,
N.T., Hong Kong, China

Anne Lee
NHS Health Scotland, Glasgow, UK

Kelly K.S. Leow
Tertiary Institution Outreach Department, Health Promotion Board, Singapore

Wong Mun Loke
Youth Health Program Development and Tertiary Institution Outreach Department,
Health Promotion Board, Singapore

Nguyen Hung Lon
Ministry of Health, Hanoi, Vietnam

Anyoli Sanabria López
UNICEF, Managua, Nicaragua

Carol MacDougall
School and Sexual Health, Perth District Health Unit, Stratford, ON, Canada

Danielle Maloney
Clinical Services and Integration Manager, Central Sydney Division of General
Practice, Sydney, NSW, Australia

Bernie Marshall
Health Promotion, School of Health Sciences, Deakin University, Burwood, VIC,
Australia

Sergio Meresman
CLAEH (Latin American Centre for Humane Economy), UNER (University of
Entre Rios), Montevideo, Uruguay

Ali Jaffer Mohamed
Ministry of Health, Muscat, Oman

Bui Phuong Nga
Ministry of Training and Education, Hanoi, Vietnam

Nguyen Huy Nga
Ministry of Health, Hanoi, Vietnam

Olusola Odujinrin
World Health Organization, Abuja, Nigeria

Washington Onyango-Ouma
Institute of Anthropology, Gender and African Studies, University of Nairobi,
Nairobi, Kenya

Avamar Pantoja
Popular Opera Center Acari, Río de Janeiro, Brazil

Peter Paulus
Institute for Psychology, Center of Applied Sciences of Health (CASH), and
MPH Program Prevention and Health Promotion, Leuphana University Lueneburg,
Lueneburg, Germany

Khatthanaphone Phandouangsy
Hygiene and Prevention Department, Ministry of Health, Vientiane Capital,
Lao PDR

Nayara Sarhan
Ministry of Health, Manama, Bahrain

Margaret Sheehan
World Health Organization, Hanoi, Vietnam

Maria Sokolowska
Methodical Centre of Psycho-Pedagogical Assistance, Warsaw, Poland

Phoungkham Somsanith
Research Institute for Education and Sciences, Ministry of Education, Vientiane
Capital, Lao PDR

Ardita Tahirukaj
World Health Organization, Pristina, Kosovo

Rose Vaithinathan
Youth Health Division, Health Promotion Board, Singapore

Raman Velayudhan
World Health Organization, Manila, Philippines

Patricia Warner
Ministry of Education, Bridgetown, Barbados

Lurenda S. Westergaard
University of the Philippines Open University, Los Baños, Laguna, Philippines

Cheryl Vince Whitman
Health and Human Development Programs, Education Development Center,
Newton, MA, USA

Barbara Woynarowska
Department of Biomedical Aspects of Development and Education, Faculty
of Pedagogy, Warsaw University, Warsaw, Poland

Cheong-Lim Lee Yee
Pre-school and Primary School Outreach Department, Health Promotion Board,
Singapore

Ian M. Young
Health Promotion consultant, Edinburgh, Scotland, UK

Section I
Introduction and Overview of Findings

Chapter 1
Introduction and Background

Cheryl Vince Whitman and Carmen Aldinger

Evolution of the Health-Promoting School Concept

Addressing the health of children in schools is not a new practice. Throughout the twentieth century and even earlier, many schools have found ways to provide health education and health services to the young people they reach. What have been new are a more holistic definition of health and the deliberate application of a public health approach to promote health in the school setting. The founders of the World Health Organization (WHO) defined health as "a state of complete physical, mental and social well-being and not merely the absence of disease or infirmity," further recognizing that "the enjoyment of the highest attainable standard of health is one of the fundamental rights of every human being" (World Health Organization [WHO], 1948).

The drive to apply public health strategies more deliberately in the education sector gained strength from the declarations made in WHO's Ottawa Charter of Health Promotion, 1986, which integrated ideas about health promotion from Canada and from WHO's European office (Young, 2005). The charter stated that "health is created and lived by people within the settings of their everyday life: where they learn, work, play and love. Health is created by caring for oneself and others, by being able to make decisions and have control over one's life and circumstances, and by ensuring that the society one lives in creates conditions that allow the attainment of health by all its members" (WHO, 1986).

Clearly, schools and educational agencies at all levels – national, state, and local – are settings where young people learn, play, and love, where adults work, and where families gather and participate in support of educational and community activities. WHO's application of these principles of the Ottawa Charter to schools became known as the concept of the *Health-Promoting School* (HPS).

This book reviews briefly the evolution of the HPS concept and its relationship to similar concepts of other United Nations agencies. Using highlights of research

C. Vince Whitman(✉)
Health and Human Development Programs, Education Development Center, Newton, MA, USA

C. Vince Whitman and C.E. Aldinger (eds.),
Case Studies in Global School Health Promotion: From Research to Practice,
DOI: 10.1007/978-0-387-92269-0_1, © Springer Science + Business Media, LLC 2009

on implementation and case studies from around the world, we see how people working in many different conditions have put the concept into practice. Their experiences come alive and we learn from them about the many methods and strategies used.

Not long after the Ottawa Charter was written, the Scottish Health Education Group, a collaborating center for WHO (European Office), assembled 150 delegates from 28 Member States at Peebles in Scotland. At this symposium, participants developed the concept of the HPS (Young, 1986). The original model consisted of three main elements: curriculum, school ethos and environment, and health and caring services.

From 1986 to the present, the HPS concept has been implemented throughout Europe, organized under the European Network of Health-Promoting Schools, with technical support provided originally by the WHO European Regional Office, until 2007. The Dutch Institute for Health Promotion and Disease Prevention (NIGZ), a WHO Collaborating Center, has now assumed responsibility for the network and changed its name to *Schools for Health in Europe* (SHE Network, n.d.).

About the same time, a similar concept, titled a *Coordinated School Health Program*, was developed in the USA. Its definition added elements, including, for example, school health promotion programs for staff and integrated school and community health promotion efforts (Allensworth & Kolbe, 1987; Kolbe, 1986). Over time, the original concept has undergone some changes but continues to be implemented by the US Centers for Disease Control and Prevention's Coordinated School Health Program (National Center for Chronic Disease Prevention and Health Promotion, n.d.). Other national government agencies in the USA have programs with similar elements. The Safe Schools/Healthy Students initiative, coordinated by the Substance Abuse and Mental Health Services Administration, is carried out on behalf of three federal agencies: the coordinator along with US Department of Education and The Office of Juvenile Justice and Delinquency Prevention (National Center for Mental Health Promotion and Youth Violence Prevention, n.d.).

In September 1995, WHO, with support from the US Centers for Disease Control and Prevention, held an Expert Committee Meeting on Comprehensive School Health Education and Promotion in Geneva, Switzerland, "to encourage educational and health institutions and agencies to coordinate their efforts to promote health through schools" (WHO, 1997, p. 1). More than a decade after the Ottawa Charter, building on the experience of Europe and North America, WHO led a movement to expand the concepts globally. The Expert Committee reviewed trends and research in school health as well as barriers and strategies, and concluded with a call to action. The Expert Committee urged all people to imagine:

a future in which schools in every nation have the healthy development of all young people as an essential part of their core mission; a world where schools take on this challenge and implement new and exciting ways to coordinate the educational process, the environmental conditions within and outside the school, and the range of available health services, in order to enhance the educational achievement and health of young people.

WHO, 1997, p. 83

Subsequently, WHO launched its Global School Health Initiative with the goal "to increase the number of schools that can truly be called 'Health-Promoting Schools'" (WHO, 1998). WHO defined a HPS, illustrated in Fig. 1, as one that:

- Fosters health and learning with all the measures at its disposal
- Engages health and education officials, teachers, teachers' unions, students, parents, health providers, and community leaders in efforts to make the school a healthy place
- Strives to provide (1) a healthy environment, (2) school health education, and (3) school health services, along with (4) school/community projects and outreach, (5) health promotion programs for staff, (6) nutrition and food safety programs, (7) opportunities for physical education and recreation, and (8) programs for counseling, social support, and mental health promotion
- Implements policies and practices that respect an individual's well-being and dignity, provides multiple opportunities for success, and acknowledges good efforts and intentions as well as personal achievements
- Strives to improve the health of school personnel, families, and community members as well as pupils; and works with community leaders to help them understand how the community contributes to, or undermines, health and education (adapted from WHO, 1998)

Since the Global School Health Initiative began in the mid-1990s, WHO has provided leadership and many services to countries to support dissemination of the HPS concept and implementation of policies and programs. With its regional

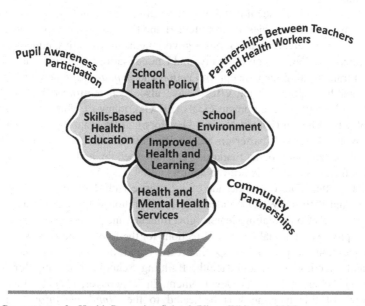

Fig. 1 Components of a Health-Promoting School (Vince Whitman, 2005)

offices and collaborating centers, WHO has prepared international guidelines and policy documents, created publications that synthesize the evidence about effective programs and strategies to address a range of health issues in schools, piloted tools for assessment and implementation, and provided in-country technical assistance to put the concept into action.

Parallel movements in education – such as *Education for All*, spearheaded by UNESCO – promoted the important link between health and education. In Jomtien, Thailand (March 1990), UNESCO's *World Conference on Education for All: Meeting Basic Learning Needs* addressed the key issues of health and nutrition as important contributors to the success of both the learner and the learning process. For the tenth anniversary of Jomtien, UNESCO and WHO joined together to prepare a 10-year retrospective of accomplishments, *Thematic Study: School Health and Nutrition* (Vince Whitman, Aldinger, Levinger, & Birdthistle, 2001). Presented and discussed at the World Education Forum in Dakar, Senegal, April 2000, the report served as a catalyst to unite United Nations agencies around the basic elements common to the models of each, under the overarching umbrella of FRESH (Focusing Resources on Effective School Health). Individual UN agencies did not give up the unique names of their own programs, but all agreed to promote and use the common elements – school health policies; skills-based health education; provision of water and sanitation – as a start for a healthy physical and psychosocial school environment and health and nutrition services. Thus, implementations of school health programs may be known by names other than the Health-Promoting School, but they still embody the same core elements of policy, skills-based health education, services, and a healthy psychosocial and physical environment.

Since the launch of the Global School Health Initiative more than a decade ago and the unity of UN agencies around FRESH and the common components of their models, many different organizations – governments, universities, nongovernmental organizations (NGOs), civil society, and United Nations agencies – have played a role in transforming the concept into action and *implementing* new or improved school health programs. Their efforts have also been reinforced by the United Nations Millennium Development Goals (MDGs), many of which align with the goals of school health (United Nations Development Programme, n.d.). The more recent WHO Bangkok Charter on Health Promotion in a Globalized World discussed globalization, product marketing to young people, and increased migration as new influences that HPSs need to address (WHO, 2005).

In 2007, after more than a decade of experience with the Global School Health Initiative and FRESH, WHO decided – in collaboration with other United Nations Agencies, WHO Collaborating Centers, governments, and professional associations – to assess progress and establish new directions for the future. The process involved the preparation of papers on specific tracks and the convening of a WHO Technical Meeting on School Health, Building School Partnership for Health, Education Achievements and Development, in Vancouver, Canada, June 2007. One track of this meeting was dedicated to the "*Implementation* of Health-Promoting School and other School Community Programs" (WHO, 2007).

The authors of the track on implementation (and of this book) are from the WHO Collaborating Center to Promote Health through Schools and Communities at EDC's division of Health and Human Development Programs. We synthesized the research on effective implementation strategies and searched worldwide for cases that illustrate how nations and local schools moved the concept into action. Given conference participants' interest in implementation and the utility of the case studies for the purpose of this book, we gathered additional case studies from various regions of the world. Our hope is that these cases, framed in the context of the research on diffusion and implementation, will inform policy makers, administrators, and decision makers about the many different approaches to implementation.

For the HPS concept to be promoted and accepted over the decade, it was necessary and advantageous to draw on the growing base of research and evaluation evidence about the link between all aspects of health and learning and academic performance. It was also important to synthesize from worldwide literature the effectiveness of various health promotion, prevention, and intervention strategies for schools and communities to address specific health conditions. As a foundation for the widespread dissemination of the HPS concept, we offer highlights from this research base.

Evidence of Effectiveness

The global movement to advance the HPS and related research made many contributions to the evidence base. Many organizations contributed to synthesizing and disseminating available research and to conducting new research and evaluation of intervention effectiveness. The evidence base generated over the last two decades advances the field's understanding of the link between education and health and of the effectiveness of policies, programs, and strategies to address health issues in school and community settings. Highlights follow.

The Reciprocal Link Between Health and Education

Research over many years has shown a reciprocal relationship between health and education: Improvements in education and features of the school as a learning environment are associated with improvements in health, and improvements in health status contribute to improvements in learning and academic outcomes. Studies in developed and developing countries alike have repeatedly shown that educated and literate people are likely to be healthier. Conversely, limited access to education has been linked to reduced health and well-being

(Nutbeam & Kickbusch, 2000). And poor quality or negative features of the school as a learning environment can negatively affect student and staff health and well-being (Awartani, Vince Whitman, & Gordon, 2008).

Relationships between *health status and educational outcomes* have been summarized in a recent publication by Jukes, Drake, & Bundy (2008). Poor health status is associated with lower school enrollment and performance. For example, children with low birth weight have poor cognitive development; stunting in early childhood has long-term effects on primary school enrollment, as stunted children enroll later in school than other children; undernutrition affects many aspects of brain development and behavioral development; iodine and folate deficiencies can lead to severe mental and physical disability; meningitis leads to severe cognitive impairment; parental infection with HIV and AIDS leads to absenteeism; and children with HIV infection perform poorly at school. Studies have also shown that food-insufficient children are more likely to receive lower math scores, repeat a grade, visit a psychologist, and have difficulty in getting along with other children (Alaimo, Olson, & Frongillo, 2001).

In addition to these more apparent and severe situations, Hough writes about what happens when these and other "louder" issues drown out attention to the quieter health problems, which often go undetected: hearing and vision problems, dental problems, anxiety, and depression. In the USA "an estimated 25 percent of students in urban schools have undetected vision problems," making "it hard for a first- or second-grader to read" (Hough, 2008, p. 28). Failure to read often leads to the child's placement in special education programs, which can be permanent (Hough, 2008).

Importantly, research has shown how improvements in health status, often delivered through schools, can lead to improved educational outcomes. For instance, malaria prevention in early childhood increases school enrollment and attendance, and school-based malaria prevention improves educational achievement. Deworming improves school attendance and the potential to learn. School feeding programs improve primary school attendance and have some modest effects on educational achievement. Preventing nutritional deficiencies promotes cognitive development; nutritional supplements and psychosocial stimulation help reverse cognitive delays (Jukes et al., 2008). Studies have also shown that physical activity is positively associated with academic performance and reduced dropout (Action for Healthy Kids, 2004; Dwyer, Blizzard, & Dean, 1996; Mahoney & Cairns, 1997; Shephard, 1997).

Girls and women, in particular, benefit significantly from the health benefits of education. Over the years, many studies – especially those from developing countries – have linked education to improved health and well-being for women, their children, and their society (e.g., Arya & Devi, 1991; Bledsoe, Casterline, Jonson-Kuhn, & Haaga, 1999; Buckshee, 1997; Caldwell, 1986; Das Gupta, 1990; Gupta, Mehrotra, Arora, & Saran, 1991; Harrison, 1997; Nussbaum, 2000; Sen, 1999). Reviews of research from around the world have shown that educated girls are healthier and more able to participate in earning income. When they become mothers, educated girls are better able to care for their children. The single most important predictor of a child's health is the mother's level of education. Education can strengthen women's ability to create healthy households, to benefit from health information, and to make good use of health services (Filmer, 1999; WHO, 1997).

A recent report, *What Works in Girls' Education: Evidence and Policies from the Developing World* (Herz & Sperling, 2004), brings together the vast scholarly literature on the benefits of girls' education. Many studies in this report show that education of girls is associated with various benefits: increased income and productivity, including farming that is more productive; healthier and better-educated families; HIV/AIDS prevention; women's empowerment, including reduced domestic violence and genital cutting; and more resources to spend on the health and education of their families.

Research also shows how many features of the school environment included in Fig. 1 – instruction, ethos, and availability of services – affect health status and learning. One of the most important conditions for learning is the school's psychosocial environment and whether or not students feel connected and part of a caring community. When students feel that they are part of the school, say they are treated fairly by teachers, and feel close to people at school, they are healthier, less likely to engage in risk behaviors, and more likely to succeed (Blum, McNeeley, & Rinehart, 2002). When students enjoy good social-emotional health, dropout and nonattendance rates are lower. There are improvements in grades, standardized test scores, and graduation rates, and improved reading, math, and writing skills (Zins, Bloodworth, Weissberg, & Walberg, 2004).

Other ways in which features of the school learning environment can positively or negatively affect health and well-being include the nature of the pedagogy, relevance of the curriculum content, and attentiveness to each child's unique attitudes and ways of learning. These features can either engage and inspire young people to stay in school and learn, or they can disaffect and alienate them, contributing to dropout, without the necessary skills to cope and succeed in life (Awartani et al., 2008).

Effectiveness of Various School-Based Intervention Strategies

Over the last two decades, many experiments to address specific health issues through schools have taken place. This research has shown that school-based health interventions, for many of the components of Fig. 1, both separately and together, can improve health and educational outcomes. Most importantly, research has shown the effectiveness of a whole-school approach that combines strategies across components to make a powerful difference (Blum et al., 2002; Lister-Sharp, Chapman, Stewart-Brown, & Sowden, 1999; Patton et al., 2006; Stewart-Brown, 2006; West, Sweeting, & Leyland, 2004). For instance, a 2006 meta-analysis that looked at the evidence of school-wide health promotion in improving health or preventing disease and especially at the effectiveness of the HPS approach found that programs that "were effective in changing young people's health or health-related behavior were more likely to be complex, multi-factoral and involve activity in more than one domain (curriculum, school environment and community)" (Stewart-Brown, 2006, p. 17). Having endorsed the HPS approach, this meta-analysis also pointed to the major benefit of addressing social-emotional and mental health through schools. These benefits were observed to be particularly pronounced when the approach included "involvement of the whole school, changes to the school psychosocial environment, personal skill development, involvement of parents and the wider community, and implementation over a long period of time" (Stewart-Brown, 2006, p. 16).

Many other studies examine the effectiveness of one or more components, such as health education and services to address one or more topics. For instance, the *Thematic Study on School Health and Nutrition*, discussed earlier, presents examples of the evidence of effectiveness of individual school-based interventions that may be combined to address a variety of health problems including safe water and sanitation, helminth infections, and nutrition, as well as lifestyle behaviors associated with STDs, HIV/AIDS, and the use of alcohol, tobacco, and other drugs (Vince Whitman et al., 2001). Since research has shown that half of all lifetime mental health disorders begin during adolescence, early identification and intervention can prevent and reduce years of suffering and harm (Kessler et al., 2007). Often, such identification is possible within the school environment where behavioral or conduct disorders become evident (Ghuman, Weist, & Sarles, 2002). Schools then are in a crucial position to influence the mental health status of millions of children. Research shows that health promotion in schools is strongest when the prevention and treatment of mental health problems are considered central to the approach (Vince Whitman, Aldinger, Zhang, & Magner, 2008).

In terms of the health education component, many studies have shown that students who participate in health education classes utilizing skills-based, participatory curricula decrease risky behaviors relative to the program (Botvin, Griffin, Diaz, & Ifill-Williams, 2001; Skara & Sussman, 2003; WHO, 2003).

A recent publication by leading researchers in school health (St. Leger, Kolbe, Lee, McCall, & Young, 2007) cites evidence of meta-analyses from published evaluations of school health initiatives for the following:

- Nutrition (Blum et al., 2002; Lister-Sharp et al., 1999; Patton et al., 2006; Stewart-Brown, 2006; West et al., 2004)
- Physical activity (Dobbins et al., 2001; Timperio, Salmon, & Ball, 2004)
- Sexuality (Kirby, 2002; Silva, 2002)
- Drugs (Lloyd, Joyce, Hurry, & Ashton, 2000; Midford, Lenton, & Hancock, 2000; National Drug Research Institute, 2002; Tobler & Stratton, 1997)
- Mental health (American Counselling Association, 2006; Browne, Gafni, Roberts, Byrne, & Majumdar, 2004; Green, Howes, Waters, Maher, & Oberklaid, 2005; Wells, Barlow, & Stewart-Brown, 2003)

In June 2007, WHO convened school health experts from around the world in a direction-setting technical meeting. Participants reviewed the evidence of school-based interventions from the past two decades and issued a call for action that includes an appeal to implement what we know to be effective and to foster the collaboration required for implementation (Tang, Nutbeam, & Aldinger, 2009). This book is one response to that call; many participants from the technical meeting contributed case studies.

Purpose of This Book

After all the efforts to invent and disseminate the HPS concept, what happened? Did governments and local schools and communities and universities put the idea into practice? How and what steps did they take and with what results? What factors influenced their process?

Our purpose in writing this book was to find examples from all regions of the world to illustrate strategies that people used to apply the concept at the national and local levels. With assistance from WHO headquarters and WHO Regional Offices, as well as the authors' networks, key people from around the world were recruited to prepare case studies about the implementation of the HPS concept. The aim was to find examples at different levels: individual school(s) or greater provincial or national scale. We identified writers and researchers from universities, ministries of education, schools, NGOs, and UN agencies. They prepared case studies, describing what took place in the context of the theory and research on factors affecting implementation. Analysis of the cases offers many insights into the feasibility of applying the HPS concept: across the spectrum of resource-rich and resource-poor situations; in different cultures; in urban and rural schools; and as a response to particular health, economic, social, or education challenges.

In preparing for WHO's Technical Meeting on School Health in Vancouver, described earlier, and writing the background paper to address Track 2 on Implementation, the authors originally collected and analyzed 17 case studies from every WHO region of the world. Given the usefulness of the cases to conference participants, we increased the number from 17 to 26. The objectives of the case analysis are to:

- Understand how the public health approach was applied to schools
- Provide learnings to accelerate and strengthen future efforts to implement school health programs
- Foster a learning community among the many players who have invested or who want to invest in or implement school health programs
- Provide guidance to WHO, FRESH partners, and countries as they shape a vision for school health toward 2015 and beyond

Methods

We conducted an extensive review of the literature on implementation research, diffusion of innovation, and education reform, using numerous databases such as

ERIC, PubMed, PsychINFO, LexisNexis, ISI Web of Knowledge, and Google
Scholar.

This review provided findings about effective implementation strategies and
informed revisions to the organizing framework, *The Wheel of Factors Influencing
Policy and Practice Change*, illustrated in Fig. 1 (under the section "Theory and
Research on Implementation" in the chapter "Framing Theories and Implementation Research"). Discussed in detail later, these factors include, for example, vision
and concept, international and national guidelines, leadership, resources, stakeholder ownership and participation, mechanisms for cross-sector collaboration, and
stage of readiness (Vince Whitman, 2005). The factors in the wheel provided the
main criteria for coding and analyzing strategies in the cases used to implement the
HPS or similar concept.

Each author of a case study was asked to address:

- Contextual background of the country situation

  - Brief introduction to the country (e.g., political system, demographics,
    educational mission and goals)
  - Social and economic indicators
  - Impetus, origin, leadership of how the HPS concept began
  - Level (e.g., national, regional, school; and primary, secondary, tertiary)

- Overview of the school health program, its impact and results

  - Date boundaries (e.g., when started, ongoing)
  - Key cast of players/agencies
  - Reach (e.g., how many schools/students reached, for implementation; in-
    crease in numbers from what to what)
  - Scope of implementation (which components or program elements were
    implemented)
  - Summary of achievements and impact (e.g., pre/post)

- Specific processes and activities in the implementation process

  - Select 3–4 strategies or methods of implementation (see Fig. 1 in the chapter
    "Framing Theories and Implementation Research") that are well-developed
    and/or unique

- Conclusion and insights

  - Recommendations and lessons learned concerning implementation

We reviewed the initial outlines and drafts of the case studies and provided
comments to case study authors consistent with the outline format (earlier), in
many cases encouraging them to elaborate on specific aspects of implementation.
Prior to the Vancouver meeting, case study authors exchanged cases with each
other to share their learnings.

Sample

Table 1 lists the regions, countries, and authors for all 26 cases.

Once we received the revised case studies, we read them thoroughly and performed an initial edit to improve readability and structure. Then we coded each case study according to the factors in the Wheel of Factors, introduced earlier. Additional codes were created for aspects of implementation that were discussed in the case studies, but were not part of the Wheel, such as advocacy, communications, infrastructure, monitoring and evaluation, and sustainability.

Table 1 List of case studies by regions

Region	Country	Author(s)
Africa	Kenya	W. Onyango-Ouma, D. Lang'o, and B. B. Jensen
	Mauritius	Odete Moises Cossa
	Nigeria	Olusola Odujinrin
	South Africa	Bruce Damons and Sean Abrahams
The Americas	Barbados	Patricia Warner
	Brazil	Sergio Meresman, Avamar Pantoja, and Carlos da Silva
	Canada	Carol MacDougall and Yvette Laforêt-Fliesser
	Nicaragua	Sergio Meresman and Anyoli Sanabria López
	United States of America	Laurie Bechhofer, Barbara Flis, Kyle Guerrant, and Kimberly Kovalchick
	Uruguay	Sergio Meresman
Europe	Germany	Peter Paulus
	Kosovo	Ian Young and Ardita Tahirukaj
	Poland	Barbara Woynarowska and Maria Sokolowska
	Scotland	Ian Young and Anne Lee
Eastern Mediterranean	Bahrain	Mariam AlMulla Al Harmas Al Hajeri, Lulwa Abd Al Aziz Al Thukair, and Nayara Sarhan
	Oman	Ali Jaffer Mohamed and Sahar Abdou Helmi
	United Arab Emirates	Mariam Al Matroushi
South and Southeast Asia	China (Zhejiang Province)	Carmen Aldinger
	Hong Kong	Albert Lee
	India	Gourdas Choudhuri, Uday Chand Ghoshal, and Elton D'Souza
	Lao PDR	Ly Foung, S. Phoungkham, and P. Khatthanaphone
	Philippines	Sheila R. Bonito, Lurenda S. Westergaard, and Raman Velayudhan
	Singapore	Rose Vaithinathan, Cheong-Lim Lee Yee, Wong Mun Loke, and Kelly Leow
	Viet Nam	Bui Phuong Nga, Le Thi Kim Dung, Le Thi Thu Hien, Bernie Marshall, Nguyen Hung Lon, Nguyen Huy Nga, and Margaret Sheehan
Western Pacific	Australia	Danielle Maloney
	Cook Islands	Debi Futter

We entered the case studies into the Atlas.ti 5.2 qualitative data management program with the assigned codes given to various sections of the case studies. The two authors of this book rated cases independently. We then exchanged cases to assess interrater reliability. From Atlas.ti, we created output by codes (which listed all sections of case studies that were coded to each particular code), and by frequency table (which listed how many times each code has been coded).

From this output, we synthesized key findings and wrote the analysis section. Case study authors reviewed their final material, which had gone through several phases of editorial review.

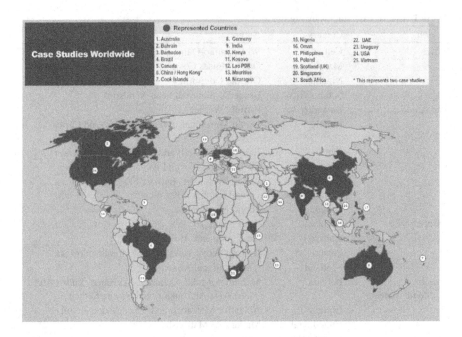

References

Action for Healthy Kids. (2004). *The learning connection: The value of improving nutrition and physical activity in our schools*. Retrieved August 27, 2008, from http://www.actionforhealthy-kids.org/pdf/LC_Color_120204_final.pdf

Alaimo, K., Olson, C. M., & Frongillo, E. A., Jr. (2001). Food insufficiency and American school-aged children's cognitive, academic, and psychosocial development. *Pediatrics, 108*(1), 44–53.

Allensworth, D.D., & Kolbe, L. J. (1987). The comprehensive school health program: Exploring an expanded concept. *Journal of School Health, 57*(10), 409–412.

American Counselling Association. (2006). *Effectiveness of school counselling*. Retrieved August 26, 2008, from http://www.counseling.org/Files/FD.ashx?guid = a60af1ec-e823-4418-b0fe-123d7af5d573

Arya, A., & Devi, R. (1991). Influence of maternal literacy on the nutritional status of preschool children. *Indian Journal of Paediatrics, 58*, 265–268.

Awartani, M., Vince Whitman, C., & Gordon, J. (2008). Developing instruments to capture young people's perceptions of how school as a learning environment affects their well-being. *European Journal of Education, 43*(1), 51–70.

Bledsoe, C. H., Casterline, J. B., Jonson-Kuhn, J. A., & Haaga, J. G. (1999). *Critical perspectives on schooling and fertility in the developing world.* Washington, DC: National Academy Press.

Blum, R., McNeeley, C., & Rinehart, P. (2002). *Improving the odds: The untapped power of schools to improve the health of teens.* Minneapolis, MN: Office of Adolescent Health.

Botvin, G. J., Griffin, K. W., Diaz, T., & Ifill-Williams, M. (2001). Preventing binge drinking during early adolescence: One- and two-year follow-up of a school-based preventive intervention. *Psychology of Addictive Behaviors, 15*(4), 360–365.

Browne, G., Gafni, A., Roberts, J., Byrne, C., & Majumdar, B. (2004). Effective/efficient mental health programs for school-age children: A synthesis of reviews. *Social Science and Medicine, 58*(7), 1367–1384.

Buckshee, K. (1997). Impact of roles of women on health in India. *International Journal of Gynecology & Obstetrics, 58,* 35–42.

Caldwell, J. C. (1986). Routes to low mortality in poor countries. *Population and Development, 12,* 171–220.

Dobbins, M., Lockett, D., Michel, I., Beyers, J., Feldman, L., Vohra, J., et al. (2001). *The effectiveness of school-based interventions in promoting physical activity and fitness among children and youth: A systematic review.* Ontario: McMaster University.

Dwyer, T., Blizzard, L., & Dean, K. (1996). Physical activity and performance in children. *Nutritional Review, 4*(2), 27–31.

Filmer, D. (1999). *The structure of social disparities in education: Gender and wealth. Policy research report on gender and development. Working paper no. 5.* Washington, DC: World Bank.

Ghuman, H. S., Weist, M. D., & Sarles, R. M. (2002). *Providing mental health services to youth where they are: School and community based approaches.* New York: Routledge.

Green, J., Howes, F., Waters, E., Maher, E., & Oberklaid, F. (2005). Promoting the social and emotional health of primary school aged children: Reviewing the evidence base for school-based interventions. *International Journal of Mental Health Promotion, 7*(2), 30–36.

Gupta, M. C., Mehrotra, M., Arora, S., & Saran, M. (1991). Relation of childhood malnutrition to parental education and mother's nutrition related KAP. *Indian Journal of Paediatrics, 58,* 269–274.

Gupta, M. D. (1990). Death clustering, mother's education and the determinants of child mortality in rural Punjab. *Population Studies, 44*(3), 489–505.

Harrison, K.A. (1997). The importance of the educated healthy woman in Africa. *Lancet, 349,* 644–647.

Herz, B. S., & Sperling, G. B. (2004). *What works in girls' education. Evidence and policies from the developing world.* New York: Council on Foreign Relations.

Hough, L. (2008, Summer). Can you hear me now? *Ed.magazine: The magazine of the Harvard Graduate School of Education.*

Jukes, M. C. H., Drake, J., & Bundy, D. A. P. (2008). *School health, nutrition and education for all: Levelling the playing field.* Oxford: Oxford University Press.

Kessler, R. C., Amminger, G. P., Aguilar-Gaxiola, S., Alonso, J., Lee, S., & Ustun, T. B. (2007). Age of onset of mental disorders: A review of recent literature. *Curr Opin Psychiatry, 20*(4), 359–364.

Kirby, D. (2002). The impact of schools and school programs upon adolescent sexual behavior. *Journal of Sex Research, 39*(1), 27–33.

Kolbe, L. J. (1986). Increasing the impact of school health promotion programs: Emerging research perspectives. *Health Education, 17*(5), 47–52.

Lister-Sharp, D., Chapman, S., Stewart-Brown, S., & Sowden, A. (1999). Health promoting schools and health promotion in schools: Two systematic reviews. *Health Technology Assessment, 3*(22), 1–207.

Lloyd, C., Joyce, R., Hurry, J., & Ashton, M. (2000). The effectiveness of primary school drug education. *Drugs: Education, Prevention and Policy, 7*(2), 109–126.

Mahoney, J., & Cairns, R. (1997). Do extracurricular activities protect against early school dropout? *Developmental Psychology, 33*(2), 241–253.

Midford, R., Lenton, S., & Hancock, L. (2000). *A critical review and analysis: Cannabis education in schools*. Sydney: New South Wales Department of Education and Training.

National Center for Chronic Disease Prevention and Health Promotion (n.d.). *Healthy schools, healthy youth!* Retrieved August 27, 2008, from http://www.cdc.gov/HealthyYouth/

National Center for Mental Health Promotion and Youth Violence Prevention (n.d.). *Safe schools/ healthy students*. Retrieved August 27, 2008, from http://www.promoteprevent.org

National Drug Research Institute. (2002). *The prevention of substance use, risk and harm in Australia: A review of the evidence*. Canberra: Commonwealth Department of Health and Ageing.

Nussbaum, M. C. (2000). *Women and human development. The capabilities approach*. Cambridge, UK: Press Syndicate of the University of Cambridge.

Nutbeam, D., & Kickbusch, I. S. (2000). Advancing health literacy: A global challenge for the 21st century. *Health Promotion International, 15*(3), 183–184.

Patton, G. C., Bond, L., Carlin, J. B., Thomas, L., Butler, H., Glover, S., et al. (2006). Promoting social inclusion in schools: A group-randomized trial of effects on student health risk behavior and well-being. *Am J Public Health, 96*(9), 1582–1587.

Sen, A. (1999). *Development as Freedom*. Oxford: Oxford University Press.

SHE Network (n.d.). *Schools for health In Europe*. Retrieved August 27, 2008, from http://www.schoolsforhealth.eu/

Shephard, R. J. (1997). Curricular physical activity and academic performance. *Pediatric Exercise Science, 9*(2), 113–126.

Silva, M. (2002). The effectiveness of school-based sex education programs in the promotion of abstinent behavior: A meta-analysis. *Health Education Research, 17*(4), 471–481.

Skara, S., & Sussman, S. (2003). A review of 25 long-term adolescent tobacco and other drug use prevention program evaluations. *Preventive Medicine, 37*(5), 451–474.

St. Leger, L., Kolbe, L. J., Lee, A., McCall, D. S., & Young, I. M. (2007). School health promotion: Achievements, challenges and priorities. In D. V. McQueen & C. M. Jones (Eds.), *Global perspectives on health promotion effectiveness*. New York: Springer.

Stewart-Brown, S. (2006). *What is the evidence on school health promotion in improving health or preventing disease and, specifically, what is the effectiveness of the health promoting schools approach?* Copenhagen: World Health Organization.

Tang, K. C., Nutbeam, D., & Aldinger, C. (2009). Schools for health, education and development: A call for action. *Health Promotion International, 24*(1), 68–77.

Timperio, A., Salmon, J., & Ball, K. (2004). Evidence-based strategies to promote physical activity among children, adolescents and young adults: Review and update. *Journal of Science and Medicine in Sport, 7*(1 Suppl), 20–29.

Tobler, N., & Stratton, H. (1997). Effectiveness of school-based drug education programs: A meta analysis of the research. *Journal of Primary Prevention, 18*(1), 71–128.

United Nations Development Programme (n.d.). *About the MDGs: Basics*. Retrieved August 27, 2008, from http://www.undp.org/mdg/basics.shtml

Wells, J., Barlow, J., & Stewart-Brown, S. (2003). A systematic review of universal approaches to mental health promotion in schools. *Health Education Journal, 103*(4), 197–220.

West, P., Sweeting, H., & Leyland, L. (2004). School effects on pupils' health behaviours: Evidence in support of the health promoting school. *Research Papers in Education, 19*(31), 261–291.

Vince Whitman, C. (2005). Implementing research-based health promotion programmes in schools: Strategies for capacity building. In B. B. Jensen & S. Clift (Eds.), *The health promoting school: International advances in theory, evaluation and practice* (pp. 107–135). Copenhagen: Danish University of Education Press.

Vince Whitman, C., Aldinger, C., Levinger, B., & Birdthistle, I. (2001). *Education for all 2000 assessment: Thematic studies: School health and nutrition.* Paris: United Nations Educational, Scientific and Cultural Organization.

Vince Whitman, C., Aldinger, C., Zhang, X. W., & Magner, E. (2008). Strategies to address mental health through schools with examples from China. *International Review of Psychiatry, 20*(3), 237–249.

World Health Organization. (1948). *Constitution of the World Health Organization.* Geneva: World Health Organization.

World Health Organization. (1986). *Ottawa charter for health promotion: First International Conference on Health Promotion.* Geneva: World Health Organization.

World Health Organization. (1997). *Promoting health through schools. Report of a WHO Expert Committee on Comprehensive School Health Education and Promotion, WHO Technical Report Series, No. 870.* Geneva: WHO.

World Health Organization. (1998). *Health promoting schools: A healthy setting for living, learning and working, WHO Global School Health Initiative* (Vol. WHO/HPR/HEP/98.4). Geneva: World Health Organization.

World Health Organization. (2003). *Skills for health: Skills-based health education, including life skills – An important component of a child-friendly/health-promoting school, WHO Information Series on School Health – Document 9.* Geneva: World Health Organization.

World Health Organization. (2005). *Bangkok charter for health promotion in a globalized world: Sixth Global Conference on Health Promotion.* Geneva: World Health Organization.

World Health Organization. (2007). *Report of the technical meeting of building school partnership for health, education achievements and development.* Vancouver, Canada: WHO.

Young, I. (1986). *The health promoting school, report of a WHO symposium.* Edinburgh: Scottish Health Education Group/WHO regional office for Europe.

Young, I. (2005). Health promotion in schools – A historical perspective. *Promotion and Education, 12*(3–4), 112–117, 184–190, 205–111.

Zins, J., Bloodworth, M., Weissberg, R., & Walberg, H. (Eds.). (2004). *Building academic success on social and emotional learning: What does the research say?* New York: Teachers Press, Columbia University.

Chapter 2
Framing Theories and Implementation Research

Cheryl Vince Whitman

Definitions

The processes for transforming a concept into health promotion and prevention policies and strategies draw on many theories in social science, public health, and education. Dissemination, diffusion, implementation, technology transfer, systems change, and capacity building are all terms used to describe various aspects of translating research to practice, but each term has a slightly different meaning. The Health-Promoting School concept has also been embedded in global education reform initiatives, such as Education for All, drawing on those methods and terminology used in transforming education systems.

Table 1 offers definitions of terms that play an important role in understanding and describing the processes for implementation. There is no broad consensus on the vocabulary and terms to describe elements of the approach.

For the purpose of this book, we define implementation as Fixsen et. al have,

> implementation is defined as a specified set of activities designed to put into practice an activity or program of known dimensions. According to this definition, implementation processes are purposeful and are described in sufficient detail such that independent observers can detect the presence and strength of the "specific set of activities" related to implementation. In addition, the activity or program being implemented is described in sufficient detail so that independent observers can detect its presence and strength.

> (Fixsen, Naoom, Blase, & Friedman, 2005, p. 5).

Most research on such programs has focused on the effectiveness of the intervention, rather than on the effectiveness of the implementation process or the relationship between implementation and outcomes. Reviews of the research offer strong support that the "level of implementation affects the outcomes obtained in promotion and prevention programs" (Durlak & Dupre, 2008, p. 327).

C. Vince Whitman
Health and Human Development Programs, Education Development Center, Newton, MA, USA

C. Vince Whitman and C.E. Aldinger (eds.),
Case Studies in Global School Health Promotion: From Research to Practice,
DOI: 10.1007/978-0-387-92269-0_2, © Springer Science + Business Media, LLC 2009

Table 1 Definitions of terms

Dissemination is defined by the US Centers for Disease Control and Prevention as the intentional spreading of innovations from the developers or originators to the intended users (Centers for Disease Control and Prevention, n.d.-a).

Implementation is a specified set of activities designed to *put into practice* an activity or program of known dimensions. It is a means of achieving an end, an instrument, or an agent.

Diffusion of innovation is the "process by which an innovation" – defined as "an idea, practice, or object that is perceived as new" – "is communicated through certain channels over time among the members of a social system" (Rogers, 1995, pp. 10–11).

Technology transfer is the transfer of ideas, information, methods, procedures, techniques, tools, or technology from the developers to potential users. Methods of technology transfer include scientific publications in peer-reviewed journals, articles in management-oriented publications, computer programs, training sessions, tours, and workshops (US Forest Service, 2005).

Systems change is the process of improving the capacity of the public health (or other) system to work with many sectors to improve the health status of all people in a community (Colorado Department of Public Health and Environment, 2005).

Education reform is a plan or movement which attempts to bring about a systematic change in educational theory or practice across a community or society (Education Reform, n.d.).

Capacity building is much more than training and includes: (1) human resource development to equip individuals with the understanding, skills and access to information, enabling them to perform effectively; (2) organizational development, including management structures, processes, and procedures, not only within organizations but also the management of relationships between the different organizations and sectors (public, private, and community); and (3) institutional and legal framework development. ("Capacity building," n.d.)

Sustainability is the ability to continue and keep a program going beyond initial, external funding and to have it become an ongoing part of an agency's program and services.

Going to scale is the process of reaching larger numbers of a target audience in a broader geographic area by institutionalizing effective programs. While there is no precise definition that identifies the amount of increased programming or coverage required for scaling-up, scaled-up programs usually reach (or provide access for) much of the targeted population within a specified area (Senderowitz, 2000; Smith & Colvin, 2000).

It is beyond the scope of this book to relate the implementation practices to the outcomes achieved as Health-Promoting Schools took root around the globe. Our primary contribution, through qualitative research and a theoretical framework, is to use case studies to illustrate the methods and strategies to put the concept into practice.

Theory and Research on Implementation

Figure 1 presents one possible framework of 12 major factors that play a role in successful implementation, *The Wheel of Factors Influencing Implementation of Policy and Practice*. Created by Vince Whitman at EDC, this framework is based on review of the extensive literature on diffusion of innovation, technology transfer, implementation research, and education reform research. The framework also draws on considerable tacit knowledge from the design and operation of large-scale training and technical assistance centers that provide services to international,

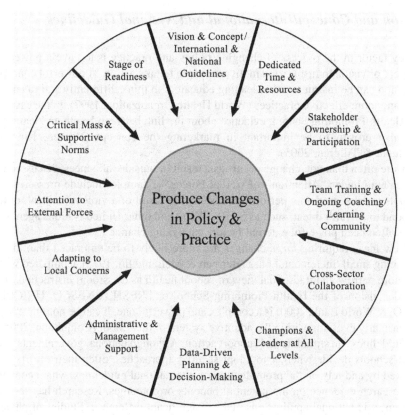

Fig. 1 The wheel of factors influencing implementation of policy and practice (adapted from Vince Whitman, 2005)

national, state, and local agencies in their implementation of innovations and evidence-based programs. Using many of these factors can also lead to sustainability and taking programs to scale.

Through meta-analyses, other researchers have identified similar factors to those depicted in the Wheel. For example, an examination of 81 implementation studies with quantitative or qualitative data on factors that affect the implementation process also pointed to a similar number of factors: "funding, a positive work climate, shared decision-making, coordination with other agencies, formulation of tasks, leadership, program champions, administrative support, providers' skill proficiency, training, and technical assistance" (Durlak & Dupre, 2008, p. 340).

Similarly, St. Leger identified a number of successful factors for starting and sustaining a Health-Promoting School, which add to those named above the celebration of milestones and the opportunity to review and refresh progress after 34 years (St. Leger, 2005).

A review of supporting research evidence for the 12 factors in the Wheel follows.

Vision and Concept/International and National Guidelines

A key factor in the process of changing policy and practice is to have a powerful concept or vision to inspire and motivate people to take action. A powerful concept or vision can be instrumental in leading educators to think differently and to adopt new and more effective practices (World Health Organization, 1997). In the case of the Health-Promoting School, evidence about the link between health and learning has also proven to be important in marketing the concept (Viljoen, Kirsten, Haglund, & Tillgren, 2005).

More often than not, change occurs as a result of outside influences, discussed in more detail under "Attention to External Forces." Examples include pressures on schools to raise academic performance, sadly the result of a violent incident, or to respond to a health threat, such as SARS. WHO and other United Nations agencies have often been powerful external factors catalyzing change.

New ideas requiring *large* changes are more likely to be embraced than ideas involving small, incremental ones (Berman & McLaughlin, 1975). Compared with the more narrow and traditional view of school health as classroom instruction, the broader vision of the Health-Promoting School or FRESH (UNESCO, UNICEF, WHO, & World Bank, 2000) is a complex and powerful one. It can be nonlinear and is constantly evolving within the adaptive system of the school (Colquhoun, 2005).

Guidelines can stimulate and support action. Although national governments and local schools decide whether to adopt specific approaches, often their efforts are sparked by and rely on the promulgation of international guidelines, which convey the research evidence on the potential benefits or outcomes. Research has shown how specific national applications make a significant difference. Studies of physician behavior in the United States, for example, have shown that dissemination of national guidelines concerning the evidence about proven clinical practice has increased by 10% the number of physicians who adopt the recommended practice (Cohen, Halvorson, & Gosselink, 1994). A study of the dissemination of the United States Education Department's Principles of Effectiveness for school alcohol and drug prevention programs found that many school districts reported that they were applying the principles and selecting research-based curricula over previously used ineffective practices (Hallfors & Godette, 2002). Further, reformers of the Russian education system working on its modernization have stated, "It must be emphasized: standards are essential" (Kuz'menko, Lunin, & Ryzhova, 2006). The effectiveness of such guidelines for influencing practice, however, has been shown to be dependent on factors and potential barriers external to their content (Trowbridge & Weingarten, 2001).

Dedicated Time and Resources

Time and resources – such as human, financial, technical, and material – are essential to ensuring change in policy and practice. There must be the workforce

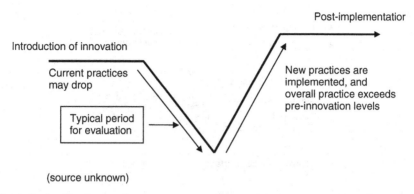

(source unknown)

Fig. 2 Cycle of implementation

with the human capacity and potential, who can dedicate adequate time to implement new programs. Sufficient time and pacing must be allowed to implement a full program cycle. One of the most common reasons a project fails is that managers underestimate how much time it will take and whether their staff and system are ready to take it on (Cohen, 1996; Rogers, 1995). Education systems must determine realistically how much time will be needed and assess staff readiness and willingness to move in the new direction.

Once implementation has begun, it typically takes from 18 months to 3 years to actually see or capture evidence of change. There must be "time for participants to discover for themselves what will and will not work for them" (Greenfield, 1995).

In the beginning, the skills of program implementers – teachers and others – often decline as they try the new skills or strategies, but they gradually surpass their former levels of competence once an innovation is established. Too often we evaluate programs early on, when experimentation is underway, as shown in Fig. 2, *Cycle of Implementation* and may fail to capture the change that is happening.

Stakeholder Ownership and Participation

Amartya Sen, winner of the 1998 Nobel Prize in Economic Science, argues that the freedom of people to participate socially and politically in shaping their lives and what they value is central to human and economic development (Sen, 1999). Sen offers many examples of how people having "agency" (the ability to act and bring about change), coupled with access to basic education and health services, can lift themselves out of poverty and transform societies. The HPS concept addresses all three factors in Sen's work.

First, central to the concept illustrated in Fig. 1 of the chapter "Introduction and Background" is the participation of parents, community members, teachers, and

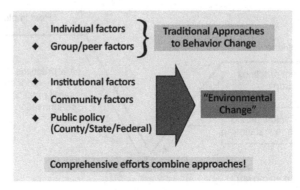

Fig. 3 Social-ecological model (Langford, 2003)

students themselves in a participatory, democratic process to shape the learning environment. Second, the HPS provides health information, skills, and access to health services. And, third, using data on the links among years of schooling, literacy, and health status, advocates of the HPS model argue that one of the most important contributors to healthy development is access to and completion of school, especially for girls.

A study of the implementation of the 1999 National Education Act in Thailand reported that community participation was one of the four essential strategies for successful implementation. Researchers reported that the schools and institutions "reaped benefits...because each community is rich in resources that provide excellent learning environments" and recommended that they "should pay attention to, and seriously plan for, action to get parent and community involvement to achieve success in learning reform" (Khemmani, 2006, p. 122).

Similarly, research on use of the *Social-Ecological Model* (Langford, 2003), illustrated in Fig. 3, reports on the importance of participation across levels and sectors in society for successful implementation of public health innovations (Glasgow & Emmons, 2007). The Social-Ecological Model takes into consideration the complex interplay between individual, relationship, community, and societal factors. Research in support of this model argues that this approach is more likely to sustain prevention efforts over time than any other (Centers for Disease Control and Prevention, n.d.-b).

Team Training and Ongoing Coaching/Learning Community

What form and type of training is most likely to result in practice change? Providing professional development and ongoing opportunities for coaching and peer leaning throughout the process of implementing an innovation are important methods to use. Until and unless enough staff, within a ministry of education or local school, are trained and committed to implementing the change in policy and practice, it is unrealistic to expect that a single person sent off-site to a one-time workshop will be able to return to his or her agency alone and create systemic practice change. For this reason, professional development needs to provide training to teams from the same agency involving *at least* three or four people from the same school or ministry, who then can benefit from ongoing coaching and exchange over time. They then can also become the critical mass that influences organizational norms. Experimental studies on training methods, including those reviewed in a metaanalysis by Joyce and Showers in 2002, "indicate that effective training workshops appear to consist of presenting information (knowledge), providing demonstrations (live or taped) of the important aspects of the practice or program, and assuring opportunities to practice key skills in the training setting (behavior rehearsal)" (Fixsen et al., 2005, p. 41).

Professional development should persist beyond the team training, to provide numerous and frequent opportunities for implementers to receive ongoing coaching and mentoring as well as support and exchange from their peers over time, especially as they try new things (Vince Whitman, 2005). The meta-analysis conducted by Joyce and Showers (2002) revealed "that implementation in educational settings occurred primarily when training was combined with coaching in the classroom" (Fixsen et al., 2005, p. 46). Similar results have been found in mental health (Kelly et al., 2000) and medical settings (Fine et al., 2003).

The literature on education reform includes many references to the benefits from creating forums for networks, where implementers participate in an ongoing exchange of ideas and experiences for continuous learning from each other (Center for Mental Health in Schools at UCLA, 2004; Eick, Ewald, Richardson, & Anderson, 2007; Lynd-Balta, Erklenz-Watts, Freeman, & Westbay, 2006; McCoy, 2006).

Taken together, the two strategies – training teams over individuals, and providing training that motivates, defines actions that make up the intervention, provides tools to perform the actions (Kealey, Peterson, Gaul, & Dinh, 2000), and enables practitioners to gain confidence – are more likely to result in practice change. Such training must be followed by ongoing coaching and mechanisms for sharing and learning from peers and others. These features of professional development are most likely to positively affect implementation.

Cross-Sector Collaboration

There is very little research on the relationship between mechanisms for cross-sector collaboration and the effectiveness of implementation. Needing multiple sectors that work together to implement an innovation adds another layer of complexity to the already complex concept of the Health-Promoting School. Created by the public health field, the HPS ideas must be led by and implemented in the education sector, with support and coordination with health content experts, in particular, and others, including nongovernmental organizations, parent groups, and universities. It is clear that education must lead. Reviewing the role of key stakeholders in school health and nutrition programs in low-income countries, Bundy et al. (2006) observed that

> In nearly every case, the Ministry of Education is the lead implementing agency, reflecting both the goal of school health programs in improving educational achievement and the fact that the education system provides the most complete existing infrastructure for reaching school-age children. However the education sector must share this responsibility with the Ministry of Health, particularly because the latter has the ultimate responsibility for health of children. (p. 1104)

Several strategies are important in the formulation of cross-sector collaboration: making clear links between the education and health outcomes; developing memoranda of understanding and a formal multi-sectoral policy that outlines the roles and responsibilities of each key sector and player; and engaging in widespread dissemination of information and consultation with the many players (Bundy et al., 2006).

Champions and Leaders at all Levels

Individuals who strongly support and advocate for a program – champions – have often been cited by education and health agencies as one of the primary reasons that they have been able to implement innovative programs. For example, an evaluation of the *Promoting Alternative Thinking Strategies* (PATHS) program for ages 6–12 found that good outcomes were associated with principal or headmaster support and high-quality implementation (fidelity, dose, duration). Without principal support, it would not have been possible to achieve the intended outcomes (Kam, Greenberg, & Walls, 2003). The leader's commitment, dedication, support, and ability to articulate the vision and motivate and inspire others are key (Kotter, 1988). A comprehensive review of 39 local school improvement efforts in the US reported that the one element a change effort cannot be without is the right type of leader. "Leaders must aim not at manipulating subordinates ... but at motivating followers, who invest themselves actively. This requires leaders who are skillful, but who are above all credible" (Evans, 1993, p. 21).

For implementing complex ideas (such as the HPS) or complex processes (such as implementing evidence-based strategies), leadership talent must exist not only at senior levels but also at every level in ministries, schools and, communities. According to Rogers (1995), the effort of the change agent – whether the leader or his or her designee – is known to predict the rate of diffusion.

Data-Driven Planning and Decision-Making

Routinely using data for planning and decision-making purposes is critical during the implementation process. As discussed earlier, data have informed the link between education and health and the effectiveness of strategies to address health promotion and prevention in schools. When planning for implementation, a range of data is useful, including:

- Health data on causes of illness, injury, and death, as well as data on risk behaviors and protective factors
- Education data on academic achievement, attendance, dropout, absenteeism, suspensions, and expulsions
- Asset and resource assessment of the human and financial capacities that systems can bring to the planning and implementation process
- Readiness data on the stage of commitment, dedication of key players, and knowledge of what is needed to create change
- Data on indicators that will be used to monitor progress over time: reach and impact

Data are essential to plan and drive the process and to inform its direction and redirection over time. As with any evaluation, identifying the many stakeholders and what data are needed to inform them over time is a key strategy within an ongoing communications strategy.

Administrative and Management Support

One of the most decisive elements affecting the success of any innovation is the availability of comprehensive and skilled administrative and management support. Without clearly assigned roles, a defined organizational structure, and close monitoring, a project may fail to achieve its prospective aims. Some have argued that inability to appreciate the effects of these dynamics on efforts to adequately plan and manage the change process may ensure failure (Fullan, Cuttress, & Kilcher, 2005). In the education sector and elsewhere, the development of a strategic plan or logic model that provides administrative and management support for carrying out activities relative to goals is routinely recognized as important in achieving outcomes. Recently, an investigation into the reform efforts of the District of Columbia public schools found that lacking "a plan that sets priorities, implementation goals, and timelines, it may be difficult to measure progress over time and determine if [a school district] is truly achieving success" (Ashby, 2008, p. 2).

By employing effective processes for communication, as well as tracking and monitoring progress according to time and budget constraints, implementers will be able to ensure accountability and the efficient use of resources (Vince Whitman, 2005). New technologies and systems for data collection and analysis are also much more likely to be used appropriately and extensively when sufficient administrative and management support is available (Wayman & Stringfield, 2004). Even with teacher buy-in to the change process, administrative support is an essential factor in success. In a study conducted in 2005 to encourage greater science instruction at the elementary level, researchers found that while teachers were generally positive, the full integration of the new program was stalled by insufficient administrative support (Kelly & Staver, 2005). Research shows that this lack of support is also one of the leading factors of higher teacher attrition rates (Gonzalez, Brown, & Slate, 2008).

Adapting to Local Concerns

All implementers must pay attention to the concerns of the users. The Concerns-Based Adoption Model has demonstrated the 80–20 rule. Unless implementers dedicate 80% of their time and attention to users' concerns, they have only a 20% chance of success (Loucks-Horsley, 1996). Beyond understanding basic concerns, ministries and schools can use the growing body of evidence on evaluated programs and strategies to help them make decisions about what to invest in doing.

But evidence of effectiveness in one setting may not apply to another. Many of the settings to which a program will be transferred are not identical to the one that produced results; the culture and ethnicity of students, the type of school system (urban, rural, and suburban), and income level of families and communities may vary. Most evaluated programs are from resource-rich areas, and their adaptation to resource-poor areas requires careful consideration. In choosing what to adapt, implementers must think through how much change or adaptation a program can undergo without threatening its ability to produce similar results. What are the core elements, dosage, and duration that cannot be changed? Research shows that attention to fidelity is critical for successful outcomes (Backer, 2001).

Attention to External Forces

Change can be stimulated and driven by a range of factors in the macro environment. For education and reform and schools, such factors can include government laws and regulations affecting education; national or international comparisons on test scores; and major economic, demographic, health, and social-political changes. Actions taken by major donors, such as United Nations agencies, foundations, and the World Bank, all influence governments in their educational priorities.

In a review of curriculum implementation in South Africa, the role of very dynamic nongovernmental organizations (NGOs), which were established in the 1970s and 1980s, was described as "able to stimulate innovation and undertake professional activities, particularly in black education, in ways that the apartheid government was either unable or unwilling to do" (Rogan & Grayson, 2008, p. 152).

Being aware of and capitalizing on a range of external factors that drive change can support various aspects of the implementation process (Rogan, 2003).

Critical Mass and Supportive Norms

A large enough number of people in any one institution or in the broader society is required to carry the message and principles forward and influence others to join the movement. A critical mass of people who share supportive norms is necessary for creating new thinking and practices within and across systems. People in groups tend to move toward normative actions, that is, toward what they believe most people are doing (Kübler, 2001). Having this critical mass can create a tipping point in supporting the implementation of innovations. Rogan (2003) writes:

> Professional forces rely essentially on convictions arising from a sense of belonging and having obligations to a professional community. Cultural and democratic forces rely on shared values and goals about teaching and learning, as well as notions about the role of education in a democratic society. A critical mass of like-minded teachers, for example, might form a "learning community", which begins to chart new ideas and practices for that school. These community-based changes ... are likely to be "deep" and enduring. (p. 1177)

Stage of Readiness

The readiness of organizations or institutions to implement changes to policy or practice is contingent on a variety of conditions, influenced by the factors described above and others. The uniqueness of each organization and situation offers many challenges to the assessment of readiness and the implementation process. Still, research suggests three general areas that affect the overall stage of readiness: strategic planning, preparation, and the organizational readiness and functioning for the actual implementation process (Simpson, 2002; Simpson & Flynn, 2007). Organizational readiness and functioning depend on several factors, such as the level of motivation among staff and the surrounding community, assessment of risks and anticipated outcomes, professional development and training, and the availability of resources and support (McKee, Manocontour, Saik Yoon, & Carnegie, 2000). By carefully addressing these concerns, readiness can be enhanced and maintained throughout the implementation process.

Overall motivation and general receptiveness and buy-in of an organization to a particular innovation or program can also be seen as closely mirroring the stages of individual behavior change originally outlined by Prochaska. This model emphasizes six distinct stages that can be used to identify the challenges to, and likelihood of, changing an individual's behavior: precontemplation, contemplation, preparation, action, maintenance, and termination (Prochaska & Velicer, 1997). For groups of individuals, progression through these stages is affected by the ability "to mobilize collective support by building and shaping awareness among organizational members about the existence of, sources of, and solutions to the organization's problems" (Backer, 1995, p. 34). Strong leadership and the availability of useful institutional resources can generate individual motivation and a supportive and receptive organizational climate that improve the stage of readiness (Saldana, Chapman, Henggeler, & Rowland, 2007).

Last, the connections among theory, research, and practice must be well understood to advance the stage of readiness (Vince Whitman, 2005). Knowledge of how to accurately interpret other experiences and research for use in a new setting can bridge these areas and help to establish workable plans for evaluation and monitoring. Benefiting from user-friendly tools and best practices models, schools, implementers, and communities can assess readiness and the feasibility of a proposed research-based program. The Organizational Readiness for Change scale (Lehman, Greener, & Simpson, 2002) and other tools can help to make the research-to-practice process much clearer and allow for more confident selection of relevant programs for implementation, particularly when supported by broader institutions (Harding & Goddard, 2000). Still, the evidence base regarding the predictive validity of these tools is just beginning to expand (Fixsen et al., 2005); although they can aid in assessing the stage of readiness, the "successful transfer of evidence-based innovations to real-world applications requires careful planning, implementation, and on-going evaluations of the progress being made" (Simpson, 2002, p. 4). If adequate readiness is not achieved and maintained throughout the process, implementers may observe lower levels of organizational and individual reliability and longer timeframe allowances, if not complete project collapse (Fixsen et al., 2005).

The 12 Wheel factors, as well as those from other models, are very important for success in the implementation process. In the next chapter, using these factors, we analyze 26 cases from around the world, illustrating and making these strategies come alive.

References

Ashby, C. M. (2008). *District of columbia public schools: While early reform efforts tackle critical management issues, a district-wide strategic education plan would help guide long-term efforts*. Washington, D.C.: U.S. Government Accountability Office.

Backer, T. (2001). *Finding the balance: Program fidelity and adaptation in substance abuse prevention*. Rockville, MD: National Center for Advancement of Prevention.

Backer, T. E. (1995). Assessing and enhancing readiness for change: Implications for technology transfer. In T. E. Backer, S. L. David, & G. Saucy (Eds.), *Reviewing the behavioral science knowledge base on technology transfer*. Rockville, MD: U.S. Department of Health and Human Services.

Berman, P., & McLaughlin, M. W. (1975). *Federal programs supporting educational change: The findings in review* (Vol. 4). Santa Monica, CA: Rand Corporation.

Bundy, D. A. P., Shaeffer, S., Jukes, M., Beegle, K., Gillespie, A., Drake, L., et al. (2006). School-based health and nutrition programs. In D. T. Jamison, et al., (Eds.), *Disease control priorities in developing countries* (2nd ed.). Washington, D.C.: World Bank.

Capacity Building (n.d.). *Wikipedia*. Retrieved October 15, 2008, from http://en.wikipedia.org/wiki/Capacity_building

Center for Mental Health in Schools at UCLA (2004). *Sustaining school and community efforts to enhance outcomes for children and youth: A guidebook and tool kit.* Los Angeles: University of California.

Centers for Disease Control and Prevention (n.d.-a). *CDC Injury Center.* Retrieved August 27, 2008, from http://www.cdc.gov/ncipc/

Centers for Disease Control and Prevention (n.d.-b). *CDC injury center: The social-ecological model.* Retrieved August 27, 2008, from http://www.cdc.gov/ncipc/dvp/Social-Ecological-Model_DVP.htm

Cohen, S. (1996). *Research to improve implementation and effectiveness of school health programmes.* Geneva: World Health Organization.

Cohen, S., Halvorson, H. W., & Gosselink, C. A. (1994). Changing physician behavior to improve disease prevention. *Preventive Medicine, 23*(3), 284–291.

Colorado Department of Public Health and Environment (2005). *Office of Health Disparities: Public Health Terms.* Retrieved August 27, 2008, from http://www.cdphe.state.co.us/ohd/glossary.html

Colquhoun, D. (2005). Complexity and the health promoting school. In B. B. Jensen & S. Clift (Eds.), *The health promoting school: International advances in theory, evaluation and practice.* Copenhagen: Danish University of Education Press.

Durlak, J. A., & Dupre, E. P. (2008). Implementation matters: A review of research on the influence of implementation on program outcomes and the factors affecting implementation. *American Journal of Community Psychology, 41*(3), 327–350.

Education Reform (n.d.). *Wikipedia* Retrieved August 27, 2008, from http://en.wikipedia.org/wiki/Education_reform

Eick, C. J., Ewald, M. L., Richardson, V. B., & Anderson, K. (2007). Building a leadership network supporting science education reform in rural east Alabama. *Science Educator, 16*(1), 8–12.

Evans, R. (1993). The face of human reform. *Educational Leadership, 51*(1), 19–23.

Fine, M. J., Stone, R. A., Lave, J. R., Hough, L. J., Obrosky, D. S., Mor, M. K., et al. (2003). Implementation of an evidence-based guideline to reduce duration of intravenous antibiotic therapy and length of stay for patients hospitalized with community-acquired pneumonia: A randomized controlled trial. *The American Journal of Medicine, 115*(5), 343–351.

Fixsen, D. L., Naoom, S. F., Blase, K. A., & Friedman, R. M. (2005). *Implementation research: A synthesis of the literature.* Tampa, FL: USF University of Southern Florida.

Fullan, M., Cuttress, C., & Kilcher, A. (2005). Eight forces for leaders of change: Presence of the core concepts does not guarantee success, but their absence ensures failure. *Journal of Staff Development, 26*(5), 54–58.

Glasgow, R. E., & Emmons, K. M. (2007). How can we increase translation of research into practice? Types of evidence needed. *Annual Review of Public Health, 28,* 413–433.

Gonzalez, L. E., Brown, M. S., & Slate, J. R. (2008). Teachers who left the teaching profession: A qualitative understanding. *Qualitative Report, 13*(1), 1–11.

Greenfield, T. A. (1995). Improving chances for successful educational reform. *Education, 115*(3), 464–474.

Hallfors, D., & Godette, D. (2002). Will the 'principles of effectiveness' improve prevention practice? Early findings from a diffusion study. *Health Education Research, 17*(4), 461–470.

Harding, W., & Goddard, C. (2000). *Assessing the feasibility of implementing a science-based prevention program: A tool for practitioners.* Paper presented at the Working Together for Prevention: Building State and Community Systems, National Conference for the State Incentive Grant and the Center for the Application of Prevention Technologies Programs, Washington, D.C.

Joyce, B., & B. Showers. (2002). *Student Achievement Through Staff Development.* 3rd ed. Alexandria, VA: Association for Supervision and Curriculum Development.

Kam, C., Greenberg, M. T., & Walls, C. T. (2003). Examining the role of implementation quality in school-based prevention using the PATHS curriculum. *Prevention Science, 4*(1), 55–63.

Kealey, K. A., Peterson, A. V., Jr., Gaul, M. A., & Dinh, K. T. (2000). Teacher training as a behavior change process: Principles and results from a longitudinal study. *Health Education & Behavior, 27*(1), 64–81.

Kelly, J. A., Somlai, A. M., DiFranceisco, W. J., Otto-Salaj, L. L., McAuliffe, T. L., Hackl, K. L., et al. (2000). Bridging the gap between the science and service of HIV prevention: Transferring effective research-based HIV prevention interventions to community AIDS service providers. *American Journal of Public Health, 90*(7), 1082–1088.

Kelly, M. P., & Staver, J. R. (2005). A case study of one school system's adoption and implementation of an elementary science program. *Journal of Research in Science Teaching, 42*(1), 25–52.

Khemmani, T. (2006). Whole-school learning reform: Effective strategies from Thai schools. *Theory Into Practice, 45*(2), 117–124.

Kotter, J. P. (1988). *The leadership factor*. New York: Free Press.

Kübler, D. (2001). On the regulation of social norms. *Journal of Law, Economics and Organization, 17*(2), 449–476.

Kuz'menko, N. E., Lunin, V. V., & Ryzhova, O. N. (2006). On the modernization of education in Russia. *Russian Education and Society, 48*(5), 5–22.

Langford, L. (2003). Using Policy as Part of a Public Health Approach, *Presentation at All-HHD Meeting, 3 Nov 2003*. Newton, MA: Education Development Center, Inc.

Lehman, W. E., Greener, J. M., & Simpson, D. D. (2002). Assessing organizational readiness for change. *Jounal of Substance Abuse Treatment, 22*(4), 197–209.

Loucks-Horsley, S. (1996). Professional development for science education: A critical and immediate challenge. In R. Bybee (Ed.), *National standards and the science curriculum*. Dubuque: Kendall.

Lynd-Balta, E., Erklenz-Watts, M., Freeman, C., & Westbay, T. D. (2006). Professional development using an interdisciplinary learning circle: Linking pedagogical theory to practice. *Journal of College Science Teaching, 35*(4), 18–24.

McCoy, M. L. (2006). Collaboration through study circles. *Journal of Family and Consumer Sciences, 97*(1), 71–73.

McKee, N., Manocontour, E., Saik Yoon, C., & Carnegie, R. (Eds.). (2000). *Involving people, evolving behaviour*. Penang, Malaysia: UNICEF.

Prochaska, J. O., & Velicer, W. F. (1997). The transtheoretical model of health behavior change. *American Jounal of Health Promotion, 12*(1), 38–48.

Rogan, J. M. (2003). Towards a theory of curriculum implementation with particular reference to science education in developing countries. *International Journal Science Education, 25*(10), 1171–1204.

Rogan, J. M., & Grayson, D. J. (2008). Towards a theory of curriculum development with reference to science education in developing countries. In M. Nagao, J. Rogan & M. Magno (Eds.), *Mathematics and science education in developing countries: Issues, experiences, and cooperation prospects*. Quezon City: University of the Philippines Press.

Rogers, E. M. (1995). *Diffusion of innovations* (4th ed.). New York: Free Press.

Saldana, L., Chapman, J. E., Henggeler, S. W., & Rowland, M. D. (2007). The organizational readiness for change scale in adolescent programs: Criterion validity. *Journal of Substance Abuse Treatment, 33*(2), 159–169.

Sen, A. (1999). *Development as freedom*. Oxford: Oxford University Press.

Senderowitz, J. (2000). A review of program approaches to adolescent reproductive health, *Poptech Assignment Number 2000.176*. Washington, D.C.: International Science and Technology Institute, Population Technical Assistance Project.

Simpson, D. D. (2002). *Organizational readiness for treatment innovations*. Fort Worth, TX: Institute of Behavioral Research, Texas Christian University.

Simpson, D. D., & Flynn, P. M. (2007). Moving innovations into treatment: A stage-based approach to program change. *J Subst* Abuse Treat 33 (2):111–120.

Smith, J., & Colvin, C. (2000). Getting to scale in young adult reproductive health programs, *FOCUS Tool Series, No. 3*. Washington, D.C.: FOCUS on Young Adults, Pathfinder International.

St. Leger, L. (2005). Protocols and guidelines for health promoting schools. *Promotion and Education*, *12*(3–4), 145–147, 193–195, 214–216.

Trowbridge, R., & Weingarten, S. (2001). Practice guidelines. In K. Shojania, B. Duncan, K. McDonald, & R. Wachter (Eds.), *Evidence report/technology assessment: Making health care safer: A critical analysis of patient safety practices*. Rockville, MD: Agency for Healthcare Research and Quality.

UNESCO, UNICEF, WHO, & World Bank (2000). *Focusing resources on effective school health: A FRESH start to enhancing the quality and equity of education*. Washington, D.C.: World Bank.

US Forest Service (2005). *Northeastern Research Station, Research and Development*: Glossary. Retrieved August 27, 2008, from http://www.fs.fed.us/ne/newtown_square/research/themes/glossary.shtml

Viljoen, C. T., Kirsten, T. G. J., Haglund, B., & Tillgren, P. (2005). Towards the development of indicators for health promoting schools. In B. B. Jensen & S. Clift (Eds.), *The health promoting school: International advances in theory, evaluation and practice*. Copenhagen: Danish University of Education Press.

Vince Whitman, C. (2005). Implementing research-based health promotion programmes in schools: Strategies for capacity building. In B. B. Jensen & S. Clift (Eds.), *The health promoting school: International advances in theory, evaluation and practice* (pp. 107–135). Copenhagen: Danish University of Education Press.

Wayman, J. C., & Stringfield, S. (2004). Technology-supported involvement of entire faculties in examination of student data for instructional improvement. *American Journal of Education*, *112*(4), 549–571.

World Health Organization (1997). Promoting health through schools. Report of a WHO Expert Committee on Comprehensive School Health Education and Promotion, *WHO Technical Report Series, No. 870*. Geneva: WHO.

Chapter 3
Overview of Findings from Case Study Analysis

Cheryl Vince Whitman and Carmen Aldinger

The concept of the Health-Promoting School (HPS) has proven to be a powerful one, capturing the attention of decision makers, teachers, and parents. It is evident that the field of school health has made significant progress in the last decade, moving from a narrow view of school health as primarily focused on classroom curriculum or health education to the broad, multiple strategies of policy, improving the school's physical and psychosocial environment and providing a range of services – all with participation of teachers, students, and the community. The 26 cases from around the globe offer inspiring examples of how the concept and research findings have been applied in everyday practice. These stories show us the passion of educators, families, and community members, striving to meet the challenges of a changing world by working toward the healthy development of individuals and of their school and community environments. By examining experiences around the globe in resource-rich and resource-poor settings, we learn about the universality of strategies that people around the world have used to put in place innovative programs that respond to their interests and needs.

Reasons the Programs Were Launched

It is most valuable to ask, across a range of settings, how and why these programs got started. What was the impetus or spark plug for action, for thinking that the HPS would improve conditions or make a difference in addressing health, social, and economic issues? This issue, related to the *external forces* factor discussed elsewhere, is important to address early on in the analysis to understand the reasons that countries and communities became engaged in the first place. The case studies confirm what has been found in the professional literature regarding some of the major reasons that moved decision makers to adopt the concept. These prior findings include the following:

C. Vince Whitman(✉)
Health and Human Development Programs, Education Development Center, Newton, MA, USA

C. Vince Whitman and C.E. Aldinger (eds.),
Case Studies in Global School Health Promotion: From Research to Practice,
DOI: 10.1007/978-0-387-92269-0_3, © Springer Science + Business Media, LLC 2009

- Data about health or education problems for youth that caused alarm among policy makers or citizens
- Increasing recognition by some policy makers of the link between health and education from several dimensions:
  - The influence of social and economic factors in health outcomes (Adda, Chandola, & Marmot, 2003; Vince Whitman, 2006)
  - The evidence base demonstrating that a student's physical, social, and emotional health is related to academic performance and test scores (Vince Whitman, Aldinger, Levinger, & Birdthistle, 2001)
  - The realization that conditions of learning (e.g., the school environment and relationships, curriculum content, and pedagogy) can negatively affect student and teacher health (Awartani, Vince Whitman, & Gordon, 2008)

- Economic or other hardships in the community and society, which spilled over to affect students and staff, leading the school to become a site for remediation and delivery of services

The model of the HPS and/or the common elements of FRESH, advanced by WHO and other United Nations agencies, became a compelling and practical way to respond. In the following section, we discuss the many ways in which the important factors influencing implementation of policy and practice (introduced in Fig. 1 in the chapter "Framing Theories and Implementation Research") have been used in the various cases to inform and design policies and programs.

HPS Components Implemented, Level of Education, and Reach

One of the innovative aspects of the HPS concept is its call that schools should place healthy development at the center of their mission and that they should use all means at their disposal as coordinated, multiple strategies to address the specific issues of healthy development that data or a community stakeholder process have identified to be important. Essentially, the HPS applies public health strategies to a school and community setting.

The cases in this book describe the degree to which various countries and schools are able to put multiple components in place, at the primary and/or secondary levels. They vary in the scale of implementation – the number of schools, teachers, and students involved. (Quotations in this chapter are all taken from the case studies that follow, unless otherwise indicated by a citation.)

For example, South Africa shares that "as we grew in understanding of the HPS concept . . . we resolved to implement all of the five pillars of HPS . . . and to adapt them to our unique conditions." The Sapphire School in South Africa implemented academic programs in the use of computers, extramural activities in sports and culture, vocational skills development, addition of security gates, and addition of an HIV and AIDS counseling center. This local-level case describes how it reached 1,022 learners, their family members, and 32 staff. The Sapphire School targeted the underlying social and economic determinants of unemployment and the specific health problem of HIV and AIDS. The school, with the leadership of a dynamic headmaster, became the community center of mobilization and problem solving.

In Viet Nam, the Ministries of Education and Health, working together, implemented various components of the HPS in 18 provinces, with the goal of reaching all 64 by the end of 2007. From the beginning, their plans included broad reach through the existing infrastructure for program delivery.

In Nigeria, the Ministries of Education and Health, working together, conducted the WHO/EDC Rapid Assessment and Action Planning Process (RAAPP) for School Health in four schools (primary and secondary) in each of 12 states. This RAAPP provides tools for ministries to come together and share a common vision with qualitative and quantitative assessment tools designed not only to identify key health challenges but also to assess capacity for implementing programs in response. Nigeria identified the many diseases caused by the lack of clean water, sanitation, and personal hygiene. As a result, these ministries implemented the installation of the borehole water hand pump, VIP toilets, and delivery of instruction on basic hygiene in a small number of schools in each state, with pre and postassessments. Thus, Nigeria used multiple strategies but concentrated on the sanitation challenge, where they could afford a modest reach and an evaluation of the results.

In China, the HPS initiative reached 51 schools, including 93,000 students and their families plus 6,800 staff, at all levels from primary through junior and senior to vocational education. Beginning with the single issue of nutrition, the Provincial Departments of Education and Health implemented all components of the HPS, addressing several different health topics and the whole development of the child. The political and community structure in communities was an asset for mobilization and broader implementation.

The United Arab Emirates (UAE) implemented all components of the HPS; in 2004–2005, there were 52 nurses and 106 doctors distributed among the different medical districts to implement the program in 745 governmental schools with a total of 287,098 students. The same staff also supervised implementation in 480 private schools with 343,535 students.

In Poland in 2007, the HPS existed in all 16 voivodships, in more than 1,400 schools of different types, mainly elementary schools, reaching about 650,000 pupils. In addition, more than 200 kindergartens in the country implemented the HPS concept in their activities.

There is tremendous variation in terms of which components of the model were implemented; what health, social, and economic conditions were addressed; reach; and scale. All cases provide valuable insights about strategies for implementation.

Insights: What Factors Supported Implementation?

Using the Atlas.ti software, a qualitative analysis of the cases was conducted, coding the strategies according to those presented in Fig. 1 in the chapter "Framing

Theories and Implementation Research." Table 1 presents the frequencies, in descending order, with which the cases describe the various factors from Fig. 1 in the chapter "Framing Theories and Implementation Research" as a method in their implementation strategy.

In this section, we discuss and present examples from the cases of how various factors were used to implement strategies that address healthy development in education settings.

Vision and Concept, International and National Guidelines (Policies)

Figure 1 (in the chapter "Introduction and Background") and the HPS definition that precedes it present the vision and concept of the HPS, created originally by the WHO European Office and European Council and then adapted by WHO Headquarters for its Global School Health Initiative. Countries around the globe found the idea to be an exciting and dynamic way to engage the many stakeholders needed to address a range of pressing health and education issues.

With the conclusion of the WHO Expert Meeting on Comprehensive School Health in 1995, WHO produced publications to promote and advocate for the HPS concept. Publications described studies on the benefits of the HPS to educational and health outcomes and offered evidence of effective strategies. WHO's Information Series on School Health summarized the research on ways to address particular health topics in schools, such as worm infections, nutritional deficits, reproductive health, and violence. Other tools were created, for example, to guide participatory processes for assessment, planning, and monitoring and evaluation at the national and local levels. WHO and the partner UN agencies provided ministries of education and health with guidelines for ways to integrate the HPS or FRESH concept into national policy, also in alignment with UNESCO's Education for All initiative.

Table 1 Frequencies of strategies mentioned in cases

Codes	Frequency
Vision and concept / International and national guidelines	151 (78/73)
Dedicated time and resources (financial, human, technical, and material)	107
Stakeholder ownership and participation	105
Team training and ongoing coaching/learning community	101
Cross-sector collaboration	90
Champions and leaders at all levels	73
Data-driven planning and decision making	73
Administrative and management support	36
Adapting to local concerns	27
Attention to external forces	18
Critical mass and supportive norms	17
Stage of readiness	9

The factors of vision/concept and international/national guidelines were first coded separately and then tallied together for the purposes of this study. Our reasons are that WHO and other organizations promoted and disseminated the vision and concept of the HPS or FRESH to countries and communities worldwide, through the international guidelines and publications that they produced. Often, countries then transformed or drew upon these international guidelines, creating their own national or regional guidelines or policies. At the national and local levels, such guidelines and policies were customized to address particular challenges and the socioeconomic and cultural context. It is difficult to untangle the vision and concept from the guidelines and policies in which the concept is embedded. For these reasons, we have clustered them together as the first factor affecting implementation; the combined total exceeds all other factors.

The following excerpts from the case studies illustrate how different countries came to embrace the concept and develop their own national or local policies to guide actions. They show how the concept was often transformed to meet local needs and how full ownership and investment could require several years, with extensive dialogue among many stakeholders.

Terms to Describe the Concept

While all the cases aimed at a comprehensive approach, the components and the names to describe a comprehensive concept varied. For instance, in Bahrain the Comprehensive School Health Initiative seeks to address three categories: instruction/curriculum, support programs and social services, and healthy physical environment. Viet Nam selected four elements, represented as the petals of a lotus flower: school facilities, health education, health services, and health policies. And in Hong Kong, the Healthy Schools Award Scheme covers six key areas: health policy, physical and social environments, community relationships, personal health skills, and health services.

Not all case studies called their schools "Health-Promoting Schools." Canada preferred "Healthy School," which they found more user-friendly than the term "Comprehensive School Health," which is used in the USA. Nicaragua reports about "Friendly and Healthy Schools," while Australia has a "School-Link Initiative," and Uruguay implements an "Education for Life and Environment" component as well as "Inclusive Education" initiatives, both of which provided an opportunity to implement components of HPS. Germany developed a new concept of "good and healthy schools," which links interventions directly to the activities that schools have to fulfill to accomplish quality criteria of good schools. Health is seen as an input and throughput factor, not an output or outcome factor.

Vision

The vision of the countries also differed to some degree. While some countries were more narrowly focused on health outcomes, others looked at a wider angle, considering the link between health and education and even envisioning the school as a catalyst for transformation.

For instance, Barbados wanted to reduce obesity, inactivity, and by extension, incommunicable diseases; and the USA saw schools as providing "an incredible opportunity to improve the current and future health and well-being of young people."

Mauritius had a bit wider view, as its ultimate project goal was that "all school activities center around the overall development of the child, s/he is the raw resource that has to be moulded into a thinking, creative being who can both integrate into, as well as transform, society." Oman stated the vision as "better health for the school community" and their mission as "working together for Health-Promoting Schools."

Brazil looked at the interrelationship between health and education:

Program organizers pursued improvements, not only in educational attainment, but also in living conditions, determinants of health, and the well-being of the children and the community. It was clear to the project team from the very beginning that it was necessary to look at all aspects of the interrelationships between health and education. The overall outcome pursued for the project was an educational one.

The concept was expressed in the school's motto,

"Transforming children into citizens of a new era," and it committed all school members to *generating an educational environment that goes beyond the school boundaries through participative solutions and the promotion of change agents and new social objectives.* [original emphasis]

The Sapphire Road School in South Africa, facing extreme poverty, massive unemployment, high rates of HIV infection, and some despair in the community, charted "a five-year vision under the name 'Let's Join and Build' ('Masibambane Sakhe')." They saw the school as a means for social transformation:

Our vision is: To ensure that the school is used as an instrument to develop not only the learners but also the parents and the community. This can be done if the school serves as the centre of educational and social transformation.

Concerning the vision and concept, they report:

Sapphire Road Primary would strive to utilize its historic educational responsibility to act as a catalyst for social "upliftment" of the community. Central to this bold conceptualization of our educational task was the actual development of the different components of the school community to a level of understanding that community members, as partners in the educational process, have an important role to play in the success of our educational objective. We managed this by initially working to change the general view of the school from a "building" to a "home away from home" owned by all.

The key question still debated is whether an educational institution should focus purely on academic education or also on the social issues of its feeder communities. The debate is good—it has propelled implementation rather than halted it.

Impetus

To implement HPSs in Oman, the concept was discussed in the joint school health committee meeting. A proposal was sent to the decision makers in both the Ministry of Health and the Ministry of Education to get approval and support. Oman adopted WHO's HPS concept in 2004–2005 and began to implement the idea in 19 schools.

In China, also,

in response to [WHO's] Global School Health Initiative, launched in 1995, and with the endorsement of the national Ministries of Health and Education, some of China's health and education agencies began implementing the HPS concept in selected schools... The recent mandate from the Chinese government for quality education calls for a holistic approach to child development and education. The WHO HPS model provided a useful structure for implementing these changes.

In Viet Nam, "interest and participation in school health promotion can be traced back to their participation in a [HPS] workshop in Singapore in January 1995." National and international guidelines have helped direct HPS in Viet Nam. The development of National Guidelines for HPS "drew on the original HPS Principles developed in 1990 by WHO and were in line with [Western Pacific Region Office] HPS Guidelines."

Similarly, a WHO expert mission introduced the concept of the HPS to the UAE, which then drew upon the WHO guidelines. Adopting the model, UAE stated its mission,

to promote, protect, and improve the health of students in UAE, through a comprehensive and coordinated school health program. The components of the program have been developed to ensure that students' physical, emotional, and social health and well-being are maintained in a state that would enable them to achieve maximum benefit from their education.

In Nicaragua, institutions and stakeholders took almost 2 years to come to a consensus on a conceptual framework and main conceptual elements of a shared vision. Implementing the concept was

not about launching new policies but about how to implement what was already on the education agenda through an innovative and coordinated strategy, avoiding duplication, dispersion, and negative competition among the different stakeholders and ongoing programs ... [The program] was inspired by the need to provide Nicaraguan children with the skills they need to address their own lives and the challenges of their changing country and region, which are embarking on a process of social and economic development.

Canada describes how it was the success at the local level that bubbled up to put policy in place at the provincial level:

Policy support (within the school boards and at the provincial level) actually occurred *after* [original emphasis] the local-level successes. It is interesting to note that policy statements were not necessary in order to achieve local commitment. Rather local-level successes actually convinced higher levels to formulate policy . . . Once policy support occurs, it does increase the profile and importance of any issue.

Dissemination of the HPS concept played a powerful role across many cases. Dating back to the Ottawa Charter, which stated that health must be created in places where people live, love, learn, and work, the application of this public health approach to the education setting began to take hold around the world. But to implement the vision and concept, along with the practical guidelines and tools for doing so, demands resources of all types, the next-most-frequently-mentioned factor.

Dedicated Time and Resources

In addition to having the time of dedicated staff and the human resources to assume responsibility for implementation, under resources we have considered financial support; human support, in terms of the availability of the workforce and in terms of their technical expertise, knowledge, and skills; and materials and tools. Taken together, these types of resources rank second in frequency of mention in the cases after the vision/concept and international/national guidelines. Later we provide examples from countries, schools, and communities of the resources they have needed in the form of the following:

- Financial resources
- Human resources and technical expertise
- Materials and tools as resources

Financial Resources

Nations, states/provinces, local schools, and communities tapped a variety of financial sources of different scales. Financial support was gained from international donors, such as WHO or the World Bank; from governments, including the ministries of education or health at national or state levels; and from philanthropists. Some cases describe financial or significant in-kind contributions from local community agencies or leaders, without which they could not have gone forward.

Yet other cases recount the fortunate circumstance of beginning with a substantial level of government support to create infrastructure, which continued through to institutionalization. Some convinced national policy makers that it was critical to tap funds for education reform as health is linked to students' academic success.

Other cases illustrate the role of small grant competitions or seed money that provided the initial catalyst for the HPS movement. This seed money often enabled countries to gain attention and then to secure additional funds, moving to a larger scale and reaching more students and schools.

A few case study authors criticize pilot funding that either started initiatives in just a few schools or experimented with one aspect of the program; they report that such pilots tended to increase disparities between the schools that had resources and those that did not. In some cases, funding of pilots never went beyond pilots. Australia shares:

Often with large initiatives rather than a complete rollout, government departments tend to hedge their bets and pilot test the initiative in a small number of areas or—even worse—in one locality. The problem is that then only a small number of sites normally receive the benefit while more money than would be the typical case is poured into these pilot sites. This level of funding is unsustainable or cannot be replicated on a large scale, which makes the initiative look too costly to the funding body. This also tends to increase the disparity between sites and create competition for funds rather than cooperation. Government departments are run on short-term cycles, and it is often the case that pilots never go beyond that, even when they show very good results. This can create disillusionment in the workforce in areas that do not receive funding, as some areas typically attract all the funding.

Other cases illustrate how program organizers pieced together monies from various national and state funding sources, with each supporting activities dedicated to specific health issues. For example, one agency might support the HIV and AIDS component; another, obesity; and yet another, violence. In one very poor community, it was the in-kind time and contributions of people in the community that made it happen.

A mix of strategies is evident for different conditions and stages of development. Most cases require a mosaic of financial resources that must be gained by persistent advocacy and determined action throughout the program cycle. Beyond the financial resources needed for country efforts, a few cases point to meeting the financial needs of the regional networks that have been so important in delivering the technical expertise through materials, training, and technical assistance, building the capacity and know-how for implementation.

The cases from Viet Nam, Canada, Uruguay, South Africa, and Singapore illustrate extensive use of small grants or seed money or in-kind community contributions.

In Viet Nam, a

small grants [emphasis added] program operated as part of Phase One and Phase Two was a key to gaining schools' buy-in to HPS.

WHO funded and or helped mobilize small grants of around $500 to about 100 schools; many schools made remarkable progress with these funds, especially in the poorer areas. The audit tool helped many schools to identify and prioritize areas in need of improvement in their schools. The grants were then used to improve the physical environment of schools by planting trees, creating garden areas, cleaning up unused space to create play areas, installing large rubbish bins, paving paths, installing or repairing wells, building toilet blocks and modest kitchens, and purchasing drinking water containers for classrooms.

The grants were an important way of involving the whole community in the project. Schools were encouraged to work with local authorities, especially the local People's Committee and Women's Union, to secure additional funds to complete the work started from the small grants. Community involvement was high in many areas, with parents being asked to volunteer their time to implement the building projects. In order to secure a small grant, schools had to submit their plans to the [Ministry of Health] for funding and approval and agree to take action in all areas of the framework, based on the audit, and to identify priority areas and develop a plan accordingly.

Demand for grants outstripped WHO's capacity to supply funds; however, WHO was able to facilitate grants from several international organizations, including the Hanoi International Women's Club, the Australian Chamber of Commerce, and the United Nation's International School in Hanoi.

The revised HPS Guidelines Booklet, developed after the demonstration project in Ha Tinh and Hai Phong, included small case studies of how the schools had used their small grants and the steps they had followed, to help guide other schools through the process.

Canada reports that

for many jurisdictions in Ontario, [Canada,] it has been the Heart Health Partnership funding that has enabled us to get Healthy Schools up and running in a meaningful way. These grants are contingent on strong partnerships across sectors, so they propel health and education to work together. The funding for Toronto enabled the central coordinating committee to provide interested schools with seed funding to help them with meeting costs and with carrying out local plans. Without this incentive, schools would be very unlikely to invest significant time or resources in comprehensive Healthy Schools work. Moreover, obtaining this significant grant brought credibility to the project and enabled both the school board and public health unit to mobilize additional internal resources and staff for training/coaching/ongoing learning and centralized planning of events.

Uruguay worked at several levels:

Between 1994 and 2005 Uruguay implemented—with support from the World Bank—a comprehensive strategy to improve its basic education system. The strategy was devoted to expanding preschool education, building institutions (particularly teacher training reform and small grants to support the implementation of quality education projects administered by schools), and introducing a full-time-school model.

Between 2002 and 2004, the program supported the implementation of an Education for Life and Environment component (or *Educación para la vida y el ambiente [EVA]*) as well as Inclusive Education initiatives in more than 250 out of the country's 4,000 primary schools. The EVA project invited schools to identify, through a situation analysis, a specific health-related issue they wanted to change. Schools then received technical assistance and a number of resources to tackle their problem and improve the health and well-being of children and teachers.

In operational terms, schools have received technical support and seed money to develop a health promotion program while making a number of tangible changes at the level of the school's physical and educational environment, involving all groups in the school community in a participative manner.

The Sapphire School in South Africa explains how

with limited financial resources, we would not have been in a position to effect our program without the assistance of social partners from outside the school environment. The Department of Health in the Eastern Cape has played a significant role in our success. They provided technical, financial, and human resource support, ranging from inoculations for our learner population to expertise and physical resources for our AIDS garden. The Rotary Club of Algoa has also been instrumental in the attainment of our vision. Through their hard work, dedication, and donation we were able to realize our academic improvement plan. Club members also assisted with material and technical support for the building of our security house and clinic.

In Singapore,

three years after the launch of the CHERISH Award, the School Health Promotion Grant was set up, making financial support from the Health Promotion Board available for schools to mount appropriate health promotion initiatives for both staff and students, enhance existing programs, or develop a more comprehensive program and improve their standing within the CHERISH Award scheme. Issued on an annual basis, the grant is used for reimbursement of up to 50% of the amount expended, up to a maximum of SG $5,000 per school per year. These funds can be used for programs or services that increase awareness or knowledge or promote behavior change. All grant recipients must take part in the CHERISH Award for that year. If a school has received the grant previously, it will be awarded it in a subsequent year only if it has shown improvement in its CHERISH Award status. The grant is publicized extensively through brochures sent to schools, training courses for teachers, HealthVine, and the Health Promotion Board's Web site. Applications should include a plan for needs assessment, evaluation, and follow-up activities to ensure sustainability. In the five years since its inception, a total of 166 schools have benefited from the grant, implementing activities such as yoga instruction or health-related training courses for teachers, fruit days or fruit breaks, health camps, treks or excursions for students, purchase of exercise equipment, conducting surveys, or relevant health screening.

In Hong Kong and Australia, we see large-scale government support to launch and support programs over time.

Although there was no earmarked funding for HPS [before 1998], the Hong Kong SAR Government had established a US$640 million (HK$5 billion) Quality Education Fund (QEF) to fund worthwhile projects to raise the quality of school education. CUHK [Chinese University of Hong Kong] and the School Councils successfully convinced the QEF that both health and education are linked to the economic performance and social cohesion of modern industrialized society. Therefore funding of US$1.9 million in 1998 and US$1.1 million in 2000 was awarded to launch the initial HPS program... QEF funding of US$2.75 million in 2001 and US$0.5 million in 2005 were awarded for Hong Kong Healthy Schools Award and Health Promoting Kindergarten (early childhood education) respectively.

In Australia, the New South Wales School-Link initiative

was officially launched in late 1999. The initial round of funding was for five years. At that time the state of NSW was divided into 17 Area Health Services. Funding was provided in the initial phase to each Area Health Service to employ a School-Link Coordinator. The Area Health Service (AHS) was to provide the operating budget for the coordinator, demonstrating its commitment to the initiative. At the end of the first five years, another three years of funding was secured to distribute to the AHSs. A small number of AHSs had absorbed these positions and made them permanent. They were able to use the extra funds provided to enhance their initiative. One AHS at this time used the extra position to pilot some work in the primary schools. Money was also invested in a formal training program for school and [Technical and Further Education] counselors and child and adolescent mental health workers.

The state of Michigan in the USA provides an example of how national health funding was given to state education agencies and the way in which they joined together funding concerning different health topics to create a large state program over time:

> The state funding for school health laid the foundation for coordinated school health, while federal Safe and Drug-Free Schools funding, provided by the U.S. Department of Education, accelerated implementation. In 1987, Michigan received additional funding from the [Centers for Disease Control/Division of Adolescent and School Health (CDC/DASH)], to develop a statewide HIV and AIDS prevention program. The funding was timely, given the national attention to this emerging epidemic and new Michigan laws that required school districts to teach about HIV and AIDS as part of their communicable disease instruction.

> The use of federal funds to support state departments of education was a novel approach at the time. State and local education agencies were a common-sense choice to have an impact on the health of young people, because they spend a considerable amount of time in school. In the United States, the educational system is an institution with its own mission, operating principles, governance structure, and culture. Like any other long-standing institution, schools are not easily influenced by external factors. The most effective school health endeavors are those that work within the educational system in collaboration with key partners to effect change in policies, programs, and practices.

> In the late 1980s, the [Michigan Department of Education] was awarded a five-year competitive CDC/DASH National Training and Demonstration grant of $250,000 to build the capacity of other states to effectively manage their HIV and AIDS grants ... In the early 1990s, the CDC/DASH increased state funding for school health with Expanded Program dollars to build the infrastructure for a state-level Coordinated School Health Program (CSHP). State departments of education received funds to work in partnership with state departments of health to build the capacity of schools to use a coordinated approach to address physical activity, nutrition, and tobacco use (PANT) and ultimately prevent chronic disease.

And Michigan, USA, has been successful in gaining funding for many other specific health topics from the agencies that address them.

> In 2004, Michigan was the first in the nation to secure a unique funding structure that allowed for state funds to be put up for federal match. In 2007/2008 this funding structure brought over $6.5 million into Michigan to help implement this component of CSHP.

> Mental health in schools is an emerging need that requires additional attention and focus. A mental health grant of more than $375,000 was recently awarded by the federal Office of Safe and Drug-Free Schools for a collaborative project between the MDE, Michigan Department of Community Health (MDCH), Michigan Department of Human Services (MDHS), and the School Community Health Alliance of Michigan (SCHA-MI). Three

school-based pilot sites will work directly with their local community mental health offices to increase access to mental health services for their students.

It is not possible to conclude from the cases that any one strategy for gaining financial resources was more effective than the other. No matter what the source or amount, more important was whether and how the program and services have become part of the ongoing way in which education and health ministries carry out their everyday work. Has the HPS/FRESH concept become the core mission of schools and the way teachers and other school staff think of their role and responsibilities in partnership with parents, the community, and health service providers? Once the concept is embraced, building the structures and costs into line items of annual budgets institutionalizes the practice. As the Michigan case poignantly says,

> American statesman Barry Goldwater said: "A government that is big enough to give you all you want is big enough to take it all away." Too often, promising programs disappear because funding is reduced or taken away.

Human Resources and Technical Expertise

The people who commit their time and effort to implement the HPS are a basic need. Even without the financial resources or, initially, even without the technical knowledge or skills, the cases illustrate how the passion of people has moved the concept forward. The technical expertise can be acquired by providing professional development for the existing workforce (discussed later in the section "Team Training") or by securing consultancies or partnerships from within or outside the country or community. Organizing the human resources into cross-sectoral committees at both national and local levels (discussed in the section "Administrative and Management Support") provides effective ways for them to work together to carry out the work.

In poor areas, several cases have underscored the importance of having the human resource of the public health nurse to provide screening and treatment services to children and adolescents.

The technical expertise requires participation of both the education and health sectors, working together. The professional literature supports the importance placed on particular knowledge and skills reported in the case studies, including the following:

- Health promotion, prevention, screening, and treatment of health issues, such as HIV, AIDS, and many others
- Social science and public health strategies, such as the following:
  - Analyzing epidemiologic, etiologic, or other data
  - Selecting targeted and evidence-based interventions
  - Knowing how to plan, implement, and evaluate program impact

- Techniques to foster participation and manage effective collaboration across sectors and with multiple partners
- Capacities in leadership, advocacy, communications, and more (Vince Whitman, 2005)

Countries found many different ways to designate the human resources or to gain the necessary technical expertise. Many refer to the important role played by international or national conferences, on-site consultations, and especially their participation in networks, such as the European Network of Health Promoting Schools. This and other networks provide technical consultations, forums for exchange and learning among peers, and valuable resources and publications. Such mechanisms within countries or regions have made possible exchange on technical issues among policy makers and practitioners. Cases also reported about school visits and "exchange trips" for sharing of best practices and lessons learned.

India writes about the importance of having the workforce and the benefits that can accrue:

> Talented, motivated manpower to create these programs and a dedicated large field force to take them to schools are prerequisites for a successful outcome. As most attitudes and habits are formed in childhood and youth, adequate investment of resources for promoting health in schools could pay large dividends in terms of good health of our future generations.

Singapore describes the value of connecting people to each other within the country:

> It is also important to provide schools with direct access to the national coordinating agency in a personal way, giving names, telephone numbers, and e-mail addresses of persons dedicated to oversee the program for their school or group of schools. Platforms for networking among participating schools to share ideas and experiences are also useful.

In countries like the UAE, the human resource provided by nurses played a powerful role. "The uneven distribution of manpower, especially in remote areas where school nurses have not been allocated to schools or have visited schools only once a week," is a problem. "Vaccination, medical examination, and health education have thus been provided by mobile teams with the cooperation of local primary care centers."

Materials and Tools as Resources

The cases provide numerous examples of the importance of materials and tools as resources, including international guidelines, curricula and training materials, and protocols for assessment, planning, monitoring, and evaluation. Often these tangible products carried the necessary technical expertise. They were disseminated broadly in print form and also available on WHO's and many other Web sites. Materials and tools played a very important role in implementation of the concept. One could argue that putting the concept into practice would not have been possible without the many different types of products that provided the knowledge, skills, and techniques for how to do it.

For policy makers and practitioners in Europe, we see how conferences and their proceedings provided guidance to many countries. In 1997, the first European Network of Health Promoting Schools conference took place in Thessaloniki, Greece, inviting representatives from all European nations. In 2002, an important follow-up conference, in Egmond-an-Zee, Netherlands, considered progress and planned forward action, which happened.

As the case study from Scotland recounts,

[The Egmond conference] included participants from 43 European countries and representatives from many of their national ministries. As a result, the publication of the Egmond Agenda was influential in many European countries in setting out the practical steps for policy makers and practitioners that were considered essential in building successful Health-Promoting School programs.

In the state of Michigan in the USA,

most impressive, was the development of the Healthy School Toolkit to assist schools in moving to a [Comprehensive School Health Program] CSHP. The toolkit contains data that make the case for healthy eating and physical activity, steps for conducting an assessment, guidance for developing and adopting policy, and ways to communicate success. More than 4,000 toolkits have been distributed and used by teachers and parents across the state.

Through teamwork, [Michigan Action for Healthy Kids] has accelerated the pace of implementing health initiatives in schools. In six short years, it has become the clearing house for reliable information, tools, and resources needed to implement a CSHP in schools and earned the status of "school health central." The fact that it is the largest [Action for Healthy Kids] state coalition, with over 500 members, representing more than 200 Michigan public and private organizations, is proof that "together we can do more." Michigan has proven that bringing together passionate, well-intended, action-oriented people will build capacity and sustainability, limit controversy, and sustain revenue streams.

Numerous examples relate how training and classroom health education materials were essential in the educational process. Lao PDR presents an interesting combination of the process to develop *and* use materials and training.

First, a review of the existing health education materials was completed. Almost 400 materials had been collected and considered, but agreement was made for improvement of the existing *Blue Box* materials, originally promoted by UNICEF. Revisions were made to modify the materials in the box, not only focusing on the issues of hygiene and sanitation, but also concentrating on malaria, diarrhea, parasite control, dengue, nutrition, dental health, and waste management. The materials in the box were revised, and some new materials were created to match the health education part of *The World Around Us.*

The number of materials in the box has increased from 13 items to 20 items. Production of the boxes was supported by WHO, UNICEF, and a non-governmental organization. Dissemination mechanisms are key to help teachers familiarize themselves with the tools and enable them to use them effectively. A training course was conducted for province and district trainers, who then conducted a course to train teachers in targeted schools. The Blue Box was distributed to all 450 schools targeted by the school health project. UNICEF and another non-governmental organization also distributed the box to additional schools. A first, rapid assessment found the materials very useful to teachers delivering health information about behavior change for students. The materials are both entertaining and educational; they create both fun and relaxation during the class.

The Philippines developed a unique Urbani School Health Kit that considers the different health needs of children at different age groups, and contains user-friendly teaching materials for each key issue:

> The kit encourages *innovative ways of teaching health*. The materials are contained in a wooden cabinet with wheels that is durable and easily transported within schools. Design considerations include: visibility (not tucked away in an office or closet), usability (appropriate, answers needs of teachers and schools), and durability (able to withstand the elements and rough handling). The box with its flip top can also be used as a platform for teaching in class. ... The learning activities are designed to allow easy implementation in a variety of contexts. Even with very limited access to resources, teachers and students should still be able to perform the activities.

In the UAE,

> the packages of training material are designed specifically to support workshops for the development of the HPS in the UAE; these training materials were developed by the UAE HPS Coordinating Committee, in collaboration with WHO. Dr. Rose Marie Erben, a consultant from Australia, located within the WHO's Regional Office in the Western Pacific Region, conducted a training workshop to train trainers on the development of Health-Promoting Schools. The training materials used in the workshops were developed after referring to the experiences and workshops conducted in Viet Nam, Mongolia, and Vanuatu. The documents of the training package include: [a] manual for facilitators; participants' workbook; [and] national guidelines for the development of Health-Promoting Schools, a framework for action. These documents provided the framework for supporting the growth and development of Health-Promoting Schools in the Western Pacific Region. The documents were edited, adapted, and published to suit the training needs of the United Arab Emirates.

Scotland notes that the country had developed training resources to respond to identified lack of capacity: "*Growing through Adolescence* was developed. When teachers made it clear that they required support in dealing with the complex mental health and social health issues concerning young people, body image, self-esteem, dieting, and eating behaviors." Scotland also suggests that the quality of teachers affects implementation. Their certification and the salaries and conditions of service play an important role.

While some countries developed materials that addressed a range of health topics, other countries developed curricula for specific health topics. Australia talks about MindMatters, a mental health program for schools with a range of curriculum materials that address social and emotional learning and Cook Islands developed a Health and Physical Well-Being Curriculum (CIHPWB).

India mentions the importance of developing interactive materials:

> Care was taken to ensure that each session was interesting, innovative and participatory in nature. The health issues were addressed through one or more of the following methods: interactive sessions, quiz programs, elocution and poster contests, audiovisual films, anti-tobacco oath-taking ceremonies, intra- and inter- school debates, articles in school newsletters, teacher orientation programs, creation of a Web site for the initiative, magic shows, rallies...

In addition to teaching materials, some case studies also reported about developing advocacy materials. Bahrain developed newsletters and leaflets, and Germany developed a leporello (folded card) and brochure.

Poland reports the importance of "social marketing of HPS concept including systematic publication in magazines for schools, manuals for schools, brochures for local governments, Web site, regional and national conferences addressed to broad audience."

Reading through the cases confirms that materials play an important role throughout the continuum of informing policy, first as tools for advocacy and planning, and then as training manuals, health education classroom curricula, and other supportive elements.

Stakeholder Ownership and Participation

A powerful feature of the HPS concept is the participation of teachers, family, community members, and students themselves in the design and implementation of the program, depicted in Fig. 1 (in the chapter "Introduction and Background"). Stakeholder ownership and participation are important implementation factors, ranking third in frequency in the cases. Having a vision and concept promoted through international and national guidelines required the ownership and participation of many constituents to move from ideas on paper to actions in schools.

At the national level, stakeholders typically involved ministries of education, health, and others, country offices of UN agencies, and civil society. At the local level, this ownership and participation ranged from engaging all community members early in the process to make the concept their own to involving teachers in the creation of programs to address their own health and to having students, for example, assume roles in program governance, participate in classroom problem-solving activities, conduct situational analyses, carry out peer education, and mentor younger students.

An important learning across cases was the need for participation to be authentic and not decorative. As we see later in the section that describes the factor of team training, many people had to learn the skills and methods to nurture participation. For example, some cases describe how government officials must let go of their authoritarian role and allow community members and parents to assume responsibility. Similarly, teachers and parents need to enable genuine student empowerment and engagement. The case from Uruguay expresses the challenge this way:

Most schools and teachers did not seem prepared to accept genuine participation. Institutional culture is a key factor: Authorities and civil servants are unaccustomed to sharing power. Public policy will have to actively pursue this cultural change, to create conditions for better long-term, real participation by children and families in health promotion in schools.

As other cases inform us, the more that stakeholders enjoy genuine participation, the more the programs seem to flourish. Such involvement provides cohesiveness between home, school, and community, contributing to the growth and sustainability of programs across time. Additional examples illustrate the benefits and values of ownership and participation.

Broad Community and Parent Involvement

From the case of South Africa, we learn:

> The crucial HPS element that enabled us to progress was community buy-in. Once the school was recognized as a social agent, it became much easier to implement some of the other elements. It took us more than two years of discussion and of convincing our community, government, businesses, and even ourselves that our course was true... While parents, teachers and learners formed the nucleus of the change process in the school, eliciting support from government departments, private sector and non-governmental organizations also played a very important role in actualizing our vision.

The evaluation conducted by their National Department of Health found that "the golden thread holding together [its] institution was community participation and ownership, a key element of the HPS concept."

From inception, Viet Nam labeled its "HPS effort a 'community project' rather than an 'education project'... Community involvement was very strong and a key to success. Parents and local authorities committed time and money to the various small works projects that positively impacted the school environment."

In Brazil, it was the leadership of the principal and teachers living in a very poor community that provided the force desiring change. This case expresses the importance of dialogue in the participation process:

> Dialogue has also been a key tool of the process. This included not only an open-minded and interactive approach to teaching and learning, but also a permanent exercise to expand the network of collaboration and find new partners for the strategy. This dialogue was essential in order to legitimate the strategy in the community and with governmental authorities. This dialogue often took place in a context of diverse ideas and philosophical or ideological backgrounds. Once again, Morin's premise was verified: "What is progressive is not an idea but the dialogue of ideas."

In Michigan, in the USA, we see how the involvement of many sectors and the collaboration between state and local levels were invaluable for advocacy and program funding:

> The process used to develop the model curriculum was as important as the product itself. A network of 115 professional and volunteer groups—representing agencies (e.g., health department, American Cancer Society), content areas (e.g., HIV education, violence prevention, physical fitness), and disciplines (e.g., nursing, school social work)—came together to develop a "road map." The partners became champions ... This collaborative ownership, with the combination of state and local-match funding and the infusion of federal funding, increased the adoption and implementation of the curriculum in a majority of school districts and schools within a few years from its inception. Collaboration among

government and non-governmental agencies has become a trademark among Michigan school health champions and continues to this day to provide the foundation for coordinated school health programs.

While the ownership and participation of those in the surrounding community is critical to implementation, so, too, is the genuine involvement of teachers and students.

Teacher and Student Involvement

To engage teachers, students, and parents, Germany used a very creative technique, implementing a Self-Evaluation in Schools (SEIS) questionnaire. Anschub.de, a nationwide program established by the Bertelsmann Foundation in 2002, believes, "One of the key points is to involve pupils more in the process of developing a good and healthy school." The other is to ask teachers and parents what they know about and how they experience the program. The SEIS is the basis of items in a questionnaire that teachers, parents, and pupils complete each spring.

There are many examples of strategies developed to involve teachers in caring for their own health. For example, in the Cook Islands, staff

decided that they wanted to address not just the physical health of their students but the other four dimensions of well-being as well. Initially, the teaching staff, the Health and Physical Well-Being Advisor, and the Public Health Nutritionist worked together to develop a health education long-term plan and a physical education long-term plan for teachers to follow. These long-term plans became the basis for teacher planning, teaching, and learning programs.

Much of the evidence in the literature regarding the effectiveness of health education or other interventions to promote positive health behaviors emphasizes the importance of participatory, active learning techniques where young people have the opportunity to practice or demonstrate specific skills (World Health Organization, 2003). Kenya, Bahrain, India, and other cases reflect this as they illustrate the importance of involving pupils deeply in the activities throughout planning and adoption.

Kenya, for example, emphasized true student participation in finding solutions to prevent intestinal worms. As a result of participatory classroom activity, teachers reported that "children took personal actions to manage their health, for example, burning and selling charcoal to get money to buy shoes, in order to be neat as well as to avoid hookworm infection." (Going barefoot is a risk for hookworm infection, which can penetrate the body through the feet.)

In Bahrain,

students have clearly articulated their desire to influence policies and services that are developed to support their safe and successful transition to adulthood. . . Policymakers and experts must continually consult with students to determine their responsiveness to and acceptance of the directions and strategies.

And, finally, in India,

> generating participation and motivation among individual students was challenging. We tried a strategy of popularizing a health promoting website (http://www.hope.org.in) for creating health awareness among students by coupling it with names and pictures of students and schools. This recognition of individuals and institutions led to a 316% increase in hit counts to the HOPE Initiative Web site.

Knowing how to manage the process of participation at all levels and knowing how to implement a concept as complex as the HPS in dynamic and ever-changing political, cultural, and economic environments demands opportunities for ongoing professional development. This factor is the next-most-often cited as important to implementation, on par in importance with stakeholder participation.

Team Training, Ongoing Coaching, and Participation in a Learning Community

Implementers of an HPS or similar model most often receive little to no formal preparation at the preservice level regarding the requisite knowledge, skills, and capacities. Therefore, continuing professional education for staff is a necessity! Team training is crucial because it prepares a group at the national or local level to go back to their organizations and to create, together, momentum for change and support for one another. Ongoing coaching is essential when staff try new practices, supporting them to overcome obstacles and to move along the path of putting the concepts into practice. And being a member of an ongoing learning community allows people to learn from peers, supported by the camaraderie of the group; to reflect on failures and successes; and to continue to experiment and try new and creative strategies in their work every day.

Through the cases, we learn that so many of the program planners needed professional development to carry out another important factor in implementation – ownership and participation. Two methods were of great value and benefit: training members from the education and health sectors together, and having training mandated so that administrators could not prevent staff from attending. Formal certification for participation in courses added to the professionalism of the investment. Opportunities to come back together for reflection made a positive difference. High staff turnover calls for mechanisms that keep training continuous, even as staff come and go.

Content of Training

Clear is the call that training must go far beyond knowledge of health topics. Several cases point out that people needed more training opportunities than were ever available. They also wanted other kinds of experiences, such as study tours and site visits to learn from and exchange ideas with experienced practitioners. Reiterating many of the general themes of successful implementation of the HPS concept as described in the professional literature (see the earlier section "Human Resources and Technical Expertise"), cases describe the range of issues that professional development must address to build capacity, such as the following:

- Basic health promotion theory and tenets of a public health approach
- Theory and underlying research of the HPS concept
- Roles, responsibilities, and competencies of different sectors
- Methods for advocacy, participation, planning, implementation, and evaluation
- In-depth knowledge about promotion, prevention, and treatment of specific health issues
- Skills to foster motivation, conflict resolution, negotiation, and communication
- Practical experience through modeling best practices, conducting class demonstrations, and designing lesson plans

And in Kenya, which evaluated the impact of student participation, the training was dedicated to having teachers move from didactic to participatory approaches for young people:

> The hypothesis is that action-oriented and participatory approaches in health education support the development of pupils' abilities to create change – their action competence ... Teachers were mostly familiar with didactic, top-down approaches; so they were struggling, in spite of good intentions, to adopt the new approach ... Given that action-oriented learning and teaching including student participation was new in the study district, the program provided technical assistance and training to teachers to help them implement the intervention. Two in-service training workshops were conducted for science teachers and head teachers in the selected schools, as well as for education inspectorate staff in the district. The workshops underscored the concepts of participation and action as key concepts in school health education. Apart from the two workshops, three of the nine schools also received continual professional support during weekly visits as part of the study design. The trainings and professional support equipped the teachers with skills and created the conditions necessary for successful implementation of the intervention.

Models of Training

From Australia, we see the value of training education and health staffs together and of mandating the training:

> The interdisciplinary nature of the training fostered an improved working relationship between the health and education sector. This training program is the first in Australia that has set out to systematically educate health and education professionals together. Coordinators are encouraged to organize the training around local child and adolescent mental health services and their cluster of local schools and [Technical and Further Education] Colleges. Approximately 2,000 health and education professionals across the state are trained with the rollout of each module. To ensure that school counselors were able to attend from State schools, the Department of Education made it mandatory for them to attend. It prevented their principal vetoing them from attending. This demonstrates a high level of commitment from education.

Regarding health and education training together in the Cook Islands, "Co-facilitating professional development helped people from both Ministries appreciate and develop a respect for one another's roles."

In Kosovo, training ethnic rivals together contributed to the process of healing and building trust after the war:

> There has been a considerable investment in professional development and training. For example, WHO organized a four-day, multi-ethnic training seminar for teachers; school directors; and representatives from the Ministry of Health, the Ministry of Education, the Ministry of Environment, the Institute of Public Health, women's associations, and the Trepca Institute. This seminar was of considerable symbolic importance, as it was the first time representatives of both communities—Kosovo Albanians and Kosovo Serbs—had trained together in any educational sphere since the conflict... It is clear that the development of joint training in health-promoting schools is one small but important way in which the two ethnic groups can work together to improve trust and relationships for the future.

The case from the Philippines speaks to the importance of team training.

> Training not just one teacher but a team composed of four teachers is part of the strategy of sustainability. The trained team are tasked to "echo" what they have learned to other teachers in their schools and to be part of a network of potential trainers for successive implementation of the Urbani School Health Kit in other regions of the country.

In Hong Kong, a training course was professionalized into a certified diploma program.

> A training course was launched at the [Chinese University of Hong Kong] in 1999, in the format of a Professional Diploma in Health Promotion and Health Education.

> In addition to acquiring essential knowledge and skills of health education, the participating teachers conducted school-based health promotion projects in groups, to gain practical experience in implementing the concept of HPS and to accept the challenge of moving away from didactic health education to a settings approach to health promotion. Those projects provided good opportunities for involvement of school staff, parents, students, and community. Most of their projects had gained the support and participation of Parent-Teachers Associations of their schools, community leaders, non-government organizations, government departments, and business companies; so a strong community partnership was established for future action. By the end of September 2004, 513 participants (from around 500 schools) had graduated from a diploma course.

In some cases training was mandatory, in others it relied on a cascade of passing on knowledge from those already trained to those not yet trained, or was offered through professional learning centers, in-service support, workshops, international consultations, or short residency programs.

Nicaragua combined a number of different models:

> Some schools started to offer short residency programs to teachers interested in learning about the model. Some others, particularly rural schools, started to act as reference centers for others in their own area, while many non-governmental organizations and private schools that learned about [Friendly and Health Schools] decided to adopt or support the model.

Participants in Training

Perhaps most important is that staff need professional development at all levels to foster engagement and participatory involvement across ministries, with parents and community, and with students and teachers in the activities themselves.

Canada writes about its training for public health nurses, drawing on many strategies for community involvement and public health methods:

During 1993–94, [public health nurses (PHNs)] at the Middlesex-London Health Unit received training on how to facilitate the engagement of school communities in becoming a healthy school. PHNs were reminded that their abilities to listen, assess, enable, and build trusting relationships were core nursing skills that would lay the foundation for facilitating the planning, implementation, and evaluation of this collaborative approach. They were expected to act as a catalyst and facilitator of the process. Over time, various tools and resources were developed to assist the school with implementation, specifically the Healthy School Profile . . ., the Healthy School Committee, a resource kit, and evaluation tools. New activities such as completing the Healthy School Profile, analyzing the data, and mobilizing a school community required additional in-service training and support. Advocacy, negotiation, and mediation skills were also enhanced through training and supervision. Health unit staff also provided workshops to educate and inform school principals and vice-principals about the process.

To combat pollution in and near Kosovo's schools, their case underscores the need to include, in the overall effort and in the training, people who are expert in the science of the content or health topic, such as pollution from heavy metals, the problem they tackled.

As part of the capacity building of local professionals who were working in the public awareness campaign, a study visit to Slovenia and Poland was organized. The purpose of the visit to Slovenia and Poland was to develop links with institutions in these countries that are involved in environmental research, environmental remedial actions, and public awareness programs.

Need for More Training

It is very important that we learn from China the need for training to provide both breadth and depth:

In one school, teachers first thought their nutrition knowledge was enough, but when the project gained in intensity, they felt a need for more professional instruction and hoped for more expert talks, though they also acknowledged that "knowledge is not enough" and that some students knew better than teachers. In another school, teachers reported a "lack of health promotion theory" and of the "health" concept. In several schools, administrators hoped WHO would provide more guidance and good examples of international HPS achievements, to help them define specific goals for themselves. School administrators also expressed a desire to visit other places with experience with health promotion. In one school, the school nurse was the only one who had psychological training. Since many students had psychological issues, they needed more teachers with this knowledge. Parents suggested offering more good training for teachers to improve the quality of the staff and introducing more advanced ideas and theories to help them toward good achievements.

Thus, while various means of training initially enabled schools to establish Health-Promoting Schools, participants requested more training, guidance, and sharing of experiences. Study results indicate that training plays an important role in effective HPS implementation.

Through the cases, we learn about many strategies that were used to train people from different sectors on a range of skills and topics. Enabling people to work across sectors, described next, is a key factor in implementation.

Cross-Sector Collaboration

Implementation of the HPS concept requires the cooperation of the education and health sectors and their collaboration with others as well. Because so many determinants of health lie outside the health sector and because programs take place in schools and communities, education must lead. In most of the cases, it was the Ministry of Health that originated the HPS initiative and then reached out to involve the Ministry of Education and more. In Poland, for example, "the national coordinator was moved from the health sector to the education sector. This was a significant achievement, which 'opened the door' for the HPS concept into the education system."

All the cases describe their methods for cross-sector collaboration, involving at least education and health, as well as other sectors at national, local, or multiple levels. Through these reports, we learn about the methods that were most effective in overcoming barriers, including the following:

- Having education serve as the lead player, connecting the effort to the core business of education, and monitoring impact according to education, as well as health outcomes
- Educating each sector about the other's disciplinary framework, language, and methods
- Capitalizing on the legal responsibility of each player for the well-being of children
- Signing official Memoranda of Understanding that define and commit players to carry out specific roles and responsibilities
- Creating both vertical and horizontal collaborating mechanisms
- Sharing both human and fiscal resources
- Including sectors beyond education to address specific issues, such as environmental pollution, or working with the private sector and mass media
- Appointing a dedicated, trusted, and skilled coordinator who will manage the cross-sectoral committee members and their work

• Having players engage in joint activities, such as training, proposal writing, and the nomination and selection of award recipients to build a collaborative team

From the countries, we gain greater insight into how they applied these methods and brought about changes in policy and practice as a result.

Mutual Agreements

The Cook Islands describes the value of a mutual agreement:

> During the development of the program, in what was a first for the Pacific, a memorandum of understanding was signed between the Ministry of Education and the Ministry of Health. This mutual agreement was fundamental in allowing the two ministries to collaborate on the project, fully utilizing the strengths of both organizations while also respecting the differences. Previously both ministries had tended to follow their own work plans without collaboration or consultation with each other. This often led to a double-up of work loads addressing similar issues, to programs unsupported (due to lack of consultation within the education), to unsuitable timing by the Ministry of Health in some of their work programs (due to the education sector having other priorities), and—at times—schools not fully supporting (due to lack of understanding) the work of the Ministry of Health ... A Memorandum of Understanding is important for defining roles and working to strengths, especially in a small nation where resources are limited. Success still depends on the right people being willing and able to work together. Leaders of organizations need to help this happen.

Similarly, the very different country of Lao PDR reports that there was no large systematic implementation until 2002, when a significant Memorandum of Understanding was signed between the Ministries of Health and Education to launch the National School Health Project, providing an immediate increase to 450 schools, a base for coordination of donor activities, and support from a Luxembourg grant through WHO. Furthermore, in Lao PDR,

> both vertical and horizontal coordination mechanisms are used to encourage collaboration and coordination between education and health sectors. The central task force is divided into four small groups; each group consists of two to three members who respond directly to coordination, monitoring, and supervision in the assigned provinces. This coordination framework encourages all task force members to participate fully in carrying out the activities with better leadership and commitment. Regular meetings among central task force members are held once a month to share and exchange experiences and information.

The UAE describes how a cross-sectoral task force has been performing the deworming of primary school-aged children since 2005. The HPS requires the "combined input of many agencies and sectors, [and] an important aspect ... lies in building partnerships and alliances among these agencies." In 2003, the Ministry of Education and the Ministry of Health signed an agreement to mark the beginning of their partnership. A high-level coordinating committee for HPS was formed with members from ministries of health, education, and nongovernmental partners responsible for planning, relationship building with the media, monitoring, and support and evaluation.

Germany's Anschub.de school health program has created a national alliance of more than 60 national institutions, organizations, associations, and prominent researchers:

> The idea is that schools cannot develop solely from the bottom up with input from enthusiastic people. Schools also need powerful and long-lasting support from the top down. Formation of this alliance is also driven by the idea that support for schools is not only the obligation of school ministries and administration; it also needs coordinated action from all the organizations that have a (legal) responsibility or that feel a social responsibility to support pupils, teachers, non-teaching staff, and schools in general. Schools thereby experience stronger and wider support for what they are doing, than through ministerial support alone.

Dedicated Resources

The cases from Australia, the USA, and Canada illustrate the importance of sharing and dedicating resources to the activity of coordination and having a trusted coordinator manage the process. Using these resources to appoint a dedicated, trusted person to manage the work of the cross-sector committees is invaluable. Australia writes:

> Another strength of the initiative is the dedicated resources allocated to coordination. This includes the time and resources given to meetings at both the state and area/regional level. Both health and education were committed at each level to contribute to the development and ongoing management of the initiative. Having a dedicated coordinator to oversee the process meant that there was someone there that could provide the type of support that is required to assist teachers and clinicians to implement mental health promotion, prevention, and early intervention in a comprehensive way.

> The coordinator needs to be of a sufficiently high position in the system to effect change. When coordinators were not given sufficient power they lacked credibility and were not able to make decisions, frustrating the process.

By engaging organizations from cross-sectors in joint activities, collaboration was enhanced. The Hong Kong Healthy Schools Award

> emphasizes the combined efforts of education and health professionals to enable the HPS program to be more comprehensive and related to school outcomes. This project shows some promising changes occurring among the students from award schools. The findings suggest that if the HPS framework is embraced comprehensively, there will be substantial gains in health and educational outcomes.

Canada found that their "successful proposal-writing process was important because a solid partnership was a prerequisite for applying; this was an automatic incentive or mechanism for cross-sector collaboration."

Participants in Cross-Sector Collaboration

In Lao PDR,

the Joint National School Health Taskforce, which consists of staff from related departments of the [Ministry of Education] and [Ministry of Health],... plays multiple roles in a cycle of school health implementation; for instance, it supports assessment and research, develops guidelines and tools, and assists provinces to plan and implement school activities.

In some instances, the problems that schools decided to tackle were highly specific, based on data about the most significant threats affecting children. These include industrial pollution in Kosovo, malaria in the Philippines, and HIV and AIDS in the Caribbean country of Barbados. In targeting these issues, their cross-sector collaboration reached out to involve players in those countries with the expertise or reach to bring added capacity to the issue.

Kosovo brought together education and health, as well as environmental and civic, organizations to address the industrial pollution affecting children. Industrial pollution from heavy-metal smelting activities is one of the main threats to health, especially to children:

> The public-awareness working group chose the Health-Promoting School approach as a main tool for raising population awareness on how to live more safely in a contaminated environment. The working group includes officials from different sectors such as health, education, environment, women's associations, the Institute of Public Health, and the Trepca Institute. Both ethnic groups, Albanian and Serbian, are represented on this working group. [The Ministry of Education, Science and Technology; the Ministry of Health; the Ministry of Youth, Culture and Sports, and the Ministry of Environment and Spatial Planning formalized their commitment in a Memorandum of Understanding.]

> This multi-sectoral method of implementation aims to improve the environment of schools through environmental health risk management activities (cleaning and greening activities).

The Philippines reached out to experts in the control of malaria and dengue fever, who became resources involved in the schools to educate both staff and students:

> Involvement of other sectors in the community such as the Kilusan Ligtas Malaria—a special private-public partnership program for malaria control involving of the Department of Health in Palawan for the prevention and control of malaria—as well as the Pilipinas Shell Foundation of Shell group of companies in the Philippines is also important in linking school health issues with their communities. Kilusan Ligtas Malaria and Pilipinas Shell Foundation were both tapped for technical experts to discuss the prevention and control of malaria. They also explained the ongoing efforts in the community to prevent and control malaria and engaged teachers to help by educating students and parents.

Barbados includes private industry and media to fund and reach beyond the schools to the community with key prevention messages:

> The HIV/AIDS component is being aided by the Ministry of Youth and Scotia Bank. The Ministry of Youth works with the schools and has produced students' work on DVDs. The message of stigma and discrimination is Scotia Bank's aim as it works in the school community with persons living with AIDS. This intervention is expected to last for three years and will reach all 45,000 students at primary and secondary level. The Ministry of Education has utilized a youth ambassador who works with HIV and AIDS groups in 12 secondary schools.

Successes of Cross-Sector Collaboration

Finally, the greatest success of cross-sectoral work has been the institutionalization of education sector policy, and even legislation, that provides ongoing support of the program.

Nicaragua writes:

> In 2005, an independent agency carried out an external evaluation of Friendly and Healthy Schools initiative (FHS) ... Results were encouraging about the impact of the model on improving the lives of school children. It is interesting to look at some of the results, which showed promising evidence of the success of the FHS model in organizing and carrying out new school-community dynamics and increasingly achieving more participation of the community. The most significant indicators [included]: increased ownership by the Ministry of Education, which opened up the possibility to influencing the general education policy, [and] *improved inter-institutional coordination.* [emphasis added]

And the most significant example of how cross-sector collaboration led to legislation is the case of Scotland.

> The experience of the [European Network of Health Promoting Schools] (ENHPS) has shown that health-promoting school initiatives are most effective when true partnership is practiced within and between all players in the process. This should include ministries, their institutions, pupils, teachers, NGOs, stakeholders, and interested parties in relevant communities. At the national level, the two most influential partners are generally the Ministries of Health and Education; in the ENHPS it is deemed that the relevant ministries commit to a formal signed agreement to support the development of health promotion in a member state's schools ...... In Scotland, after relatively modest progress in the 1980s and early 1990s, developments accelerated to a level where national legislation has now been set out on health promotion in schools and on nutritional standards in school food.

Cross-sectoral collaboration is essential. Bahrain has noted, "Among the significant potential benefits of collaboration is the enhanced capacity to tackle and resolve complex health and social problems that have proven impossible for individual sectors." Furthermore, the case of Bahrain summarizes the reasons for cross-sector collaboration very completely:

> The Health-Promoting Schools program in Bahrain is a collaborative effort between the Ministry of Health and the Ministry of Education. In 2000, a high-level joint committee between the Ministry of Health and Ministry of Education was formed to put into place a strategic plan for school health in Bahrain: "The Bahrain national school health program." The school health program started in 2002, when the Ministry of Health and the Ministry of Education reached an agreement to establish a comprehensive school health program for Bahrain.

> The Ministry of Health collaborates with the Ministry of Education in a Joint Committee, as well as with the Gulf Council Committee (GCC) and with the World Health Organization, Eastern Mediterranean Regional Office (WHO/EMRO).

Bahrain has renewed its emphasis on finding ways to link the various sectors that influence the development of children and adolescents. This intersector collaboration is essential because of the following:

- Intersectoral action makes possible the joining of forces, knowledge, and the means to understand and solve complex issues whose solutions lie outside the capacity and responsibility of a single sector.
- There are many opportunities to engage health, education, social services, recreation, housing, culture, and justice sectors in joint strategies to achieve shared goals.
- Among the significant potential benefits of collaboration is the enhanced capacity to tackle and resolve complex health and social problems that have proven impossible for individual sectors.
- "Children deserve love and respect for who they are." They are central to Bahrain's investment in its future and must be acknowledged and involved in shaping change and development of the population's health.
- The social services sector is an important partner, particularly in its role to support youth who are experiencing difficulties in family life.
- Each sector has a unique responsibility for initiating discussion, offering its perspective, communicating with its constituents, and providing leadership to engage others in collaborative efforts to better meet the needs of children.
- Most youth spend a significant portion of their time in the school environment. The Ministry of Education has a particularly important role to play in the healthy development of children and is a key partner in developing strategies for youth and their families.
- Focusing on the determinants of health, the Ministry of Health is well positioned to act as a catalyst in the identification of policy, planning, service delivery, and research needs related to child and adolescent health and development.

Though many cases recount the difficulties and barriers of cross-sectoral collaboration, some cite this factor as one of the most important in moving implementation to a larger scale or institutionalizing the program into policy and legislation. In dealing with collaboration, countries have typically needed to spend additional time and resources to work with more players, to clarify roles and responsibilities, to overcome rigid institutional agendas, and to mediate when some individuals or agencies try to impose their singular ideas on others.

Champions and leaders at all levels, as discussed in the next section, were very important for this process.

Champions and Leaders at all Levels

Few cases use the term *leadership* in describing important factors. Yet almost all report that leadership, commitment, and political will are required – from the government, key officials in health and/or education, principals, teachers, and community leaders – for this initiative to become reality. It is also clear that the leadership of WHO and the United Nations agencies, which participated in defining and promoting this comprehensive approach to school health, has been most instrumental in convincing and persuading national-level government leaders to adopt and implement the concept. In many instances, cases refer to the leadership of WHO's introduction and consultancy on the HPS and the value of international guidelines.

At the country level, it was, most often, the leadership of the Ministry of Health that began the work, often supported by researchers in universities to provide the data. Health ministries soon found that their leadership could go only so far unless embraced and joined by leaders in the education sector.

Scotland describes three phases of leadership: The first phase, *Early Experimentation*, was initiated by the health sector. The second phase, *Strategic Development*, occurred when the education sector began to perceive the benefits of meeting social and educational needs in schools and communities and played a more significant role. The third phase, *Establishment*, was reached when the innovations became embedded in the normal ways of working of the school. Scotland also recognizes that implementation does not progress in a simple linear way:

> It is now recognized . . . . that educational reform frequently includes unpredictable shifts and fragmented initiatives. It would be misleading to suggest that progress usually occurs in a simple linear way and in steady increments. Progress is, of course, highly political: Rapid progress is theoretically possible when a strong political will exists; when the political priorities change, the process can stall or go into reverse.

The vigilance of leadership in paying attention to issues was reported to be substantial. China comments:

> Implementing HPS started with strong support from the leadership—in the province, municipality, and school. This included "paying attention"—or giving priority—to the HPS project as well as obtaining financial support. As one teacher said, "everything can be done if the leadership pays attention to the issues."

The Role of the Principal

From the Philippines, India, and Brazil, we learn about the influential leadership role of the principal, which, as research has also documented, makes a difference in the implementation of new programs. The case from the Philippines shares that

> the support of the school principal is key to the successful implementation of the Urbani School Health Kit and its broader vision of helping schools become Health-Promoting Schools. The principals who were supportive of the teachers' efforts to find innovative ways of teaching and integrating healthy habits in their courses had the most energetic and creative teachers as well as students. Principals can be primarily concerned with academic achievement of the students. By emphasizing the significant role of health in the child's learning, it is not difficult to point out that the goals of education and health are the same: children who are healthy and able to reach their full academic potential.

Project HOPE, in India, notes that

while students were easy to enthuse and stimulate, teachers often proved difficult. Many lacked enthusiasm and energy to experiment with anything new and often viewed HOPE activities as wasting time (meant for formal lessons) on a low-priority topic of health.

Leadership proved to be very vital; the enthusiasm of the principal was reflected in the behavior of the teachers.

In Brazil, a principal deeply embedded in the life of the community made a powerful contribution:

The project started in 2000 and is still progressing. Professor Avamar Pantoja, who has been teaching and living in the community area for many years, is the headmaster who leads the project. She joined the Alexandre de Gusmão School first as a teacher and then as a teachers' coordinator, before being chosen as the school principal in 1999. She has been re-elected for this role three consecutive times. She has lived in the neighborhood since 1975 and also worked in a neighboring school for seven years before moving to Alexandre de Gusmão. In many ways, this project reflects her personal process of learning from and commitment to the community, which has developed over the years.

Implementing the principles of a global school health strategy in a context of such complex conditions, such as those faced by the Alexandre de Gusmão school in Rio de Janeiro, does not happen without contradictions and different points of view between regional managers and people on the ground. Disagreements on the process and clashes of interests and leadership have been common. The role of the school's principal as a leader and facilitator in creating a consensual plan of action has helped to solve conflict and provide strategic orientation each time these contradictions have challenged the process.

Leadership Across Levels

Several cases include examples of leadership across levels. For example, Bahrain's Joint National Committee of Health and Education met with community leaders to engage them in the ideas. The Committee established team leaders of interested people from the schools and community responsible for implementation.

Oman illustrates the leadership and commitment across levels that were so important for what they did:

Many factors played a role in the success of HPS in Oman. First is the commitment and support of higher authorities in [the Ministry of Health], [the Ministry of Education], and international organizations. Second is a sense of ownership and partnership of health and education sectors, schools, communities, and students. Third is the presence of school health services with objectives and activities. Fourth is the effective role of the Omani community and their participation in health issues. Fifth is the presence of effective parents' councils in all schools.

Viet Nam shares examples of the importance of leadership from the ministry to the teacher level:

Critical to the success of the project was that eight to ten champions of the program sprang up, including key central figures in both [the Ministry of Education and Training] and [the Ministry of Health], two young enthusiastic teachers in the pilot province of Ha Tinh, and the Deputy Director of the provincial health centers in Ha Tinh and Hai Phong, whose enthusiasm for the program helped extend its reach and deepen its effectiveness.

The energy, commitment, and passion of leaders, whether in formal designated roles with titles, or through their actions and deeds to bring about change, have proven to be important factors in the implementation process. Leaders rely on and use data for all types of decisions doing this work. The next section gives examples of how data were used in many different and important ways to propel the movement forward.

Data-Driven Planning and Decision Making

In the field of public health, in particular, data drive and inform the types of health promotion and disease prevention strategies selected to target specific populations for identified health issues. To successfully target, implement, and evaluate the HPS model, social science, education, demographic, and economic data also play an important role. Data from these various fields enable planners to:

- Identify prevalent health and mental health patterns of illness, injury, and death among students, staff, family, and community members
- Examine school enrollment rates, retention, completion, academic scores, absenteeism, expulsions, and truancy
- Understand the social, economic, and environmental factors contributing to health and education outcomes
- Advocate for and influence political will to address these issues
- Assess the capacity and readiness of the systems to respond and implement solutions, including careful attention to the factors presented in Fig. 1 in the chapter "Framing Theories and Implementation Research"
- Inform progress at all stages of development to make course corrections and program improvements
- Track who is reached with what program or strategy, for what duration, and for what health and education outcomes

At the beginning of this chapter, we have seen clearly how many cases relied on and used data as the impetus or driving force to launch the HPS initiative. Examples of ways in which data were used to mobilize action and resources, along with other purposes, follow.

Scotland, which has succeeded recently in passing legislation to incorporate health promotion for schools into the mission of education, worked closely with researchers over many years to demonstrate not only the health threats, but also their impact on academic performance:

> The HBSC [Health Behaviors in Scottish Children] study provides a unique data set on the health of adolescents in Scotland over a 16-year period. The study takes a broad approach to examining young people's health in the context of social factors including family, peers, school and socio-economic status, and the developmental process of puberty. As an example of the kinds of intelligence supplied, consider the example of gender. Gender

and socio-economic inequalities are evident in many aspects of health behavior and well-being; in general, girls are less positive about their own health and well-being, suffering more frequently from self-reported health complaints, including feeling low. These findings and other relevant trends are presented in Scottish HBSC Briefing Papers... and in the HBSC international reports Young People's Health in Context... This research has played a part in the identification of the specific needs for health promotion among young people in Scotland, leading to specific developments in practice, policy, and legislation...

While there have been few large-scale research programs on the specific impact of health schools on health behaviors, one important longitudinal study... followed over 2,000 children from age 11 years to age 15 years, investigating possible school effects on smoking, drinking, drug use, and healthy diet. The results showed considerable variation in the rates of these health behaviors among 43 secondary schools. After adjusting for prior (age 11) behavior and socio-demographic characteristics, the analyses showed that, with the exception of diet, school-level variation (school effects) remained, meaning that these factors did not account for the differences.

School effects were stronger for smoking and drinking alcohol than for illegal drugs, the effect remaining in a cross-classification analysis of school and neighborhood. Using data from pupils, together with three independent measures, higher levels of smoking, drinking, and drug use were found in schools containing more pupils who were disengaged from education and knew fewer teachers, also in larger schools independently rated as having a poorer ethos. The authors concluded that these results were compatible with the attention given to school ethos in the Health-Promoting School model.

Similarly, in Germany, students' relatively low scores on the PISA (Program for International Student Assessment) test, together with a discrepancy of scores for pupils from low-income and migrant families, prompted the Bertelsmann Foundation to launch *Anschub.de, The Good and Healthy School*. With a national alliance of more than 40 organizations, including the education and health ministries, the program is organized around the central question, "How can improvements in the health of students and staff improve educational outcomes?" Germany's prior experience with HPSs on a smaller scale had demonstrated the need for framing the concept more in terms of benefits to education, rather than using the school as a setting to promote health.

In Hong Kong, a large-scale surveillance study of 26,000 students of age 10–19 from 48 primary and secondary schools reported 14% of students feeling that their physical and emotional health had interfered with their normal daily activities most of the time; 15% admitted to being regular smokers. Older students reported more physical and psychological problems than younger students, and few adopted healthy lifestyles. These data, coupled with the SARS outbreak, produced support from the Center for Health Education and Health Promotion of the Faculty of Medicine of the Chinese University of Hong Kong and the School Councils because they recognized that "both health and education are linked to the economic performance and social cohesion of modern industrialized society. Therefore funding of US$1.9 million in 1998 and US$1.1 million in 2000 was awarded to launch the initial HPS program."

Lao PDR, in 2000, launched the HPS in 30 schools, recognizing that poor nutrition contributes to half of all child mortality and that poor sanitation and personal hygiene contribute to the high incidence of helminths among children. In the Cook Islands, in 2002, alarming health statistics for youth and indicators of school performance served as a catalyst. The UAE cites rapid changes in immigration and economic development, increases in chronic disease, and concern for rising health care costs as reasons to expand health promotion in schools for young people. China witnessed the success of a WHO/HPS intervention that successfully reduced parasitic infections among youth in rural schools. These data stimulated the governments in another province to adopt the model to address student tobacco use and nutritional problems, as well as injury prevention.

In Nigeria, in 2003, with WHO and EDC, the Federal Ministry of Health and the Federal Ministry of Education conducted the RAAPP for School Health. The RAAPP is a process of qualitative data collection to assess children's health problems and the capacity of ministries to respond. Through the RAAPP, Nigeria identified significant gaps in federal-level management, policy, and capacity to provide school health programs. Even though very few data are actually available on the specific health issues of Nigerian schoolchildren, the coming together of the two ministries, identifying their lack of capacity, was enough stimulus to drive action.

In the Eastern Cape of South Africa, the conditions of 90% unemployment, abject poverty, and escalating rates of HIV infection motivated the schools and community to come together creating a vision, *Masibambane Sakhe* (Let's Join and Build). Uruguay, in 2002, experienced a severe economic crisis, drastically increasing the number of children living in poverty to one-third of the population. The conditions in the lives of children and families overflowed into the public school system, creating a need for policies and social safety net-type programs to be implemented through the schools (typically, more children receiving meals). In Brazil, the Alexandre de Gusmão Municipal School is located in a low-income project in which 50% of the houses are shanties, bordering an extremely polluted stream, which creates precarious and hazardous living conditions. These "miserable living conditions make drug trafficking the most attractive income-generating alternative for young people." Yet the Alexandre de Gusmão's health promotion project "applies a popular education approach, in which the school is the center of social action and education and serves as *an instrument* for stimulating and enabling the future of children."

These cases of South Africa, Uruguay, and Brazil argue that health promotion is even more important in conditions of economic hardship, as the methods of public health provide the means to empower people to gain control of the determinants of their living conditions. Thus, not only data about health or educational indicators, but also data about social conditions may support the establishment of school health programs.

Administrative and Management Support

Many cases did not amplify procedures or structures for administrative or management support. The common feature across many countries was the use of a HPSs planning committee, illustrated by China:

A further factor in implementation is administrative and management support. Schools set up special *HPS planning committees* [original emphasis]. Principals and/or vice-principals led or co-led these committees. Committee members included administrators and teachers with authority from various areas throughout the school (e.g., morality education, physical education, logistics, teaching, student works, school health service, counseling), selected according to the positions and roles they already held, so as to attach the project to their regular work systematically throughout the school. In some cases, students, parents, and/or community members also served on this committee. The committees discussed the policy to carry out, made a plan, and discussed details and assignments of tasks and strategies to carry out the plan. They set up and perfected various systems in the school, made modifications to the school policy, and took responsibility for project implementation. They developed a work plan, based on their regular work, integrating HPS interventions and making them part of the overall school responsibility.

Popularizing [original emphasis] the HPS concept through various means of communication also played an important role in the administrative and management support of this project. Schools used wallboards and bulletins for propaganda, students passed on materials to parents and community members, and schools held parents' meetings and sent letters to parents. One school reported using news media and the Internet for publicity.

This combination of special HPS committees with frequent and various communication to popularize the HPS concept and interventions seemed to ensure that the HPS concept and interventions could be spread efficiently throughout the school and to the community.

Similarly, Nicaragua describes its use of a committee or project team to oversee management and administration:

Each participating school and community set up a project team composed of the school principal, community leaders, representatives of the student government and school council, teachers, parents, and children.

This team follows the "HPS implementation cycle": (1) information and awareness-raising in the community, (2) participant commitment, (3) participatory self-diagnosis, (4) work plan, (5) monitoring, and (6) evaluation and certification. In Bahrain,

all schools were asked to form committees for health promotion. The head of each committee should be the second person in the school (deputy of the school principal); representative members should include the teacher of physical education, food canteen coordinator, school councilor, and school nurse... Regular meetings of these committees should be conducted with the leaders in the Ministry of Education about the plans and implementations.

From Hong Kong, we learn that
at follow-up evaluation, 98.2% of the participating schools had set up a working group or committee for school health promotion and education whereas only 53.4% of the participating schools had such kind of working group at the baseline assessment.

Similar to Germany, which has regional coordinators for the Anschub.de program, Canada realized the need for coordinators or consultants:

Within public health, there was, originally, one central Planning and Policy School Health Consultant. It was soon recognized that this central coordination, internally within the health unit and externally with school board partners, was crucial, so four School Health

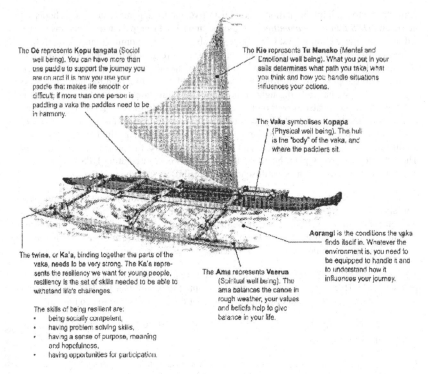

The Oe represents **Kopu tangata** (Social well being). You can have more than one paddle to support the journey you are on and it is how you use your paddle that makes life smooth or difficult; if more than one person is paddling a vaka the paddles need to be in harmony.

The Kie represents **Tu Manako** (Mental and Emotional well being). What you put in your sails determines what path you take, what you think and how you handle situations influences your actions.

The **Vaka** symbolises **Kopapa** (Physical well being). The hull is the "body" of the vaka, and where the paddlers sit.

Aorangi is the conditions the vaka finds itself in. Whatever the environment is, you need to be equipped to handle it and to understand how it influences your journey.

The twine, or Ka'a, binding together the parts of the vaka, needs to be very strong. The Ka'a represents the resiliency we want for young people, resiliency is the set of skills needed to be able to withstand life's challenges.

The skills of being resilient are:
- being socially competent,
- having problem solving skills,
- having a sense of purpose, meaning and hopefulness,
- having opportunities for participation.

The **Ama** represents **Vaerua** (Spiritual well being). The ama balances the canoe in rough weather, your values and beliefs help to give balance in your life.

Fig. 1 Adapting WHO's definition of well-being to Cook Island culture

Coordinators (now called Consultants) were put in place, linked to the School and Youth Teams of liaison nurses working with schools. A large part of the coordinators' role has involved in-servicing front-line PHN [Public Health Nurses] and health promotion staff.

The need for leadership and coordination of a committee or task force is confirmed by the case study from Lao PDR:

Currently—as several partners are carrying out the health promotion activities in schools—the task force needs strong leadership to identify a coordination and collaboration mechanism, planning and implementation, and information flow management. Good leadership can ensure effective sector-wide collaboration and avoid duplication.

Thus, the cases that mention administrative and management support illustrate the need for and value of a coordinator, planning committee, or task force for school health, with members from various areas throughout the school.

Adaptation to Local Concerns

The HPS concept is a broad one, allowing for and encouraging national local adaptations. Many of the products and tools provided by WHO and other UN agencies were developed to guide implementation, as well as to provide and encourage processes for adaptation in response to local culture and a wide range of other conditions.

The case study from the Cook Islands provides a beautiful example of adaptation of the central concept of health and well-being to the culture of the South Pacific, using the elements of their traditional boat. Figure 1 illustrates this unique translation. The Cook Islands represent the four dimensions of health in the Ottawa Charter. They also add a fifth dimension of environment: Mental and Emotional, Physical, Spiritual, Social, and Environment.

Other cases illustrate the need for adaptation to address particular health, education, or community issues; capacity, structure, and ability to deliver services; differences in resource-rich and resource-poor, urban and rural environments. One case argues that adaptation must begin with the basic indicators that will be used for measurement and the importance of customizing those indicators to the local situation. Examples of these reasons for adaptation follow.

China addresses specific issues, explaining that

> vocational school students previously experienced failure, so they needed to develop confidence. In rural schools, students and families had lower basic educational levels, so they needed to learn about basic safety and injury prevention. In urban schools, students experienced a lot of pressure to achieve high academic scores, so they benefited from psychological consultation. Some schools were concerned about *balancing health and academics*, especially when parents were worried that the HPS project might have a negative impact on their child's academic education.

Developing a work plan tailored to each individual school helped to adapt the HPS project to local needs and concerns.

Viet Nam demonstrates the need and ways to adapt to address resource differences:

> The model was successful in that it could be applied in different socioeconomic areas. However significant differences in implementation, needs, and success were observed between urban and rural settings. The project had a very significant impact in the poorer provinces that were coming from a lower base of physical infrastructure and teaching capacity. In many poorer schools there had been virtually no teaching materials to support the curriculum. In the wealthier provinces, HPS helped to refine and elaborate the curriculum already in place and helped schools focus on what environmental improvements were needed. In Hai Phong, for example additions of health rooms and nutrition programs were popular.

Beyond content, adaptation for structure and delivery was necessary, as Australia points out:

> While the three focus areas of the initiative are consistent across the state, there is scope for flexibility in how each Area Health Service implements School-Link. This flexibility is necessary as not all areas have the same services and structures. Geographical distances can also alter the way the School-Link Coordinator might be able to interact with schools. For example an inner city coordinator may be able to have more direct contact with schools and provide more in-services, whereas due to large distances a rural coordinator might not be able to develop relationships in the same way and may not have access to the same services for young people. The flexibility also allows coordinators to address needs of specific commu-

nities in their local area; for example, some might have higher culturally and linguistically diverse populations, while others may have higher Indigenous populations, others may have highly affluent populations, and others may have more socially disadvantaged populations.

Finally, we learn from Hong Kong about the importance of developing local indicators:

> Each country was encouraged to develop indicators to meet the local needs. The indicators and guidelines developed were evidence-based and have a broad range of objectives. They were designed to be relevant, adaptable, and achievable, so they can be used to develop good practices...

As these examples show, adaptation can take many forms, from adapting the health concept to the local context, to adapting the HPS to socioeconomic conditions of the learners, to giving flexibility in services and structures, and developing indicators to meet local needs. This adaptation is necessary to make school health initiatives relevant to the local context and conditions.

Attention to External Forces

External forces were also major reasons for ministries and schools to adopt the HPS approach; the health, economic, social, and political forces having an impact on children and families inspired people to use this approach as an opportunity to make necessary changes.

In China, the one-child policy was the larger context influencing motives to take on this HPS approach:

> China's one-child policy, introduced in 1979 and underpinned by a system of rewards and penalties, allows one child for urban residents and, with some restrictions, two children for rural residents... The effects of this policy played a role in implementing the HPS project in two aspects.

> First, because the government permits parents to have only one child, parents have an intense desire for that child to succeed and prosper and often have very high academic expectations for their child. Parents transfer these high expectations to their child, often creating serious pressure for the child to do very well in school. School administrators, teachers, students, and parents in this study all seemed to agree that students are under much pressure to succeed in school. The pressure extends beyond the children to their teachers, as families expect teachers to enable students to succeed.

> On the other hand, teachers, parents, and students repeatedly noted that because parents have only one child, children wield tremendous influence in their families. They indicated that parents and grandparents are likely to follow the suggestions and advice from their child and grandchild. They consider the child "the little emperor." Indeed, parents seemed to make behavior changes, especially reducing or quitting smoking (mostly fathers or grandfathers) and changing dietary habits (mostly mothers) after the child shared new knowledge and expectations. Grandparents seemed to be especially responsive to their grandchild, whom they reportedly "spoiled." For example, grandfathers told us they stopped smoking after their grandchildren convinced them to do so.

These observations indicate that the one-child policy contributes the risk factor of academic pressure that resulted in stress and affected mental health, but also contributes the success factor of effective outreach to family members and convincing them to change unhealthy behaviors.

Capitalizing on a move to democracy and freedom, the HPS provided opportunities for countries such as Poland and Kosovo.
In Poland,

[the] HPS project was implemented in the first five years of the political, social, and economic transition, when an explosion of enthusiasm of Poles and readiness to introduce changes was observed. Many schools recognized the HPS concept as attractive; its dissemination started very soon and continued for the next 15 years.

In Kosovo, people hoped after the conflict that they could come together to solve the larger health problems created, especially for children, by industrial pollution:

The conflict in the Balkans in 1999 and also the gradual deterioration of conditions left Kosovo with severe problems in its infrastructure, local capacity, and relationships among the main ethnic groups. Environmental pollution has left a legacy of severe heavy metal contamination in specific, heavily populated industrial areas.

As a response to the environmental contamination and its impact on human health, WHO, in collaboration with local institutions, worked towards establishing sustainable structures to implement a comprehensive program of activities that will raise awareness of and decrease exposure to the complex problem of pollution from metal lead and other poisonous heavy metals.

Even wealthier countries facing change found that the external factors of modernization and resulting lifestyle changes were important factors to implement the HPS model. The UAE illustrates these modern day challenges:

The per capita income exceeded Dh61,000 in 2005 and is considered to be one of the highest in the world. The high income has facilitated rapid socioeconomic development, as well as the establishment of a modern infrastructure of health and educational services. This rapid change has also affected the disease patterns as a result of changing lifestyle. Cardiovascular diseases, cancer, diabetes, and other chronic diseases have emerged as the leading causes of morbidity and mortality. The ever-rising cost of health care has led to a revision of prospective health strategies, placing a greater focus on risk management and disease burden reduction, as recommended by WHO. . . . All of these factors have been taken into consideration when developing and revising the school health program.

As these case examples illustrate, conditions in the larger political context, such as specific policies, conflict, democratization, as well as modernization and lifestyle changes are important external forces that can propel the establishment of HPS.

Critical Mass and Supportive Norms

Many cases used multiple strategies to create a critical mass of people who embraced the HPS idea, becoming part of a movement to propel it forward and to put program elements in place. These strategies, often used in combination, included involvement of many sectors and stakeholders (discussed in detail under that factor), professional development of teachers and school staff in groups, use of popular media to reach community members and parents, and the inclusion and deployment of influential opinion leaders or schools as leaders to spread the concept to others.

An example from Germany elaborates on how the cultivation of partners has contributed to creating a critical mass in support of implementation:

> The "Alliance for sustainable school health and education" creates a movement of big national partners who will form an association to promote the good and healthy school. These partners are GOs and NGOs, combining resources from both these fields and also from educational, health, and private sectors.
>
> Now decision makers from school administration and education or health-related organizations and associations at the state and federal levels, as well as private companies, are invited. Accordingly, Anschub.de acquires political power, and the decisions that are made influence and change school health promotion much more than before, because the level of action is different. These are strategic partners in an endeavor to support schools.

Kenya describes the important role of professional development in gaining a critical mass:

> Teachers used the skills and knowledge they acquired during in-service to implement the interventions during ordinary classroom teaching to pupils. This process created a critical mass of pupils who had developed visions about how to improve their health, their learning, and their home and school environments. Through participation and action in everyday activities the intervention pupils interacted with other pupils who were not part of the intervention in school and in the community, thereby creating another critical mass of knowledgeable people as regards health matters in the district. The project successfully created a critical mass of health actors within the school environment (teachers and pupils) and the home/community environment (children and adults).

India's case informs us of their strategy to use the influential leadership of the school principal, combined with the power of the media:

> Also, the Principal of La Martiniere College, the most prestigious and popular school in Lucknow, lent his support to this venture by becoming one of the founders of HOPE Initiative and joined in the launching of the first phase of activities in his school. The tremendous response received from this school, and the positive publicity that the initiative received through the local media, gave birth to the idea of promoting health awareness in schools throughout the city. As a result, an organization by the name of HOPE Initiative was established in November 2004.

Finally, Canada points to the very important need for a critical mass of students as leaders in an effort that is intended to promote and protect their health and well-being:

> We have also learned that a critical mass of students on a committee is essential to mitigate the power imbalance that can occur when adults and children are members of a committee together. PHNs and principals have been mindful of encouraging meaningful student and parent participation. As staff and principals have moved to other schools, they have championed the initiative in their new schools. Students who graduate from elementary school often continue their involvement on a committee throughout high school.

Thus, creating a critical mass is important on various levels, including national organizations that lend support and a critical mass of pupils who can move the vision forward at school level, even when they transfer to other schools.

Stage of Readiness

Very little in the cases addressed the many aspects of readiness. Examples were provided of perceived need, demand, incentives, and motivation to begin a program. Less attention was dedicated to describing other factors of readiness, such as the capacity to handle the program, knowledge and skills of practitioners, acceptance and commitments of key players, or competing initiatives or demands. As mentioned earlier in this book, the reasons that countries or cases gave for beginning the program were typically emerging data about significant health or education issues or an economic or social crisis in a country or community.

In some cases, implementation began with a situational analysis. Other cases describe how implementation proceeded slowly or not very successfully in the early years. Over time, people began to recognize the need for partnerships between health and education to make the program work, but for many countries this realization was not evident at the start. Once formed, the cross-sectoral commitments, advocacy, and training led to extended reach and results.

Because of the newness and breadth of the concept, however, many places were probably not entirely ready for implementation or did not grasp fully ahead of time what would be involved, but went ahead anyway. Knowing exactly what training might be needed, where to find it, the cost, etc. may not have been an integral part of the early planning for implementation. In fact, the case study from India reports that "health promotion in schools was unknown in schools in Uttar Pradesh," and Cook Islands found that "change of practice takes a long time, especially when *content* and *pedagogical* strategies are both new." [original emphasis]

The cases provide interesting examples of what readied them to move forward.

In some cases, it was a demand and need for capacity and services not available in the school to address critical problems. Australia tells us:

Mental health is an area in which schools have consistently asked the health sector for support, rather than the health sector trying to convince schools that they need to address a particular health issue. Commonly health issues that we are addressing in the school setting are about changing student's behaviors that will have an impact on their health into the future, but the impact in mental health is much more immediate. Schools globally are experiencing difficulties with students who are disengaged from schools, bullying and harassment, disruptive behavior and suicide. In stepping into the School-Link role some coordinators were inundated with requests for help from schools. This was quite different from having to knock on doors of schools and encourage them to participate.

Often, schools may not have been ready but took on the program to assess and address their problems and then grew it as they could. For Nicaragua, the development of [Friendly and Healthy Schools] was not fast. It grew out of the progressively increasing interest of communities and teachers as the program's reputation among Nicaraguan schools disseminated and grew. The certification of the first five schools as healthy and friendly on the basis of their ability to respond to the needs identified in the situation analysis and the priorities agreed with the community was an important incentive to other schools. Since 2006, the initiative has already been numerically significant, reaching 387 schools and 35,000 children.

Even though the cases imply that there might not have been full readiness in the capacity or resources needed to implement school health programs, the challenges at hand demanded action. Thus, readiness was reached over time and a lack thereof at the beginning did not hinder successful implementation – most likely since the other factors of the Wheel of Factors Influencing Implementation of Policy and Practice were more strongly prevalent and apparently compensated.

Conclusions

The cases illustrate beautifully the many ways that the HPS and similar concepts have succeeded in capturing the imagination of staff in ministries and local schools and communities as a way to respond to their needs in education, health, economic, and social conditions. The HPS concept has been shown to offer a purposeful and powerful way to adapt a basic approach and strategies to meet the particulars of specific challenges, culture and context.

The Wheel of Factors Influencing Implementation of Policy and Practice

Though there was no manual prescribing effective strategies for implementation, the 26 cases demonstrate clearly how leaders at the national and local levels used many factors similar to those in the Wheel of Factors Influencing Implementation of Policy and Practice (illustrated in Fig. 1 in the chapter "Framing Theories and Implementation Research"), all drawn from research on diffusion of innovation and implementation.

Looking at the strategies and factors that enabled countries and local schools and communities to put the concept into practice, we see clearly how WHO's Global School Health Initiative has rippled throughout the world, inspiring people with a vision to use the concept and methodology for change. It is evident that the power of ideas in charters, frameworks, and international guidelines, if disseminated broadly, can have a major influence on policy and practice. The ways in which the Ottawa Charter advocated that health must *not* be limited to the health sector, but applied to people's everyday life, where they learn, work, play, and love gained transference. This essential idea, applied to schools, originally by the WHO European Regional

Office, has gained much appeal. Then through the development and dissemination of technical products and consultations, the ideas began to take hold in many places.

Countries, through their ministries of health and education, as well as local schools and communities, found a variety of ways to garner the financial, human, and technical resources to move from idea to action. No matter what initial method was used to gain financial support – broad-scale government funding, modest funding, or philanthropy for pilots, in-kind contributions of people's time and expertise – each initiative found a way to put the ideas into practice at some level of scale. Due caution was given about funding for pilot projects, which in some cases never went beyond that level. Beyond financial support, the technical expertise and know-how about the many health topics and processes and methods needed were most significant. People's passion, commitment, dedicated time, hope, or belief in solutions was probably one the most prized and somewhat intangible human resources of all. The publications from WHO and other agencies, country consultations, training, and technical assistance all proved invaluable in knowledge and skill building to gain the resource of technical expertise. The regional networks and Web-based support, relatively new mechanisms in the 1990s, enabled countries to gain access to materials and people in new and exciting ways.

A very important factor in the success of implementation was the participation of multiple stakeholders across sectors and disciplines. Participating in and having the agency to influence the process happened at many levels. The cases illustrate the multisector participation among health, education, media, and others at the national level. At the local level, a similar pattern occurred, along with the deep involvement of school and community-level leaders with parents, teachers, and students themselves. Such participation took place, for example, in teachers' attention to their own health, in using media to educate and inform parents and the community, and in students' active participation in the classroom or their active engagement in the community. Students themselves actively found solutions to the health threats they were facing. In one case, in an entrepreneurial way, children sold charcoal to earn money to buy their own shoes as a means to prevent intestinal worms.

Given the newness of applying a public health approach to an educational setting, professional development was essential for planners in ministries, as well as for administrative staff and teachers. Professional development had to go beyond training and technical assistance on health topics to cover many of the methods of using data or fostering cross-sector collaboration. Joining health and education staff together in training proved to be very valuable, as did the use of experts in such topics as industrial pollution that went beyond the bounds of what education or health could provide. Training people together in Kosovo, for example, provided a poignant opportunity to begin healing the wounds from war as people united in a common purpose for their children.

Many of the health and education problems are so complex that they require collaboration, at least across the education and health sectors, and often more. Having a skilled and dedicated person to manage the collaboration proved to be important to it working well. Across the cases, the health sector typically took the lead, but realized very quickly that it needed the education sector not just to be involved but to lead for real progress to happen. Such collaboration was often enhanced through joint activities such as training, fund raising, or proposal writing. From Scotland to Nigeria and Cook Islands, we learn the necessity of cross-sector collaboration to achieve legislative support to institutionalize the commitment to programs over time. Given the importance of cross-sector collaboration, more research and study must be done to understand and deepen strategies for its effectiveness, such as the formulation of agreements or role clarification.

Champions and leaders, who vigilantly paid attention to the implementation process across stages of early experimentation, strategic development, and establishment, proved invaluable. Many cases speak to the essential role of the school principal at the local level if the HPS concept is to be fully applied. This is especially the case because teachers often needed the added encouragement or support to try something so new. In addition, it was the leader's deep knowledge of and caring for the community – its children and the people – that resulted in the adaptation and finding of consensual ways to put interventions in place. Leadership across levels, from the ministries to the local level leaders in the schools, in turn, provided them with the commitment from higher authorities.

Data often provided the reason or impetus for the effort, informing health and education officials about serious issues in society, as well as demonstrating the power of interventions to improve not only health status, but also academic performance. Whether they were a country's low scores on academic performance through the PISA or other instruments, surveillance data reporting high levels of student depression or obesity, or data on levels of unemployment and rates of HIV infection, data played a powerful role in galvanizing attention and commitment to action. Baseline data were often gathered, as well, through such tools as the RAAPP or other forms of situational analyses to understand the capacity for implementation or the barriers to it. However, it was not only data about health or educational indicators that contributed to the establishment of HPS, but also data about social conditions, poverty, and economic crises that overflowed into the school system and created a need for schools to address these issues, in some cases utilizing schools as a means for social transformation.

Cases did not describe their administrative or management support mechanisms in great detail, but almost all had a dedicated HPS planning and implementation committee, at either the national or local level. This committee was made up of representatives across sectors and institutions. In China, for instance, principals and/or vice-principals led or co-led these committees. Committee members included administrators and teachers with authority from various areas throughout the school.

It was very important to countries and local schools to be able to adapt the concept to fit their particular circumstances, whether it was local culture and customs, socioeconomic circumstances, particular issues, or their structure available for program delivery. The case study from the Cook Islands, for example, provides a beautiful example of adaptation of the central concept of health and well-being to the culture of the South Pacific, using the elements of their traditional boat.

School health programs were also utilized in response to external forces, such as health, economic, social, and political forces that have an impact on children and families. For instance, in China, the one-child policy and a government mandate for quality education were the larger context to take on the HPS program. In Poland, HPS was introduced when the country was ready for change during the political, social, and economic transition, and in the UAE, changes in disease patterns and lifestyle were taken into consideration when developing and revising the school health program.

Many cases illustrate how they gained a critical mass of people to become involved. Such strategies ranged from creating a national alliance of public and private organizations to become involved, as in the case of Germany, to creating a critical mass of pupils with a vision for health, as in the case of Kenya. India uses the overlapping roles played by the school principal, local media, and the Internet to engage and involve the entire community. Students, also involved extensively on committees in Canada, championed the concept throughout their schools, creating a critical mass of young people who carried the ideas forward.

Readiness to implement the HPS or similar concepts was one of the factors mentioned least often. It is probably likely that in many circumstances a country or community may not have been all that ready, but the problems and challenges demanded action. Had institutions gone through an extensive readiness assessment, they might have lost precious time, or the reality of what was not in place might have been too daunting. In many instances, people plunged in with the motivation of improving conditions for the health, teaching, and learning of young people– the driving force supporting their effort to respond to factors demanding immediate attention.

Monitoring and Evaluation

This book has focused on the methods and factors in implementation and not on the evaluation results of national and local efforts. Yet we cannot end our discussion without acknowledging countries for their examples of monitoring and evaluation (M&E) efforts and highlights of results. The M&E techniques address process evaluation, often documenting the number of schools, teachers, and students reached with various products and services. For example, Singapore documents how its reach has increased from 84 schools in 2002 to 276 schools in 2006 – covering 148 primary and 131 secondary schools with about 400,000 students. In Zhejiang Province, China, the initiative reached 51 schools – representing 93,000 students and their families and 6,800 school personnel – including all levels from primary through junior and senior high to vocational schools, located in rural and urban areas throughout the province. In 2007, Poland describes regional networks of HPS in all 16 voivodships, in more than 1,400 schools of different types, with elementary schools dominant, reaching 650,000 pupils, plus more than 200 kindergartens.

Additionally, M&E describes intermediary results, for example, the capacities that ministries and schools developed to be able to deliver the program, the number of teachers trained or curricula distributed. For example, Canada reports the number of schools with a Safe and Healthy School Committee in place, principals' engagement, and the financial support received from the public health unit, as well as the adoption of tobacco-free policies. Often these criteria and indicators of capacity building or intermediate outcomes are the basis for awarding schools a gold, silver, or bronze prize, according to their ability to deliver a HPS program. For example, Lao PDR developed an accreditation system for schools, a checklist that sets forth standards at gold, silver, and bronze levels for schools to achieve consistent with national policy. Singapore's elaborate award system records the increase in the number of schools receiving the Silver and Gold awards from 49% in 2002 to 83% in 2007.

Yet others tapped student and teacher satisfaction with the effort. Germany's extensive SEIS survey, administered to teachers and students, reports every 2 or 3 years. This survey, for example, shows how interventions gradually became more directed to improving school climate and ethos, identified as key issues. Other cases move beyond process and satisfaction to report on the health or education outcomes of students either pre and postprogram or in comparison with students and schools not involved. Kenya documented environmental changes of placing hand-washing facilities near latrines, building new rubbish pits, installation of drying racks for utensils – all resulting in more sanitary behaviors among students. Hong Kong found statistically significant differences in self-reported behaviors in health and hygiene and in students' satisfaction with life. Through surveys, Canada's evaluation found improvement in students' ability to discuss issues and to problem-solve, agreement on the value of working together in resolving issues, and an increase in students' ability to speak out and take action on identified health and social issues. The cases themselves provide much more detail on the methods and their results.

In conclusion, one of the most dramatic and important results of implementing the HPS or similar concept was the change in the community's attitude toward the school from a pure educational institution to one that more broadly addresses the changing lifestyles and conditions for all, expressed so well by the South Africa case: "We managed this by initially working to change the general view of the school from a 'building' to a 'home away from home' owned by all."

Recommendations

The case studies portray powerful examples of ways in which education and health, working together, can make a profound difference in the healthy development and learning of young people as well as the health and well-being of the surrounding community. In looking ahead to 2020 and the challenges facing schools and communities worldwide, it is imperative that these and similar efforts continue and expand. To support that effort, we make these recommendations:

1. International agencies, such as WHO, UNESCO, UNICEF, and the World Bank, along with nongovernmental organizations, should revitalize and reinvigorate their commitment to Focusing Resources on Effective School Health (FRESH)

and continue to provide the leadership, country consultations, technical documents and tools for countries and local communities to address ever-changing situations. Materials and tools have been invaluable to implementation.

2. Schools should include health and well-being as part of their core mission, as physical, social, emotional, mental, and spiritual health affect learning and school performance.

3. More and more countries should take leadership to examine the role of schools as social agents for development. Schools reach out to communities and school staff and, as appropriate, take the lead in addressing prevalent issues of social development, which will, in turn, contribute to better health and school performance.

4. Financial support should be available and directed to large-scale efforts from the start, so that the excitement and momentum of pilot efforts do not fade and die out when they have the potential for such positive results.

5. Cross-sector collaboration should be elevated as a topic of research and study, professional development, and creation of tools and materials that foster understanding and ways to make it as effective as it can be.

6. Professional development materials and modules, including Web-based courses, should be developed to support staff at the national level of ministries and at the local level of schools and communities, especially teachers. Training is essential, and many of the cases note that what was offered was inadequate. There must also be moves to create professional development that includes the concepts, methods, and content at the preservice level, where the link between health and education and strategies and ways to address their interdependence is virtually ignored. Professional development must address public health concepts and methods, content of specific health issues, and a range of strategies for participation at all levels, including the use of participatory methods in the school and classroom.

7. Networks, which have proven to be a powerful way to provide countries with the technical expertise and support for implementation, themselves should receive financial and collegial support, as they can have broad reach and impact.

The compelling progress of implementing HPS and similar concepts during the last decade that these case studies illustrate – in resource-poor and resource-rich countries – gives great inspiration for even more significant change to occur in academic achievement, health, and social development – through schools – when countries follow these recommendations and draw on the lessons learned presented in this book.

References

Adda, J., Chandola, T., & Marmot, M. (2003). Socio-economic status and health: causality and pathways. *Journal of Econometrics, 112*, 57–63.

Awartani, M., Vince Whitman, C., & Gordon, J. (2008). Developing instruments to capture young people's perceptions of how school as a learning environment affects their well-being. *European Journal of Education, 43*(1), 51–70.

Vince Whitman, C. (2005). Implementing research-based health promotion programmes in Schools: Strategies for Capacity Building. In B. B. Jensen & S. Clift (Eds.), *The health promoting school: international advances in theory, evaluation and practice* (pp. 107–135). Copenhagen: Danish University of Education Press.

Vince Whitman, C. (2006). *Framework for health promoting schools to address social and economic determinants: A discussion paper*. Paper presented at the Technical Meeting, WHO Collaborating Centres for Health Promotion, 16–18 Feb 2006, Singapore.

Vince Whitman, C., Aldinger, C., Levinger, B., & Birdthistle, I. (2001). *Education for All 2000 Assessment: Thematic Studies: School Health and Nutrition*. Paris: United Nations Educational, Scientific and Cultural Organization.

World Health Organization (2003). *Skills for health: Skills-based health education, including life skills – An important component of a child-friendly/health-promoting school, WHO Information Series on School Health – Document 9*. Geneva: World Health Organization.

Section 2
Case Studies

Chapter 4
Kenya: Action-Oriented and Participatory Health Education in Primary Schools

W. Onyango-Ouma, D. Lang'o, and B.B. Jensen

Contextual Introduction

Brief Introduction to the Country

Kenya lies across the equator in East Africa, on the coast of the Indian Ocean. It borders Somalia to the east, Ethiopia to the north, Tanzania to the south, Uganda to the west, and Sudan to the northwest. While the last census conducted in 1999 estimated the population to be about 29 million inhabitants, 2006 estimates put the population at about 34 million. The population growth rate is about 2.6%, while the life expectancy is about 55 years and in some areas as low as 40 years. The literacy level was estimated to be about 85% in 2003; however, this varies across regions, with some regions having very low literacy levels. The GDP is about $41.36 billion (2006) with a per capita income of $1,200, while the unemployment rate is high. Although only 8% of total land is arable, Kenya is mainly an agricultural country, relying on cash crops such as coffee, tea, wheat, and a variety of subsistence crops.

The government is a republic, comprising a central government and decentralized administrative units, while the political system is based on multiparty democracy. The languages spoken include English (official), Swahili (national), and numerous indigenous languages.

Impetus and Origin of the School Health Program

The school health program was implemented at the regional level in primary schools in one district. The program was implemented under the umbrella of the Kenyan-Danish Health Research Project, an interdisciplinary project dealing with

W. Onyango-Ouma(✉)
Institute of Anthropology, Gender and African Studies, University of Nairobi, Nairobi, Kenya

C. Vince Whitman and C.E. Aldinger (eds.),
Case Studies in Global School Health Promotion: From Research to Practice,
DOI: 10.1007/978-0-387-92269-0_4, © Springer Science + Business Media, LLC 2009

a range of health issues, including micro-nutrient supplementation, control of intestinal helminths, and maternal and child health in Bondo District, western Kenya. It was initiated following research findings that intestinal helminth infections were prevalent among schoolchildren in the district, causing substantial morbidity. Bilharzia (*Schistosoma mansoni*) was also found to be prevalent at different levels depending on the distance from the nearby Lake Victoria (Ouma et al., 1996).

Globally, school-aged children have both the highest rate and the highest intensity of helminthic infections. Intestinal helminthic infections are responsible for loss of blood, growth retardation, and impairment of school performance; treatment may reverse these effects with a very fast return to normality (World Health Organization, 1995). In the long term, intestinal helminth infections cannot be controlled by mass treatment alone; an integrated approach, involving behavioral, educational, and environmental factors, is required to ensure a sustainable control. As a result of international advocacy for school health education, many countries, Kenya included, are currently exploring strategies to plan, implement, and evaluate comprehensive health programs. The school health program took the foregoing issues as its starting point.

Overview of the School Health Program

The school health program was conducted from 1999 to 2002 in nine primary schools[1] in one district. The program consisted of two main research strands or components: research in parasitology and research in health education. The two elements are closely linked in pupils' and schools' lives, as successful health education leads to an improved health status among schoolchildren, while good health conditions improve the learning possibilities in schools.

The school health education component aimed at specifying the conditions for an efficient health education leading to better health – in the short and the long run – focusing on geohelminth and schistosomiasis infections. The main concepts and principles within the health education activities developed were *participation* and *action*. Pupils' participation is considered to be the most important precondition for developing ownership among the pupils and thus also for affecting pupils' daily actions and behavior (Jensen, 1997; Simvoska, 2004).

The hypothesis is that action-oriented and participatory approaches in health education support the development of pupils' abilities to create change – their action competence (Jensen, 2000). This means that an action-oriented health education embraces pupils' own actions as important and integrated elements. The actions could be targeted

---

[1] The research project came to an end in 2002. Since then, the schools have continued to work with the Health-Promoting School concept, implementing various aspects of the research project on their own. The schools have also embraced new dimensions, including HIV/AIDS, which has ably captured health promotion for staff and pupils.

at pupils' own life, the environment at the school, the pupils' families, or the local community (Onyango-Ouma, Aagaard-Hansen, & Jensen, 2005).

The key actors in the program were researchers, pupils, teachers, education inspectorate staff, trainers of trainers in action-oriented health education, and community members. The different actors played different roles that were complementary to the implementation of the program.

The program was spread out across nine schools with similar characteristics in one district. The initial implementation was limited to pupils in classes 4 and 6 in the respective schools, giving a total of 536 pupils. However, these intervention pupils engaged in health education activities that targeted the entire school population. Each of the nine schools had an average student population of about 250; thus the program reached additional pupils.

Apart from pupils, teachers were also trained as part of the project and were specifically responsible for the implementation of the intervention in their respective schools. A total of 18 teachers (two in each school) and 9 head teachers were trained in the district. The role of teachers was to teach the pupils on intervention topics and thereafter to serve as facilitators to the pupils, offering support during the implementation phase. In addition, education inspectorate staffs at the district were trained to help them understand the project objectives and potential benefits, so as to facilitate program implementation.

Although the program had an impact at the community level, the result was not documented beyond the homesteads of the 536 intervention pupils. The program aspects that were implemented in the school and home environments included improved sanitation, through construction and maintenance of clean latrines and safe water drinking practices. Although these improvements were reported in homesteads of the 536 pupils and other pupils, there was no systematic follow-up to report the figures.

Scope of Implementation

The school health education program comprised three interventions:

1. The use of flip charts as an interactive tool in the school's health education
2. Establishment of an extracurricular health club
3. In-service training in the form of continual professional support

The nine schools were divided into three groups of three, each receiving a different set of interventions. In the first group, only flip charts were used; in the second group, only health clubs were introduced; the third group received a combination of health club and flip-chart interventions. In addition, one school in each of the three groups received continual professional support in the form of fortnightly visits consisting of observations, discussion, and advice from researchers. None of the schools had previously been involved in health education programs.

Prior to interventions, a baseline study was conducted to establish pupils' level of knowledge of worms, as well as their visions, commitment, and motivation about healthy lifestyles. The baseline created a benchmark against which to conduct process and final evaluations.

Two teacher-training workshops of two days each were organized to set the ground for the implementation of interventions, by building the capacity of teachers to participate effectively in the school health program. Teachers were introduced to key health education concepts including participation, action competence, and the IVAC (Investigations-Visions-Actions-Change) approach (Jensen, 1997). They were also exposed to the school health program interventions (including treatment, flip charts, and health clubs), to help them take ownership of the form and content of the interventions. Knowledge of worms in terms of their life cycles, vectors, associated morbidity, and transmission aspects, as well as prevention and control strategies were also included in the training.

Different Intervention Forms Implemented

Flip Charts

This intervention activity developed flip-chart teaching materials, in collaboration with the learners. The use of the flip charts aimed at bridging the gap between folk knowledge and scientific understanding of how worms are transmitted and what could be done to reduce infections and reinfections. The flip charts also called for pupils' participation in school and in the local community. For instance, pupils were assigned to discuss what they could do, in their class and in their families, to make sure that "worms stay away."

The teachers trained in each school used the flip charts to teach about transmission and prevention of worms during ordinary classroom lessons with pupils in classes 4 and 6 in all the nine schools. Teaching was action-oriented – as opposed to the traditional didactic approach – so as to evoke pupils' participation. Pupils were involved in investigations to find causes and sources of infection as well as actions to be taken to prevent transmission in the school and in the community. Since the charts were developed with the learners, they generated a lot of interest and fun that were key to pupils' commitment and participation. Teaching was done throughout one school term (three months).

Health Clubs

The second type of intervention was the establishment of extracurricular health clubs in schools. The new, innovative approach was to link the work done in a health club to the concepts of action and participation. Health clubs stimulate and motivate pupils as they play a major role in the activities. Although the structure of the health club – via the notion of participation – was to be developed in cooperation with the partners involved (pupils and teachers), it was defined as a group of people outside the classroom situation, who have decided to come together to share ideas on health issues, with a view to promote their own health and that of their families and communities. Pupils themselves formed the health clubs and decided on the form of membership, although the teacher acted as a patron.

Health-club meetings were organized weekly in the participating schools, where they discussed health issues pertaining to transmission and prevention of worms. The meetings focused on the knowledge and identification of tangible actions that club members could take to change the health conditions in the school and at home. Club members went farther, with actions such as putting in place hand-wash facilities and ensuring that pit latrines were in a clean state. The role of the health club was to enhance the promotion of health and the prevention of diseases, at school, within the community, and at home. The major difference between a health club and the typical class situation was that pupils in a health club were the main decision-makers, while the teacher served primarily as a facilitator.

Continual Professional Support

The third type of intervention was continual professional support, giving teachers focused and intensive support during the program implementation. The intent was to learn whether intensive in-service support was necessary for the introduction of new and challenging teaching approaches into the Kenyan school system to succeed. This support was provided in the form of regular miniseminars, two or three hours long, in schools, where the current developments and difficulties were presented and analyzed. The teachers kept logbooks, in which they described their own experiences, evaluations, and observations. Teachers received support from a consultant who visited the schools fortnightly to strengthen their skills and competencies for implementing the program.

Overall, teachers and pupils had the freedom to determine their implementation time frame, that is, either during or after regular school hours. Researchers observed, discussed, and recorded not only the implementation of activities either in or outside class, but also the changes effected by the school and the surrounding community, such as personal hygiene, sanitation, and environmental management.

The Health-Promoting School Concept

The interventions that were implemented addressed two elements of Health-Promoting Schools – a healthy school environment (physical and psychosocial) and outreach to families and community. The interventions developed pupils' action competence through action and participation in health matters in school and home environments. With regard to a healthy school environment, the interventions addressed both physical and psychosocial aspects. Changes in the physical health conditions included actions such as making hand-wash facilities, ensuring that pit latrines were cleaned, cleaning the school compound and classrooms. These actions were aimed at maintaining the school's environmental hygiene and preventing transmission of worms. Flip-chart and health-club interventions facilitated the development of pupils' action competence to take action along these lines. Health clubs also addressed psychosocial concerns by developing life skills in children, giving them a sense of responsibility, raising their self-esteem, and recognizing their efforts.

Outreach to families and the community was achieved through children's participation and action in activities aimed at promoting hygiene and sanitation to prevent the transmission of worms in the home environment. These actions included the maintenance of personal hygiene, putting in place new latrines to improve sanitation, and environmental hygiene (e.g., appropriate refuse disposal).

The school health program also incorporated school health services. The health services involved mass treatment of pupils against *Schistosoma mansoni* and intestinal helminths. The mass treatment was conducted at the beginning of the project, and teachers were trained to conduct the deworming every six months.

Monitoring and Evaluation

Baseline studies were conducted as a basis for future evaluation. The studies focused on potential barriers and possibilities for the development of action-oriented and participatory health education in schools. Standardized questionnaires were administered to pupils to elicit information on components of action competence, motivation for becoming involved in action-oriented health education, common knowledge regarding worms/diseases, and possibilities and motivation for collaboration between school and community.

The evaluation of the project was carried out as both process and outcome evaluation, involving quantitative and qualitative methods. During process evaluation, barriers and possibilities for developing action-oriented and participatory health education were identified through structured observations and recorded by teachers, pupils, and researchers. Simple quantitative counting of social and physical health-promoting changes (e.g., new latrines) in the schools was also done. During health-club meetings, pupils recorded their activities within the school and home environments. In the final evaluation, pupils' knowledge regarding worms as well as their visions, commitment, and abilities to take action and facilitate change were assessed through standardized questionnaires. The development of pupils' and teachers' opinions, knowledge, and commitment about participatory-learning issues were assessed through in-depth interviews.

Summary of Achievements

- Generally students possessed a high degree of action competence, that is, their ideas about how to improve health, and their commitment to taking concrete action in the health field.

- Of the three intervention forms, the health club had the greatest impact on students' competence and knowledge, probably because the more informal climate encouraged students to participate and take ownership.
- The other two intervention forms – the flip charts and the continual professional support – did not make any remarkable difference when they were used as the single intervention in a school.
- The schools where health clubs were combined with flip charts had the greatest impact, probably because the use of the flip charts added more time to the projects as a whole.
- A number of conditions were identified that facilitate participatory teaching/learning approaches:

  - A positive, creative, and explorative attitude among teachers
  - Availability of methods such as the IVAC model and materials such as flip charts.
  - Good teacher/student relationship through reduction of power imbalance by creating informal settings in the extracurricular health clubs.

- A number of factors were identified that hinder participatory learning approaches:

  - Teacher training: From their initial training, teachers were mostly familiar with didactic, top-down approaches; so they were struggling, in spite of good intentions, to adopt the new approach.
  - Staff turnover: Frequent transfers, deaths, maternity leaves, and the like made it difficult to maintain continuity in the project.
  - Punishment traditions: In some schools, the teachers' authority was manifested through punishing students, which militated against the introduction of participatory learning/teaching approach.
  - Language: The use of English created communication barriers between students and teachers especially in the lower classes.

- Remarkable changes were observed over time in pupils' personal and environmental hygiene choices. Hand-wash facilities (leaky tins) were placed next to the pit latrines in schools. Pupils ensured that the tins had water at any given time and were willing to spend time and energy getting water for the tins, as water is a scarce resource in the district. Compost heaps and rubbish pits were established and effectively used where none had existed before. Dish racks for drying utensils were put up in the homes near the intervention schools, indicating that pupils, either alone or in partnership with parents/guardians, translated what was learnt and practiced in school into regular, practical, health-enhancing actions at home.
- Actions also encouraged and fostered creativity and resourcefulness among children. In all the nine schools, teachers reported that children took personal actions to manage their health, for example, burning and selling charcoal to get money to buy shoes, in order to be neat as well as to avoid hookworm infection.

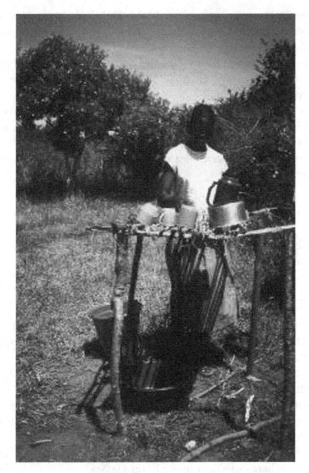

Picture 1   Students participate in creating a dish rack for drying utensils on health project

Specific Aspects of Implementation

Vision

The program implementation focused on the development of visions and commitment among pupils. The program assessed whether pupils developed visions and commitment on how they could improve their health, learning, and school and home environments. This was considered fundamental for changes in the disease dimensions of the school health education program, such as knowledge of worm transmission and prevention. The development of visions and commitment was also considered as an important precondition for pupils' participation in the program.

Training

Given that action-oriented learning and teaching including student participation was new in the study district, the program provided technical assistance and training to teachers to help them implement the intervention. Two in-service training workshops were conducted for science teachers and head teachers in the selected schools, as well as for education inspectorate staff in the district. The workshops underscored the concepts of participation and action as key concepts in school health education. Apart from the two workshops, three of the nine schools also received continual professional support during weekly visits as part of the study design. The trainings and professional support equipped the teachers with skills and created the conditions necessary for successful implementation of the intervention.

Critical Mass

The initial in-service courses created a critical mass of teachers, head teachers, and education inspectorate staff that were equipped with knowledge and skills regarding the design and implementation of action-oriented and participatory school health education intervention programs. Teachers used the skills and knowledge they acquired during in-service to implement the interventions during ordinary classroom teaching to pupils. This process created a critical mass of pupils who had developed visions about how to improve their health, their learning, and their home and school environments. Through participation and action in everyday activities, the intervention pupils interacted with other pupils who were not part of the intervention in school and in the community, thereby creating another critical mass of knowledgeable people as regards health matters in the district. The project successfully created a critical mass of health actors within the school environment (teachers and pupils) and the home/community environment (children and adults).

Resources/Local Adaptation

The implementation took place in a resource-poor setting, so the program had to make do with what was available. Two major constraints in the area were inadequate reliable water supply and shortage of infrastructural facilities such as latrines. Although these were potential barriers to the implementation of the program, the challenge of dealing with them or devising alternatives was considered as a great step toward developing a vision and commitment to healthy conditions. As a result pupils brought water for drinking and cleaning latrines in schools, while in the home environments they built pit latrines and dish racks where they were lacking, in partnership with adults. Because of pupils' commitment and motivation, the project was adapted to the local situation despite the lack of resources and necessary facilities in the school and home environments.

Conclusions and Insights

The action-oriented and participatory health education strategies had impact on key variables (vision, commitment, participation, and knowledge of worm transmission and prevention); effects varied depending on the intervention strategy applied. Overall, the presence of the health-club intervention had the greatest impact, especially where it was combined with the flip-chart intervention. The combination of the health club and the flip chart gave pupils more time to engage in project activities. The content of the flip chart was more knowledge-based; during the health club sessions, children explored what they had learned earlier in flip-chart lessons, thus gaining more time to reflect on appropriate health actions.

Recommendations

1. Teacher training:
   - Teachers need to develop competence to teach with participatory approaches without feeling "loss" of their authority and control.
   - Preservice as well as in-service training of teachers should integrate action-oriented and participatory teaching and learning approaches in more systematic ways.
   - In-service training and professional support should be made available to teachers who are committed to explore and further develop more student-centered teaching and learning approaches as part of their normal practice.

2. Collaboration between school and the community:
   - Authentic, action-oriented teaching approaches, where pupils take action in the community as integrated parts of their teaching and learning, help to build their action competence and commitment in the health area. Consequently, closer links should be established between the school and the local community.
   - Health clubs could be valuable starting points for supporting an action-oriented approach among pupils where concrete heath problems in a community can be addressed.

3. Learning materials and models:
   - Materials and models (such as flip charts and IVAC-approach) with a built-in action-oriented and participatory approach should be developed and disseminated to teachers.

4. The curriculum:
   - The current curriculum, which is overcrowded and encouraging didactic approaches, is inefficient. A more flexible curriculum that allows students to influence the teaching processes should be developed.

- As inspiration for future revisions of the national curriculum a number of case studies and within and between schools should be initiated. These cases should be supported, followed, and documented by trained educational researchers.

Acknowledgment   This project had financial support from the Danish International Development Assistance (DANIDA) through the Kenyan-Danish Health Research Project (KEDAHR).

References

Jensen, B. B. (1997). A case of two paradigms within health education. *Health Education Research 12*, 419–428.

Jensen, B. B. (2000). Health knowledge and health education in relation to a democratic health promoting school. *Health Education 100*, 146–153.

Onyango-Ouma, W., Aagaard-Hansen, J., & Jensen, B. B. (2005). The potential of schoolchildren as health change agents in rural western Kenya. *Social Science and Medicine 51*, 1711–1722.

Ouma, J. H., Magnussen, P, Thiong'o, F. W., Muchiri, E., Luoba, A., & Adoka, S. O. (1996). Kenyan-Danish Health Research Projects. Unpublished report.

Simovska, V. (2004). Student participation: A democratic education perspective—experience from the Health-Promoting Schools in Macedonia. *Health Education Research 19*, 198–207.

World Health Organization. (1995). *Health of school children: Treatment of intestinal helminths and schistosomiasis*. Geneva, Switzerland: World Health Organization.

Chapter 5
Mauritius: Health Promotion for Youth

Odete Moises Cossa

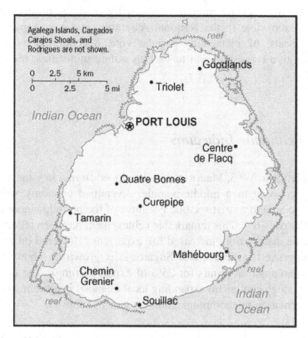

Picture 2   Map of Mauritius

Contextual Introduction

Brief Introduction to the Country

Mauritius, a volcanic island of lagoons and palm-fringed beaches in the Indian
Ocean, with a total area of 2,040 km^2 (788 sq miles), has a reputation for stability
and racial harmony among its mixed population of Asians, Europeans, and Africans.
The island has maintained one of the developing world's most successful democ-
racies and has enjoyed years of constitutional order.

O.M. Cossa
World Health Organization, African Region, Harare, Zimbabwe

C. Vince Whitman and C.E. Aldinger (eds.),
Case Studies in Global School Health Promotion: From Research to Practice,
DOI: 10.1007/978-0-387-92269-0_5, © Springer Science + Business Media, LLC 2009

A stable democracy with regular free elections and a positive human rights record, the country has attracted considerable foreign investment and has earned one of Africa's highest per capita incomes. The total population is 1.3 million, with life expectancy of 70 years for men and 76 years for women (UN, 2009).

The country's political structure includes a cabinet (or Council of Ministers) appointed by the president on the recommendation of the prime minister; a president and vice president elected by the National Assembly for 5-year terms (eligible for a second term); a prime minister and deputy prime minister appointed by the president, responsible to the National Assembly; and a unicameral National Assembly (70 seats; 62 elected by popular vote, 8 appointed by the election commission to give representation to various ethnic minorities; members serve 5-year terms).

Social and Economic Indicators

Since independence in 1968, Mauritius has developed from a low-income, agriculturally based economy to a middle-income, diversified economy with growing industrial, financial, and tourist sectors. For most of the period, annual growth has been in the order of 5–6%. This remarkable achievement has been reflected in more equitable income distribution, increased life expectancy, lowered infant mortality, and a much-improved infrastructure. Sugarcane is grown on about 90% of the cultivated land area and accounts for 25% of export earnings. The government's development strategy centers on expanding local financial institutions and building a domestic information telecommunications industry (Table 1).

Impetus, Origin, and Leadership

Aware that the school is an important setting for the improvement of people's health in general and young people's health in particular, the World Health

Table 1 Selected social and economic indicators

GDP	US $6.4 billion
GDP per capita	US $5,124
Literacy	84%
Urbanization	42%
Population growth rate	0.8%
Maternal mortality rate	15 per 100,000 live births
Infant mortality rate	14 per 1,000 live births
Under-5 mortality rate	15 per 1,000 children

References: (UN Statistics Division, 2009; WHO Statistics Division, 2009)

Organization (WHO) Regional Office for Africa (AFRO) has embarked on a long-term program to promote health through schools. It is believed that this is one of the best models to enhance both health and the capacity of young people to learn; therefore, any school within a given country in the continent that embraced this concept is commonly called a Health-Promoting School.

According to WHO AFRO, "a health promoting school strives to provide a healthy environment, health education, school health services, along with school/community projects and outreach, nutrition and food safety, programmes, opportunities for physical education and recreation, programmes for social support, counselling and mental health promotion" (WHO/AFRO, 2002).

The Health-Promoting Schools project in Mauritius was initiated by the then-named Ministry of Education, Science and Technology.

In 2006, the Ministry of Education and Human Resources launched a curriculum reform initiative in line with major socioeconomic and technological changes at both the national and international levels (Mauritius Ministry of Education & Human Resources, 2006b). The goals of the national curriculum include, among others, the following relevant objectives in Health Promotion: (1) to promote an all-round development of the individual – physical, intellectual, social, and emotional – leading to a balanced, active, healthy, and productive lifestyle and (2) to promote a culture of lifelong learning for greater access to an ever-changing job market.

The program targeted primary and secondary school levels.

Overview of the School Health Program

Dates Boundaries

Mauritius is one of the African countries that have embraced the concept of Health-Promoting Schools through the Ministry of Education and Human Resources. The health promotion experience herein reported dates back to 1997, and coincides with the WHO AFRO start-up of a project to help member states implement the Health-Promoting Schools initiative.

The Mauritius School Health Program started in 1997 through a phased approach implemented by the then Ministry of Education, Science and Technology. The project had a national reach and coverage. Initially, it targeted students of the primary sector, mainly standards I, III, and V; subsequently, it was extended to all classes.

A new health program for secondary schools was launched, involving 158 secondary schools and some 28,000 students of Form III and Lower VI, through a collaborative venture between the Ministry of Health and Quality of Life and the Ministry of Education and Human Resources.

Key Cast of Players

The main players included the Ministry of Education and Human Resources and the Ministry of Health and Quality of Life.

Reach

The program is currently ongoing. It targeted 60 primary schools and has been extended to reach 156 secondary schools and a total of 28,000 students, according to the Ministry of Education and Human Resources. The program now targets all schools. However, staff constraints have prevented officers from conducting regular visits to 130 of the schools.

Scope of Implementation

The preproject was implemented in phases (Beeharry, 2001).
   Phase I included several procedures:

- Designing and printing of a health booklet to cover a minimum of 12 grades
- Identification of schools, meeting with head teachers/deputy head teachers (HTs/ DHTs) and parents through Parent-Teacher Associations (PTAs), to familiarize them with the advantages of the project
- Training of teachers, administrative staff, and caretakers
- Creating a proper environment in the school
- Preparation by a nutritionist of guidelines for balanced meals
- Adoption of classes by class PTAs to help in the implementation of the activities
- Adoption of the appropriate formula for a balanced diet to the students
- Screening and follow-up of students

   In *Phase II*, the same procedures were applied to reach all primary schools and to cover the totality of the school population.

Medical Checkups

Mauritius has provided numerous medical checkups to primary school children. In a bid to improve the quality of life and prevent complications, the medical check program is now extended to the students of secondary schools. Recently the School Health program has been expanded to include the so-called *three earlies* program, comprising early screening, early diagnosing, and referral actions as early as possible aiming at removing barriers to learning and implementation of proper actions (Mauritius Ministry of Health and Human Resources, 2006a).

The *medical check program* provides the following:

- Full medical checkup, including dental examination, and follow-up, in Standards I and V and additional dental examination in Standard V
- Polio drops provided to all at school entry
- Vision testing in Standards III and VI
- Booster doses of tetanus vaccine in Standards I and VI
- The "three earlies" program comprising early screening, early diagnosing, and referral actions
- A balanced diet
- Physical exercise/movement education
- Distribution of pamphlets on general health information
- School Health Club, through which health promotion activities are conducted to ensure the full participation of students
- Designing and printing of a health booklet
- Training of teachers, administrative staff, and caretakers
- Preparation of nutrition guidelines for a balanced meal
- Adoption of the appropriate formula for a balanced diet to the students

Summary of Achievements and Impact

The Mauritius experience on Health-Promoting Schools has not yet been formally evaluated to produce evidence of the program's achievements and their impact on the lives of learners, teachers, and the school community. Overall, it can be said that the program has reached a large number of school-going children, with effects on both their health lifestyle and their learning outcomes. Teachers who have undergone training sessions and who have been primarily responsible for the implementation of the program have also changed their attitudes toward their own health and have transferred this knowledge to their communities and family members as well.

The success of the program is also shown by the fact that it evolved considerably to higher levels and is now focusing on performance improvement.

Moreover, the Ministry of Education and Human Resources is now considering a Comprehensive Holistic School Health Program, with an eye to the direct impact on the student's overall performance in school as well as on the adult he or she will become.

Specific Aspects of Implementation

Goal/Vision

The Government of Mauritius considers that an essential part of an effective school health service is to ensure that children are healthy and are able to learn.

"Equipping young people with knowledge, attitudes and skills through health education, is like giving them a vaccination against health threats" (Faugoo, 2007).

The Mauritius project's ultimate goal was that "all school activities center around the overall development of the child, s/he is the raw resource that has to be moulded into a thinking, creative being who can both integrate into, as well as transform, society" (Beeharry, 2001).

The main premises of the project were that it was essential to nurture students – from the very beginning of the school cycle – so thoroughly that they can remain healthy throughout the years of study and beyond.

Good health implies a high level of cognitive, physical, and moral development, which will have a direct impact on the student's overall performance in school as well as on the adult he or she will become, hence the society that will emerge.

Scaling Up

The Ministry of Education and Human Resources is considering a Comprehensive Holistic School Health Program. The program will focus on the following: (Gokhool, 2006)

- Healthy physical school environments
- Services and mechanisms in schools to ensure healthy development of the student
- Comprehensive, holistic health education across the levels from preprimary through secondary schooling

Health education will deal with knowledge, understanding, and value-oriented skills in several areas:

- Education of the body: systems of the body, the related organs, their functioning and malfunctioning or diseases, and proactive skills and techniques for a healthy lifestyle
- Education of the heart: emotional stability, through studying feelings, emotions, blockages, etc.
- Education of the mind: development of an alert, scientific mind that uses logical and critical thinking

The secondary education level will adopt a consistent, sustainable approach to include active student participation; training teachers for knowledge and skills; follow-up, monitoring, and a collective support system; and enriching the school environment.

Health education will also entail a social program aimed at addressing students' aggressive behavior, attitudes toward sexuality, personality conflicts, and emotional problems acquired in earlier life experiences.

Proactive skills will be coupled with therapeutic skills to ensure that students grow healthily. The curriculum reform launched in late 2006 will be a critical

Table 2 Curriculum reform components

Level	Content
Primary	Health and physical education
	Development and understanding of basic scientific concepts, environmental issues, and values that lay the foundation for a healthy living
	Body awareness
	Sex education
Secondary	Promotion of creativity, artistic dispositions, physical health, and fitness
	Sex education
	Physical education
	Drug education
	Health education

(Mauritius Ministry of Education & Human Resources, 2006)

opportunity for scaling up what the Mauritius Government has attempted to do in the past in the field of School Health. The curriculum will be structured to include relevant content on school health (Table 2).

Positive aspects of the implementation include the following:

- The integration of school health/health education parameters in the performance measurements.
- The consideration of a Comprehensive Holistic School Health Program rather than a piecemeal and project-based program.
- *Targeting all schools*. This is unique; other countries have not yet achieved it.

Conclusions and Insights

The Mauritius Government school health program has advanced significantly over the last few years. The introduction of health into the formal primary school curriculum, together with regular health education sessions in both primary and secondary schools, has significantly contributed to the welfare of school-going children across the country.

Acknowledgment The author had support from the WHO AFRO.

Reference

Beeharry, D. (2001). Mauritius Country Profile: Health Promotion in Schools: Promoting a Heathy Lifestyle. Washington, D.C.: American University. Available from: http//www.american.edu/academic.depts/cas/health/iihp/iihpcpmaurtius.html.

Faugoo, S. (2007). Address by the Health Minister at the Launching Ceremony of the Secondary School Health Programme. Moka, Mauritius: Ministry of Health.

Gokhool, D. (2006). Address by the Minister of Education and Human Resources at the Launching of Rehabilitation and Health Society. Réduit, Mauritius: Ministry of Education and Human Resources.

Mauritius Ministry of Education and Human Resourses. (2006a). Project Document to Improve the Level of Educational Achievement in Primary Schools in Deprived Regions. Geneva: UNDP. Available from: http//un.intnet.mu/UNDP/downloads/info/SOCIAL_DEVELOPEMENT/ZEP/Pro.Doc/ZEP%20Project%20Document.doc.

Mauritius Ministry of Education and Human Resources. (2006b). Towards a Quality Curriculam: Strategy for Reform. Phoenix, Mauritius: Republic of Mauritius. Available from: http://www.mieonline.org/home/articles/469/1/Towards-a-Quality-Curriculum-Strategy-for-Reform-Nov-2006/Page1.html.

UN Statistics Division. (2009). World Statistics Pocketbook: Mauritius Country Profile. Geneva: UN Statistics Division. Available from: http://data.un.org/CountryProfile.aspx?crname=Mauritius.

WHO Statistics Division. (2009). WHO Data: Mauritius. Geneva: WHO Statistics Division. Available from: http://data.un.org/Data.aspx?q=mauritius+literacy&d=WHO&f=inID%3aSDEC11%3bcrID%3a109.

WHO/AFRO. (2002). A special health promotion project: The health promoting schools initiative. Retrieved March 23, 2009 from www.afro.who.int/healthpromotion/project.html.

Chapter 6
Nigeria: Health-Promoting Schools[1]

Olusola Odujinrin

Contextual Introduction

Country Situation

Nigeria, the tenth largest country globally and the fourth largest economy in Africa, lies on the west coast of Africa and occupies approximately 923,768 km^2 of land bordering Niger, Chad, Cameroon, and Benin. Nigeria is the most populous country in Africa, with a population of 140 million (NPC, 2006) and one of the ten mega countries in the World Health Organization (WHO) mega country school health project. One out of every five Africans is a Nigerian. About 64% of the population lives in rural areas with the balance of 36% living in urban areas. About 70% of the population is under the age of 30 while those under 15 make up 44%.

Nigeria has more than 350 ethnic or linguistic groups. The country is divided into 36 states plus a Federal capital territory (FCT), as shown in Fig. 1. The states are further divided into 774 local government areas (LGAs) and the FCT into 6 area municipal councils. Military leadership has dominated the postindependence period (since 1960) with the recent 8 years being the longest period of democratic governance in a stretch. The health indicators are typical of those for developing countries: maternal mortality rate is 800/100,000 live births; infant mortality is 100/1,000 live births, and under-5 mortality is 201/1,000 live births.

[1]HPS team in Nigeria: Dr. Taiwo Oyelade, World Health Organization, Abuja, Nigeria; Dr. Babatunde Segun, Federal Ministry of Health, Abuja, Nigeria; Mrs. Modupe Akerele, Federal Ministry of Health, Abuja, Nigeria; Mrs. Adenike Etta, Federal Ministry of Health, Abuja, Nigeria; Mr. David Ajagun, Federal Ministry of Health, Abuja, Nigeria; Mrs. Rakiya Idris, Federal Ministry of Health, Abuja, Nigeria – Family Health, Department of Public Health, Federal Ministry of Health, Abuja, Nigeria.

O. Odujinrin
World Health Organization, Abuja, Nigeria

C. Vince Whitman and C.E. Aldinger (eds.),
Case Studies in Global School Health Promotion: From Research to Practice,
DOI: 10.1007/978-0-387-92269-0_6, © Springer Science + Business Media, LLC 2009

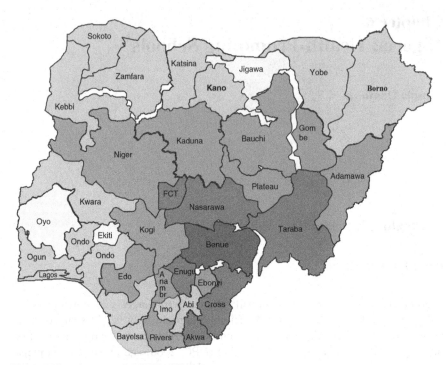

Fig. 1 Thirty-six states plus FCT of Nigeria

School Enrollment

There has been a general increase in school enrollment of up to 44% in 2003. This was due to the commencement of Universal Basic Education in 1999, which included attendant sensitization, mobilization, advocacy, and strong political will led by the Federal Government. This response is contributing immensely to the attainment of Millennium Development Goal 2, the achievement of universal primary education. The achieved progress is judged "good" for primary school enrollment and completion, while the literacy rate among ages 15–24 is rated as "fair" by in-country MDG assessment.

Overview of the School Health Program

Coordination of School Health Activities in Nigeria

The Federal Ministry of Health (FMOH) in Nigeria is the apex body responsible for the health of the citizenry. Nigeria operates a three-tier level of government – federal, state, and local government – with ministries of health at the state level and departments of health at the local government level. The federal level formulates policies, sets standards and guidelines, develops training documents, etc., while the state and local government levels implement and replicate. The Adolescent and School Health unit of the FMOH is concerned with the development of the healthy child, with particular attention to children in school. The unit is responsible for policy formulation and for monitoring of programs aimed at the health of the school child.

Rapid Assessment and Action Planning Process (RAAPP)

Nigeria was one of the countries that participated in this school health project in 2001, in collaboration with WHO and Education Development Center. Through this assessment, the gaps in federal level management of school health at FMOH and the Federal Ministry of Education were identified. The RAAPP also identified the need for a section on school health to be part of the school policy; it also set the foundation and sowed the seed for the introduction of the Health-Promoting School (HPS) initiative in Nigeria.

School Health Service in Nigeria

The Nigerian school health service aims at promoting positive health and preventing disease; offering early diagnosis, treatment, and follow-up of defects; awakening health consciousness in schoolchildren; and providing healthful school environments. With 28.8% of the Nigerian population being between 5 and 14 years (which constitute the core of the school age), school health deserves an important place in the national health system, agenda, and programs (NPC, 1998). While the school health system focuses on the physical, social, and mental development of school-age children, it also addresses relevant health needs of teachers and other school health personnel. There has been a huge decline in the health system, and the school health component was not spared. Many of the original provisions are now ruments of the past, and structures are either dilapidated or bare.

While school health services have been part of Nigeria's public health and educational system for decades, very little is known about the current state of the system – its functioning, coverage, and effectiveness. Also, very little is actually known about the health status of Nigerian school children, which the school health service is supposed to primarily focus on. This urged us to seek funding and carry out a survey of the school health system, even after Nigeria was dropped from the Global School-Based Student Health Survey (GSHS) in 2003.

The National School Health System Assessment

As part of the overall objective of strengthening the school health system in Nigeria, and to provide relevant data for program management, the FMOH in collaboration with the Federal Ministry of Education and with the collaboration of the WHO initiated a rapid assessment of the school health system in March 2003. The results of the assessment were to provide opportunities for development of evidence-based policy and program interventions. Appropriate tools were developed; interviewers were trained on how to conduct physical examinations on school children, to assess visual acuity, using the Snellen chart, and to assess hearing loss. Orientation on the assessment of the classrooms and the school environment was part of the training to ensure uniformity.

The study covered 12 randomly selected states – Adamawa, Bayelsa, Ebonyi, Edo, Ekiti, Gombe, Imo, Jigawa, Kogi, Kano, Osun, and Plateau. The assessment of the school health system was carried out through administration of structured questionnaires by trained data collectors to three groups: heads of schools (head-master/headmistress/principals), students, and parents of school-aged children. Four schools were selected in each state: two primary and two secondary schools. Equal numbers of schools were selected from the urban and rural areas. Sixty students were to be selected in each participating school, from the entry, mid-period, and graduating classes. Thirty parents of school-aged children were also selected per state within the environment of the selected schools.

The study revealed, among other findings, that many of the public schools lacked water and toilet facilities, and about a quarter of students had low body mass index (BMI), suggestive of undernutrition. This prompted the introduction of the HPS initiative, which seemed the best option for improving the quality of the health of the Nigerian school children and the school environment.

Specific Aspects of Implementing the HPS Initiative in Nigeria

With support from WHO, the HPS initiative was introduced in 2005.

Objectives

The objectives of the HPS initiative are as follows:

- To create awareness of key environmental risk factors
- To develop positive attitudes toward adoption of personal hygiene norms by children of age 6–18
- To mobilize children to participate in environmental sanitation actions
- To develop leadership skills in keeping safe and healthy environments among children of age 6–18.

- To improve community attitudes and skills regarding the development and use of simple, resource-effective, and culturally appropriate environmental sanitation facilities
- To develop life skills among children of age 10–18 to enable them cope with the challenges of adolescence

Preintervention Advocacy Visit and Community Mobilization

Two working days were set aside for site preparation and advocacy visits to key stakeholders and policy makers at both state and LGA levels. FMOH and WHO officials paid advocacy visits to the officials of the state Ministries of Education and Health, and to school management bodies in the state for primary and secondary schools, following on earlier communications on the project. Those visited were asked to accept responsibilities and ownership of the project.

Community leaders were also visited and informed of the project and its benefits to them and their children. The schools' parent-teacher associations were also duly informed. Through these visits, support was solicited and acquired.

Trainings

A training manual was developed by FMOH and WHO to train teachers, students, and school food vendors on the concept of HPS, safe food, hygienic food vending, safe water, personal hygiene, healthy habits and lifestyle, environmental sanitation and waste management, and life skills. A 5-day training was conducted for the teachers as counselors, plus a 3-day training for pupils as environmental health marshals, and a 2-day training for the food vendors. Various teaching techniques were used for the training; these included brainstorming, demonstration and return demonstration, lecture/discussion, and field visits. The language of delivery was a combination of English and local dialect as found appropriate for effective communication. Pre- and posttests were administered to the teachers and pupils to assess learning uptake.

Water and Sanitation

In addition to the training, a borehole well with hand pumps was sunk, and two sets of three compartments of VIP toilets were constructed in each school to support training on environmental sanitation.

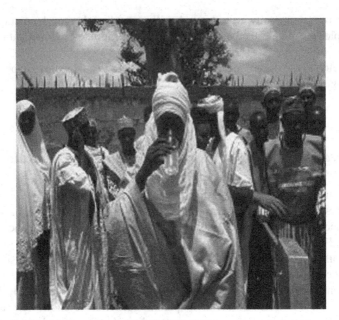

Picture 3   Drinking clean water as result of water pump

Commissioning of Borehole and VIP Toilets

A commissioning ceremony of the facilities took place on completion of the constructions of the borehole and the VIP toilets. This allowed for inspection of the facilities by community leaders and parents, as well as for their identification with the project, giving them a sense of ownership.

Expected Follow-Up School Activities

The schools' HPS teams were charged with the responsibility of setting up school health clubs, where the counselors (the teachers) were expected to offer health club members in-depth health education on the various topics covered during their training, as well as regular health talks to the school population at school assembly and similar forums. The marshals (pupils) were expected to ensure that all students keep the school environment clean, participate in school environmental health activities, and maintain the facilities. School authorities were also encouraged to allow the HPS marshals to give 5-min health talks on the assembly ground on topics such as healthy habits, environmental sanitation, personal hygiene, safe water, safe food, refuse and waste disposal management, food vending, skills-based health education, and livelihood skills. The LGA environmental health officer is supposed to assist in the maintenance of the school facilities and environment; the school health nurse is expected to run the health service for the pupils and see to the provision of adequate nutritious school meals; the food vendors cook under hygienic conditions and serve balanced diets to the pupils.

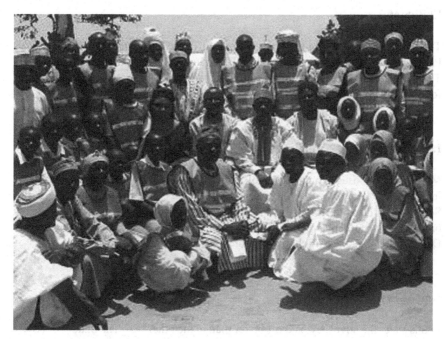

Picture 4   Teamwork on HPS planning

Memorandum of Understanding

At the completion of the training, a memorandum of understanding (MOU) was signed for each state by key stakeholders – FMOH; WHO; state commissioners/permanent secretaries of health, education, water resources; Water and Sanitation (WATSAN) officer; local government chairmen; headmasters/principals of the schools. The MOU indicated the roles and responsibilities of all concerned.

Monitoring and Evaluation

Semiannual or annual visits were scheduled, funds permitting. A baseline assessment instrument was developed late in Phase 1 and used thereafter for capturing baseline data.

Phase 1 HPS

The project was supported in the 2004–2005 biennial plans and implemented in three of the twelve states that participated in the School Health survey. These were Ekiti, Gombe, and Imo States. Two schools from the list of schools that were surveyed (one primary and one secondary) had the intervention. The selected schools, categories, and number trained for Phase 1 are described here.

Ekiti State

The two schools were United High School, in Ilawe Ekiti, and St James Anglican Primary School, in Igbara Odo, both in Ekiti South West Local Government Area. Twelve teachers (6 from each school), 20 students (10 from each school), and 10 food vendors were trained.

Imo State

More than the usual complement of trainees attended the training: 22 teachers, including teachers from four other schools, 33 pupils, 4 staff of the School Health Service unit of the State Ministry of Health, and 13 food vendors. Only the two schools originally slated for intervention, Sam Njemanze Primary School and Comprehensive Development Secondary School, had boreholes and VIP toilets constructed.

Gombe State

In this state, the advocacy paid off better than in the other two. The State WATSAN agreed to fence the facilities for security. The two participating schools were Gombe Junior Secondary School, in Patami, and Bogo Science Primary School, in Kumo. Forty-two participants were trained in total, comprising 12 teachers, 20 students, and 10 food vendors.

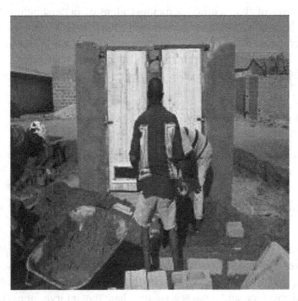

Picture 5 VIP toilet

Phase 2 HPS

Four states benefited under Phase 2 in the biennium 2006–2007 – Bayelsa, Kogi, Jigawa, and Oshun.

Kogi State

The project in Kogi started in 2006. The participating schools were Model Primary School, in Igbaruku, and Egbe Comprehensive High School.

Bayelsa State

The process had to be suspended in Bayelsa, because the state wanted motorized pumps for the borehole and the State WATSAN was demanding far more monetary resources than were given to other states. During the site preparation/advocacy, it became obvious that the state would need to share the costs of the borehole and VIP toilet. Representation was made to the policy makers in charge.

The state finally agreed to augment the budget to cover the costs prevailing in its state. The project resumed after the national election in April.

Overall, about 160 primary and secondary school pupils/students and 72 teachers in primary and secondary schools have been reached in six states. We are planning to be in four states this year and proceed similarly until we cover all the states.

Conclusion

We learned several lessons:

- It is possible for government ministries and agencies to work together effectively and synergistically.
- Community involvement from the beginning – at the planning stage – can result in project ownership and contributions, in both kind and cash.
- Pupils can acquire skills for environmental risk reduction.
- Information sharing and involvement can make health workers and non-health workers more committed, better performers, even in the absence of monetary remuneration.
- With advocacy, adequate information, diplomacy, and firm resolve, government can be made to live up to its responsibility.

It is highly desirable that interventions should be introduced in all states in many of the schools surveyed. This may be possible in the next one or two WHO biennial periods. An evaluation will follow to assess the effect of the interventions. If outcomes are positive, a case will be made for programmatic reflections of these interventions for the improvement of the health of the Nigerian schoolchild.

References

National Population Commission (NPC). (1998). *1991 National population census. Analytical report*. Abuja, Nigeria: Author.
National Population Commission (NPC). (2006). *National population census preliminary report*. Abuja, Nigeria: Author.

Chapter 7
South Africa: Sapphire Road Primary

Bruce Damons and Sean Abrahams

Contextual Introduction

Introduction to Country and Province

Sapphire Road Primary School is situated in South Africa, in the city of Port Elizabeth, in the province of the Eastern Cape, which has a population of about 7.5 million people. The Eastern Cape Province is one of the most rural provinces in the country. It is also one of the largest provinces geographically and the third poorest of all nine provinces. Here, the daily struggle for a better life is waged more intensely because even after the advent of democracy in 1994, the sting of our apartheid history remains highly visible in many spheres of civil society.

Social and Economic Indicators

Our feeder population is characterized by 90% unemployment, conditions of abject poverty, and many of the social challenges prevalent in economically challenged communities, such as HIV/AIDS, substance abuse, lack of nutrition, and low literacy.

Level

Sapphire Road Primary is a primary school serving learners from grades 1 to 7. In 2007, we had 1,022 learners enrolled, supported by 27 educators and 5 nonteaching staff members working in the school. The average size of a household is about four

B. Damons(✉)
Sapphire Road Primary School, Port Elizabeth, South Africa

C. Vince Whitman and C.E. Aldinger (eds.),
Case Studies in Global School Health Promotion: From Research to Practice,
DOI: 10.1007/978-0-387-92269-0_7, © Springer Science + Business Media, LLC 2009

persons; thus, we have contact with more than 4,000 people. However, we reach considerably more people through our community outreach programs under the Health-Promoting Schools (HPS) model.

Impetus, Origin of Rebuilding

The school convened a meeting of all stakeholders in 2000 to chart a 5-year vision under the name "Let's Join and Build" ("Masibambane Sakhe"). From this assembly, a new direction for the school emerged: In the future, Sapphire Road Primary would strive to utilize its historic educational responsibility to act as a catalyst for social "upliftment" of the community. Central to this bold conceptualization of our educational task was the actual development of the different components of the school community to a level of understanding that community members, as partners in the educational process, have an important role to play in the success of our educational objective. We managed this by initially working to change the general view of the school from a "building" to a "home away from home" owned by all. This change in outlook enabled us to mobilize the community members to take responsibility for their children's education and also to utilize the school as an important opportunity for their own self-development. The key question that was and is still debated around our vision is whether an educational institution should focus purely on academic education or also on the social issues of its feeder communities. We argue that these two areas are not mutually exclusive. In fact, we believe that in a transformed South African society, every institution should play a much greater role in educating not only the learners placed in its care, but also their parents and the broader community. Our challenge is to strike an equitable balance between the educational demands of the learners and the social needs of the parents and the community.

Overview of School Health Program

We began the process of school transformation primarily as a response to the social conditions peculiar to our feeder communities. When we were introduced to the HPS concept through the Health Department of our government, in 2006, we were already well on our way to actualizing our vision. As we grew in understanding of the HPS concept, it was evident that the vision for our school and the HPS principles intersected on many levels. Although we identified areas of convergence, our self-analysis also revealed areas of difference in approaches. We resolved to implement all of the five pillars of HPS (services, policy, environment, community, and skills-building) and to adapt them to our unique conditions. In the process of our school development thus far, we have learned that there is no magic blueprint for success and no single theory that guides us to our set objective. Instead, we have striven to create a flexible, elastic organization that can adapt and respond proactively to the dynamic demands of our communities. In 2000, for example, our focus was on unemployment and lack of skills, while in 2004 our focus changed to HIV/AIDS and health. Thus, we need a flexible plan based on solid principles rather than a rigid, prescribed plan to direct our developmental course. While parents, teachers, and learners formed the nucleus of the change process in the school, eliciting support from government departments, private sector, and nongovernmental organizations also played a very important role in actualizing our vision. Without these stakeholders, our progressive momentum would not have been possible. The crucial HPS element that enabled us to progress was community buy-in. Once the school was recognized as a social agent, it became much easier to implement some of the other elements. It took us more than 2 years of discussion and of convincing our community, government, businesses, and even ourselves that our course was true. After 3 years, we are only beginning to see the fruits of our endeavors. Even in our success, we still have detractors and skeptics at all levels of civil society. Patience in leadership was the key. Of all the theoretical factors, we believe that community ownership and broad stakeholder participation were the most critical to our success. Developing our own sense to identify challenges and respond to them was in line with the general ethos and culture of our feeder communities and was critical to our success.

Achievements

The following notable achievements of the 5-year vision plotted in 2000 were accomplished from 2003 to 2008.

Academic:

- Teachers are part of an international pilot program that focuses on improvement of teaching practices.
- Introduction of new reading and health approaches in 2008.
- Weekly training of teachers in the new reading approach.
- Integrating the personal wellness of learners into the learning process.
- Use of unemployed parents as volunteers in the classroom, assisting teachers.
- No school fees for 2006.
- Strong extramural programs that include rugby, soccer, netball, mini cricket, choir, and arts and culture.
- Exposing learners to field trips.
- Constant training and retraining in programs related to the curriculum.

Skills development:

- Ongoing training of unemployed youth and parents in basic skills such as welding, computer literacy, sewing, and carpentry. Since the inception of the school, it has trained more than 300 unemployed members of the community.
- Building of a security house on the premises of the school, using bricks that were made by unemployed parents.

- Security gates to protect the school, installed by unemployed parents trained at our skill school.
- Repairs to school furniture and securing of neighboring schools' buildings, using our skills school.
- Making of our entire sport kit by the sewing section of the skills school.
- Moral regeneration program included as part of skills development.
- Opening of an accredited training center for the unemployed, on the premises of the school, which will train the unemployed from ten other communities.
- Adult Basic Education and Training (ABET) classes for parents to teach reading skills – launched in 2007.

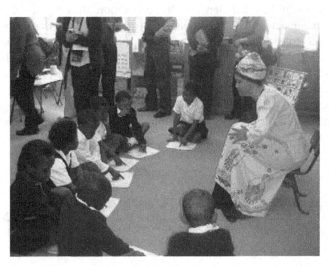

Picture 6 Teacher in the classroom

Health:

- Unveiling of an AIDS ribbon at the entrance of the school and piloting of the "We Care" HIV/AIDS awareness program with Family Association of South Africa (FAMSA).
- Opening of a counseling center on the premises of the school, to help the community deal with social issues, including HIV/AIDS. The center is manned by peer counselors who do advocacy as well as home-base care.
- Establishment of a vegetable garden that is run by the school. The produce from this garden is given to the more than 30 families that are either infected or affected by HIV/AIDS.
- Running a pilot sweet potato project that provides an income for unemployed parents.
- Regular health talks by local clinics and NGOs that focus on prevention and cure, for example, on tuberculosis, nutrition, and substance abuse.

- Building a clinic and a counseling room on the premises of the school in 2006, which was done by parent volunteers. The clinic opened officially in February 2007 and will serve the community and school. Ten parents and a supervising doctor volunteer in the clinic. The school program will start with health screening of all learners.
- Personal wellness programs for teachers, featuring fabric painting, meditation, and stress-coping mechanisms.
- Mass tuberculosis testing program on the premises of the school, beginning in May 2008. Of the 713 community members tested, 8 were positive.

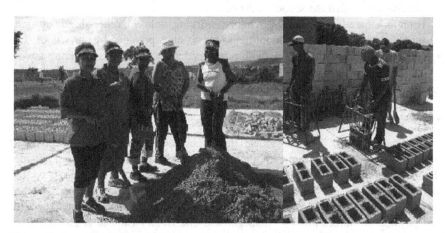

Picture 7 Community volunters building clinic

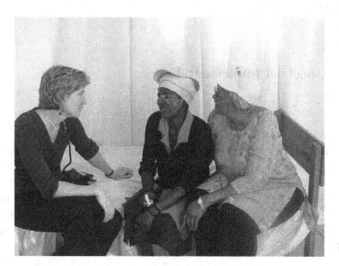

Picture 8 First patients examined by visiting USA Doctor Sue Taylor

Community outreach:

- Opening of a gym by the weightlifting association of South Africa to promote weightlifting development in the area. Two of the learners from these classes won gold medals at the national weightlifting championships in 2005.
- The school is used by five different churches from the surrounding area to hold services on the weekends.
- The school's sports field serves as a home venue for the local soccer club.
- Recognition for work done by the president of the country as well as receiving the Batho Pele award from the premier of the province. The deputy president of our country visited the school in 2006.
- Founding member of Active Schools, working with 11 other disadvantaged schools to ensure that they adopt the same vision expounded by our school.
- Developed outreach programs with other feeder communities, including advocacy as well as development programs.
- Adopted parent and teacher charters that recommit us to providing quality education to the most vulnerable sector of society.
- No vandalism since 2003.

As a school with limited financial resources, we would not have been in a position to effect our program without the assistance of social partners from outside the school environment. The Department of Health in the Eastern Cape has played a significant role in our success. They provided technical, financial, and human resource support, ranging from inoculations for our learner population to expertise and physical resources for our AIDS garden. The Rotary Club of Algoa has also been instrumental in the attainment of our vision. Through their hard work, dedication, and donation we were able to realize our academic improvement plan. Club members also assisted with material and technical support for the building of our security house and clinic.

Specific Aspects of Implementation

Vision

Our vision is to ensure that the school is used as an instrument to develop not only the learners but also the parents and the community. This can be done if the school serves as the center of educational and social transformation.

We have adopted the vision that our school should be the center of the entire community, fostering social and academic upliftment. We have made sure that our programs reflect this vision, which is essential if we want to be able to tackle the various challenges that confront us daily.

Our vision is built on the following rationale:

Academic:

- The ultimate objective of the school is academic learning. However, because of our challenges, we want to use this tool as a mechanism to "liberate the mind from mental inferiority."
- Encourage educator learning at local, national, and international levels.
- Recognize the fact that no constructive learning and teaching can take place without a stable social and educational environment.
- Ensure that we develop all our learners holistically.

Skills development:

- Critical for school growth is the growth of the community surrounding the school.
- High levels of unemployment contribute to many of the evils of society.
- School has the infrastructure to make a meaningful difference not only in the lives of our learners but in the lives of the community they come from.
- Communities tend to have more respect for institutions that make meaningful contributions to their development.
- Skills school is presented on the premises of the school.
- Unemployed people acquire basic skills that they then can use for themselves or for the benefit of the school.

HIV/AIDS:

- Include learners and parents living with the virus.
- Government needs assistance with challenging the pandemic.
- The only way to defeat the ignorance around the pandemic is by constantly running capacity building programs.
- The clinic on the school grounds will allow us to monitor the health of our infected families as well as to deal with some of the other health issues that confront us on a daily basis.

Community outreach:

- It is important that the school plays a central role in the development of the community in general.

Further Development

After the Vancouver conference (WHO, 2007), our principal, Mr. Damons, was really moved by the amazing amount of work that WHO does, globally and centrally, to deal with health challenges. It also made him realize that we have to start taking responsibility at all levels of society if we want to see sustainable change in our communities and countries. He also realized the need to hear voices from developing countries, particularly on the successes of programs being implemented to deal with various challenges confronting institutions. He also became acutely aware of the need for data generated by persons who are citizens of those countries.

Consequently, Mr. Damons presented the proposal of six pillars, which he was introduced to at the Vancouver conference, to seven schools in our city and encouraged these schools to adopt the proposed model as a tool to address the challenges confronting us at an institutional level. He submitted a document that had the six pillars of HPS as its core but included an additional pillar, quality education. We have gathered tremendous support for this program, now named the Intsika 7. (Intsika means pillar in Xhosa, one of our traditional languages. It is the center of the hut and keeps the hut from falling in.) Ironically, we are seven schools; our model has seven pillars, and 7 is regarded as a lucky number. Our government has been extremely encouraging in the pilot of this program, and the schools have been doing amazingly since its implementation in 2008. We have already won two awards, one local and one provincial, and we are in the process of being nominated for a national award.

The seven schools involved are all primary schools. We serve about 8,000 pupils in total and an even larger community base. The profiles of these schools are very similar to Sapphire Road Primary, and in some cases the conditions are worse.

Intsika (Pillar) 7 Model

This is the model we are piloting in seven schools in our country: The first pillar is the one we introduced, and the six other pillars are the pillars from the HPS model. We are already experiencing amazing feedback, and our government has given the blessing for the pilot. This approach was recommended by Mr. Damons after the Vancouver Conference. Figure 1 (at the end of this chapter) provides a brief summary of the model.

Objectives:

- We recognize the need to build on what we have already achieved, not only to improve the quality of education to our learners but also to develop the communities that our learners come from.
- We do not want to reinvent the wheel, but we can continue the existing programs that are working and introduce new programs that will achieve the government's objective of "A better life for all!"
- We use the proposed seven-pillar model based on the WHO health promotion program (six pillars) and adding the seventh pillar and naming it pillar 1: quality education. For HPS to make sense, we need a clear link between academic progress and implementation of the health pillars.

- We do not have a final document, rather a dynamic fluid document that must be adapted to suit local contexts.
- The pilot group will experiment as a model that can be refined and scaled up or duplicated in poor areas.

Community Participation (Stakeholder Ownership and Participation)

Central to change or even improvement in any community is the community buy-in and ownership of the change and improvement. We have successfully managed to change our school from just an academic institution to a place that is central to community upliftment and development. Communities should have a say in what programs are run at the school. In poor communities, schools become important centers for intellectual development; at the same time, they must reflect the positive ethos of these communities. Developing a long-term, integrated vision with the community allows for ongoing, sustainable development that can take place through the school.

In the words of one of our community members, "Although we are unable to read, we know what we need to improve our lives." Schools can fill that important gap by providing literacy training together with structured programs such as HPS to deal with the many challenges confronting poor communities. These communities have amazing stories of resilience and "ubuntu" – humanness – that we can learn from. Our communities have attended the "University of Life!"

Champions and Leadership

In our seven-pillar model we have coined the term "seed champion." The seed champion is the principal of the school. We believe that it is critically important for the visionary to take the lead from the onset. He/she must be able to replicate leadership in order to manage the vastness of the programs needed to see true qualitative growth. In the seven-pillar model that we introduced, the seed champion has to assist and coordinate the activities of all seven pillars. To facilitate leadership growth, each pillar has its own champion/leader. The joint vision for all the programs is crafted by everyone but the administration. Supervision and implementation of these programs is the responsibility of the pillar champions. The coordination and implementation of the programs into a cohesive plan for the organization is the responsibility of the seed champion.

Leadership development and support of the pillar champions is critical for the success of programs. Personal belief in the success of the program, commitment,

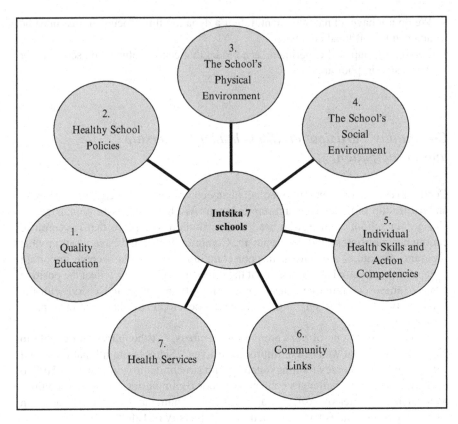

Fig. 1 Intsika (Pillar) 7 model:

Pillar 1:
- Quality of teaching and learning that takes place in the school
- Teacher development
- Curriculum development
- Extra- and cocurricular activity
- Optimal utilization of teaching time
- Educational policies
- Various researched techniques
- Work on a 5-day period using Monday to Friday
- 60% Reading across learning areas = 18 periods
- 20% Math = 6 periods
- 10% Life skills = 3 periods
- 10% Health = 3 periods

Fig. 1 (Continued)

• Thursday day ends at 12.00 pm for all learners, teacher group training 12.30–3.30

Pillar 2:

•Developing policies that are implementable and in a language that our communities can understand

• General Health Policy Statement for all schools – common approach

• Related integrated specific health policies, e.g., HIV/AIDS, nutrition, antitobacco, environment

Pillar 3:

• Neatness of surroundings of school

• State of buildings, grounds, and play space

• State of toilets and availability of clean running water

• Attention to "green" environment of the school

Pillar 4:

• Relationship among staff

• Relationship among learners

• Relationship among parents

• Relationship between staff and learners

• Relationship between staff and parents

• Relationship between learners and parents

• Relationship between school and wider community

Pillar 5:

• Capacitate learners to deal with challenges related to health according to their age cohort

• Capacitate educators to deal with challenges related to health for themselves and the learners they serve

• Capacitate community to deal with health challenges to themselves and to the welfare of their children

• Programs to deal with health challenges

Pillar 6:

• Consultation with local community structures

• Relationship with surrounding community that might not be parents at the school

• School's social responsibility to deal with social challenges of surrounding community

Pillar 7:

• Partnerships with health services at all levels

• Creation of on-site health services

personal sacrifice, hard work, and belief in the possibility of making a difference should motivate the leader. Personal growth, making a difference, recognition, networking, and personal opportunity are all positive spin-offs of commitment to the improvement of lives.

Conclusion and Insights

We believe that we have far exceeded the objectives we set in that meeting in 2000, and this is reflected in our profile. This is further endorsed by a recent evaluation by the National Department of Health of the activities of our school. It found that the golden thread holding together our institution was community participation and ownership, a key element of the HPS concept. We were congratulated for having actual and concrete proof of community involvement as opposed to theorizing about the concept. In reflection, as leaders in a poor institution, we are of the view that the delivery of quality education is rendered ineffective unless all the social elements that impact on education are addressed. Schools should transform from being regarded as ivory towers to being strong social organs capable of satisfying the needs of their communities, particularly in impoverished areas.

Reference

WHO. (2007). Report of the Technical Meeting of Building School Partnership for Health, Education Achievements and Development. Vancouver, Canada: WHO. Available from: http://www.jcsh-cces.ca/upload/WHO%20Technical%20Meeting%20Report.pdf

Chapter 8
Barbados: School Health Case Study

Patricia Warner

Contextual Introduction

Barbados is the most easterly of the islands of the Lesser Antilles. This tiny 21-mile-long by 14-mile-wide island is surrounded by the Atlantic Ocean on the northeastern end and by the Caribbean Sea on the southwestern side.

The island historically was under British leadership from 1625 until its independence in 1966. It has a population of about 270,000 persons with approximately 96% blacks of African descent, 3% white of British descent, and 1% of Asian descent.

Political, Social, and Economic Indicators

Barbados has enjoyed political stability from the postcolonial times. It is reputed to have the third oldest parliament in the Caribbean.

Since 1966, the island has been governed by a two-party system. The system has led to a stable economy. The economy has moved from one of indentured labor with a dependence on cotton to a sugar-driven economy and, more recently, a tourist-oriented economy. This has led to a vibrant offshore business sector, which enhances the island's social growth and economic profile.

Barbados's desire is to become a developed country by 2020. One of the aims is to have a healthy population through accessibility to free health care and knowledge that would lead to healthier lifestyles, thus providing the base for a sound and sustainable economy.

P. Warner
Ministry of Education, Bridgetown, Barbados

C. Vince Whitman and C.E. Aldinger (eds.),
Case Studies in Global School Health Promotion: From Research to Practice,
DOI: 10.1007/978-0-387-92269-0_8, © Springer Science + Business Media, LLC 2009

Education System

The island has free compulsory education from nursery to secondary level. The government subsidizes tertiary level. Students at the nursery and primary level benefit from a school-feeding program. Students at secondary level are assisted with textbooks while tertiary level students are asked to pay 2% of the total tuition cost. The government oversees just over 85% of the schools. These are 82 primary and 22 secondary government-managed schools, 16 privately managed schools, 1 polytechnic for technical and vocational education, 2 colleges – a Teachers' Training and a Community College – and 1 branch of the University of the West Indies, namely, the Cave Hill Campus.

Overview of the School Health Program

Date Boundaries/Key Players

Since 2002, persons in the Health and Education sectors have raised concerns about the health of the Barbadian people. As Barbados becomes globalized, there has also been the increased awareness and adoption of other lifestyles. Lifestyle changes include eating habits that are somewhat detrimental and children who are constantly involved in technology but not exercise. Travel, too, is often by car or bus and not by walking. The result has been a population increasingly susceptible to health risks.

The results of the Barbados Food Consumption and Anthropometric Survey revealed that 24.2% men and 37.5% women were diagnosed with non-communicable diseases (FAO, 2005). The World Health Organization Report states that Barbados has the 12th fattest persons of 194 countries surveyed. In 2005, a local consultation on the strategy for the prevention and control of non-communicable disease for Barbados recognized that more work with the entire population was needed.

Prior to 2006, the Central Government made efforts to look after the well-being of its school-aged population. A school-feeding program was introduced for all primary students at a cost of 10 cents per day or at no cost for those who could not afford to pay. This school-feeding program was a component of the free education policy for children of age 5–16. It intended to address students' nutritional deficiencies and increase academic performance. In addition, there has been a *Healthy Lifestyles* Week in school and an annual healthy lifestyle fair, which are corporate ventures. *Physical education* and *health and family life education* are also compulsory subjects on the schools' curriculum with *physical education* being examinable at the Caribbean Examination Council's level.

In 2006, the Ministry of Health invited all stakeholders to join in the fight against the rising illnesses associated with poor health choices. That ministry took the lead in setting up goals for the entire population. One aim was to reduce the incidence of obesity and, by extension, of non-communicable diseases, beginning as early as possible, with the school population.

The Ministry of Education responded and formed an internal committee; after internal consultations, the schools' health initiative was launched and witnessed by 3,000 students on May 18, 2007. All partners were invited to join in the drive to combat the negative fallout of poor health. The partners involved persons in the private and public sector and in NGOs, together with sports persons who have contributed significantly to the island.

Specific Aspects of Implementation

The implementation phase was simple and targeted the school level. The Ministry of Education, Youth Affairs and Sports used its technical staff to work on ensuring that schools and community groups were sensitized. The sports persons led the way by visiting schools and sharing their experiences as they spoke of the importance of healthy bodies. Students identified with these persons, since they are cricketers or other outstanding sports persons who have made representation at national and international level. The schools also selected former students to help with this process.

Another effort was to partner with the private sector, especially the print media. The local newspapers published articles and promoted sporting events more. The hallmark of the activity is the monthly magazine on health, which can be purchased for a small cost. Local actors and actresses were also able to assist in the promotion of healthy practices, through skits on garbage disposal, safe food-handling practices, and keeping safe sexually. The lone television station must be credited for its ongoing work on health-related matters. Programs of public interest are telecast on areas of personal as well as community health.

These ventures may be lost to some students, who may not capture what is presented in the media; therefore, efforts were made to offer student-friendly activities. Schools are now directly involved in two events that are coordinated by the public and private sectors but funded mainly by private sector entities. These are the schools' healthy lifestyles clubs competition and the Nation Newspaper's annual fun walk. Schools are acknowledged for participating and receive trophies and prizes. The healthy school competition tests the number of different paces used in a choreographed routine, and zonally the best teams are selected for the final. The schools enter the fun walk for a small fee per person. In both events, the schools are rewarded and given publicity.

In addition, the Ministry of Education recognized that schools were involved in the sale of food, including snacks that were unhealthy and of little nutritional value. The then Minister of Education addressed this matter by writing to all schools, encouraging the use of healthier snacks with more nutritional value, beverages with less sugar content, and food with reduced sugar and salt content. It was also the intention of the ministry to ensure that all members of the schools' staff were aware of the initiative and embraced aspects such as exercise in the everyday programming of students. Schools were circularized after discussions were held, and this was the agreed upon method.

It must be clear that this is not a project but a conscious effort by the Government of Barbados to reduce obesity, inactivity, and – by extension – non-communicable diseases in the school-aged population and the entire society. The approach is an entire island effort with the school playing its role. Of interest, too, is that the island has conducted its own research; these findings were responsible for the initiatives.

The school health initiative has recognized that the component of mental and sexual health could not be ignored. The areas being incorporated are violence prevention and HIV/AIDS. Praises must be given to UNICEF (Barbados) for ably conducting a study on: "Creating a safe school environment, the whole school approach to discipline." This study is research-based and attempts to examine all aspects of health that can affect student performance. At present, a number of primary schools and one secondary school are involved in this comprehensive study, scheduled to end in 2009.

The HIV/AIDS component is being aided by the Ministry of Youth and Scotia Bank. The Ministry of Youth works with the schools and has produced students' work on DVDs. The message of stigma and discrimination is Scotia Bank's aim as it works in the school community with persons living with AIDS. This intervention is expected to last for 3 years and will reach all 45,000 students at primary and secondary level. The Ministry of Education has utilized a youth ambassador who works with HIV and AIDS groups in 12 secondary schools. These students are creating videos to assist other students.

Summary of Achievements

There have been incremental achievements since May 2007. Most schools have implemented parts of the initiative because the principals share the sentiments of the Ministry of Education. One principal remarked that the initiative started 3 years ago at her school. The students there were not allowed to bring unhealthy snacks; she kept any that were unhealthy and returned them to the parents. At that school, fitness is of utmost importance, and there has been an existing parent group for the last 2 years. This school shares the philosophy that a healthy body leads to a healthy mind and that student performance will increase in all areas.

Other success stories have been achieved through principal and parent collaboration. Schools with vibrant parent-teachers' associations and community outreach programs have done well. Schools have formed health clubs and cheerleaders' groups, expanded the physical activity program to include areas such as African, line, and ball room dancing, drum-beating, stilt walking, and, of course, dancing to the calypso beat and engaging in healthy lifestyle days. The synergies between school and community volunteers have been most pleasing.

Students have shared their opinions at focus groups and individually over the weeks from February 25 to March 14, 2008. These are examples of the comments:

- "I don't want to miss Fridays, we have so much fun at health club."
- "I have to keep letting my Dad know that I need healthy snacks."
- "I love water days at my school. We can have only water and now I don't need so many beverages even at home."
- "Being a body builder was always my dream, I now have the opportunity through the school's program."
- "My teacher is a fitness freak!"
- "I have a new appreciation for persons with HIV and AIDS."

Children have been reading food labels and questioning the content of their meals; this has challenged parents. One parent says that she allows the child to read and make a decision on what she wishes to eat. Even the school-feeding program has increased vegetables, fruits, and low-calorie meals on its menus.

Physical Education is also transitioning, and students attest to enjoying the activities more since everything is not just competitive but also fun.

Conclusions and Insights

Some Drawbacks

Any initiative that is intended to be as broad and as far-reaching as this will suffer drawbacks.

Some of these are that training will be needed for all school vendors. The guidelines are being revised, in hopes of guiding the vending policy of all schools and for all school events. Vending will be an insurmountable challenge, since all schools have vendors either on school grounds or on the outskirts of the schools' compounds.

Monitoring and evaluation has been implemented, though this has not been done as effectively as it should be. However, the aim is to engage principals in a self-administered tool and verify some of the submissions with visits to the schools. Some schools need greater guidance, and in the near future the Ministry of Health, the NGOs, and the Department of Youth will be utilized to assist in areas of need.

The Way Forward

As the initiative expands, individual schools will need budgets to execute their activities. It is good for the Central Government to assist at the onset, but funding for aspects such as safe schools must be sourced outside of regular annual budgeting and must be considered as important for continuity.

Of note, too, is assistance in resource development; schools cannot be executing this project on their own. Teacher training must be broadened and include the development of manuals for creating and sustaining healthy schools and healthy students.

Acknowledgment   The study was written with support from Colin Clarke (Senior Youth Development Officer).

Reference

Food and Agriculture Organization of the United Nations (FAO). (2005). *The Barbados Food Consumption and Anthropometric Surveys 2000*. Rome: FAO.

Chapter 9
Brazil: Addressing the Social Determinants of Health: The Experience of a Municipal School in Rio de Janeiro

Sergio Meresman, Avamar Pantoja, and Carlos da Silva

This kid looks just like his parents!
But he's got no father nor mother
So, what does he looks like?
The face of forgiveness or revenge?
The face of despair or hope?
Homeland that gave me birth!
Which was the homeland that gave me birth?!

Gabriel O Pensador, Brazilian rapper

Introduction

This essay documents an experience of the ABC & Art Project, a participative school management and health promotion initiative in the Municipal School Alexandre de Gusmão, located at the Columbia Park-Acari Housing in Rio de Janeiro (Brazil).

The Alexandre de Gusmão school team is composed of a majority of teachers who live in the community and work *full time*. With most schools in deprived areas in Brazil as well as in other Latin American countries, teachers tend to have at least two different jobs in different places. They sometimes live in yet a third neighborhood. The different roles and locations of teachers influence their understanding of the community, Alexandre de Gusmão, the neighborhood, its dynamics, and the people who live there. These multiple roles of teachers affect their commitment to the community and vice-versa.

S. Meresman(✉)
CLAEH (Latin American Centre for Humane Economy), UNER (University of Entre Rios), Montevideo, Uruguay

C. Vince Whitman and C.E. Aldinger (eds.),
Case Studies in Global School Health Promotion: From Research to Practice,
DOI: 10.1007/978-0-387-92269-0_9, © Springer Science + Business Media, LLC 2009

The project started in 2000 and is still progressing. Professor Avamar Pantoja, who has been teaching and living in the community area for many years, is the headmaster who leads the project. She joined the Alexandre de Gusmão School first as a teacher and then as a teachers' coordinator, before being chosen as the school principal in 1999. She has been reelected for this role three consecutive times. She has lived in the neighborhood since 1975 and has also worked in a neighboring school for 7 years before moving to Alexandre de Gusmão. In many ways, this project reflects her personal process of learning from and commitment to the community, which has developed over the years.

The Brazilian Context

Brazil is South America's largest country, known internationally for its outstanding football achievements, its beautiful music, and its endemic social disparities.

While Brazil is a very rich country in natural resources (with the largest forest in the world, the Amazon), its unequal distribution of income (the most unequal globally according to UNDP) has contributed to huge health problems. For instance, 90% of urban homes and just 25% of rural homes receive water from general distribution. It is estimated that only 35% of water is potable, while 60% of garbage is disposed of inappropriately. In some municipalities of the Amazonas, 90% of children and adolescents are born in poor families, compared with less than 2% in some municipalities in Rio Grande do Sul. With regard to education, children in Brazil complete an average 6.1 years of study. Virtually everyone enrolls in school, but only 84% of young people finish elementary level; 57% finish secondary school. Illiteracy is extremely high in the adult population.

Nearly 400 students attend the Alexandre de Gusmão Municipal School, in two shifts. The school is located in the Columbia Park area in Rio de Janeiro and is part of the Acari neighborhood, a low-income project that houses a population of 40,000 people.

The area is a tough one to live in. Approximately 50% of these houses are shanties, bordering the Acari River, an extremely polluted stream, which creates some of the most precarious and hazardous living conditions in existence. Floods affect the area regularly and transmissible diseases are a constant concern.

Miserable living conditions make drug trafficking the most attractive income-generating alternative for young people – as carriers, sellers, and gunmen. The financial, social, and cultural exclusion of this community can also be expressed in numbers: Human development index, 0.573; population density, 179 inhabitants per square meter; life expectancy, 56–58 years; literacy rate, 80–84% (IBGE, 2000).

This discouraging environment reinforces negative messages to the children and adolescents of Acari – a lack of appreciation and respect for life, with little hope for a dignified future. The community's environment is also a barrier to the development of personal projects, such as succeeding in school or looking after one's health, as even the most lucky can only dream of a very low-paid job in the informal market.

Aspects of Implementation

Addressing the Determinants of Health and Education

The Alexandre de Gusmão's health promotion project applies a popular education[1] approach, in which the school is the center of social action and education and serves as *an instrument* for stimulating and enabling the future of children. Transforming society becomes a major goal and a way to develop awareness and promote action, with the potential to triumph over the social and economic determinants and living conditions of the community, which influence the health of all.

From the beginning of the project, the need to address the structural, social, and economic determinants of health and well-being of the children was very clear to the school team. I asked Avamar, "How was the program started? What were the reasons, causes? What was your inspiration?" She answered me right away, "Throughout my professional career ... from being in contact on a daily basis with the students and their families, I came to understand that a profound lack or inadequateness of social and health policies in our community was preventing us from getting good results from all the efforts we made to educate our children in the schools. At the same time, poor education was an important determinant for the permanent reinforcement and worsening of living conditions of the people in the community."

Teachers like Avamar and schools like the Alexandre de Gusmão are in a good position to tackle the intertwined determinants of education and health through comprehensive approaches. They gain legitimacy from their ability to deal with very profound social variables in the community life, such as relationships among family members, and their knowledge of the needs and interests of the most relevant stakeholders. Also, schools and teachers are often the only remaining presence of a public institution, in a context from which the state has progressively withdrawn as a guarantor of social protection and collective will.

Coordinating with Health Services to Provide Basic Care

In the context of very deprived areas of the city and the limited access of the community to health care, it was critically important that the project acknowledged the need to provide basic health services. The school team went to the health professionals, working in the nearby health posts and hospital, for help and solidarity.

---

[1]Based on the teachings of Paulo Freire, author of *Pedagogy of the Oppressed* and internationally recognized as an educator and social scientist. See http://www.paulofreire.org/

A partnership with the Carlos Chagas hospital was launched, which provided access to training of teachers and voluntary mothers. Initially, the training focused on how to protect and promote oral health at school age. Mothers and teachers chose the topic because they felt that it provides an opportunity to address a very important issue of child health through "tangible" interventions. In some places, bad oral health is a direct signal that a person is poor and lives in a poor neighborhood. Such associations often stigmatize people and contribute to their own low self-esteem. At the same time, addressing oral health problems offers a very valuable entry point for health education and promotion of healthy habits.

Another agreement was made with a health post that is responsible for emergencies in the area. A nurse was designated to be the liaison person with the school, and a referral system was established for students to access oral and mental health services.

However, there are still many gaps and difficulties regarding access to basic health services. The health post and its professionals are overwhelmed with the volume of people seeking care. There are also difficulties related to getting to the heath post, which is located quite far from this community, requiring patients to afford transportation. The school team shares with the health staff the idea that preventive measures, such as teeth-brushing or learning about healthy foods and hygiene habits, should be taught and carried out by the parents at home rather than at the school where it takes place today.

Introducing Art as an Educational and Health-Promoting Tool

In the Alexandre de Gusmão School, art and literature have been powerful tools for mobilizing children and families in a health-promoting and empowering experience. In its very "Freirean" way,[2] the Acari project used reading as a way to promote communication and critical-thinking skills, two important health- and life-related competences. The school initiated a Home Reading Project, which developed into a small network composed of three other schools, two churches, and a community strategy that involved teachers and voluntary parents in teaching reading. The Home Reading lends books, organizes reading gatherings, and encourages and supports children to engage in research projects. Home Reading also organizes visits to museums and libraries to stimulate children in reading. These activities expanded the scope of social interaction for the children and families and generated new and positive referents for them.

The project used music as another avenue to engage children in workshops and after-school classes. Besides expanding the preparation of the children for future

---

[2]"Reading Is Changing the World," P. Freire.

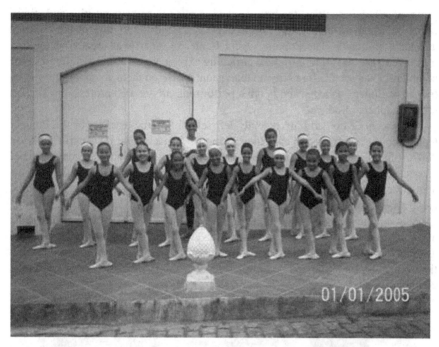

Picture 9 Young dancers prepare for a ballet class, one of the ten work shops and courses offered by the Popular Opera Center of Acari. The project was initiated in the Municipal School Alexandre de Gusmão and today to the community

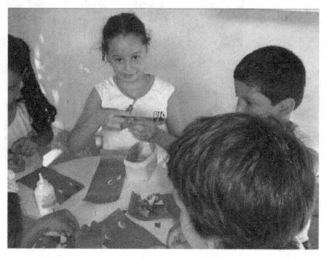

Picture 10 Students participate in a workshop to stimulate reading

professional opportunities, the arts program worked to create a positive and stimulating environment that would rescue citizenship and the dignity of the children and the community. The Popular Opera Center of Acari was created as another initiative of the school to introduce enriching experiences that most children in the community had seen before only on television; it offered them an opportunity to be trained as singers, dancers, and in other performing-arts-related professions, such as escenographers, producers.

Adolescents who had only recently left school became teachers of the Popular Opera project and started to earn their living from teaching at the Acari Center. In 2007, some of the best students created the Acariocamerata and recorded a CD of classical music. The excellence of their music earned them a nomination for the Tim Prize of music. Together with their singing students, they are preparing the first Acari Opera, in which the community is actively engaged.

Recognizing that self-esteem, self-efficacy, participation, self-determination, and self-expression contribute to healthy development and well-being, the design and delivery of these important arts activities are seen as making a major contribution to health promotion and countering many of the negative social factors in the community.

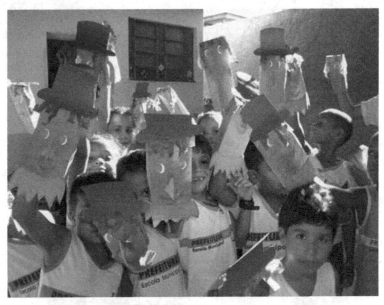

Picture 11 Students show the handcrafts that were produced by than in the *Reading Corner*. Eight hundred children take part of reading stimulation activities every month

Addressing the Subjective Dimensions of Power

Teachers agreed that what generates and permanently reinforces their feeling of impotence is not just seeing children who are obviously suffering from anemia, parasitosis, or so many other maladies of poverty. It is not the frequent complaints of the children who are assaulted by toothaches or earaches, without resources to see a doctor. What actually makes teachers and school personnel feel paralyzed is having to deal with the apathy of children and the passivity of parents who seem to have given up and who accept conditions of extreme suffering as if they were normal. Furthermore, the state or government authorities are largely absent, apart from the permanent presence of security forces.

Introducing music classes in the Alexandre de Gusmão School was – most importantly – a way to expand children's experiences, provide a means for self-expression and joy, introduce positive referential models, and improve the expectations that teachers and parents have from their children. The offering of music and the other arts generated a climate of developing personal resources, of giving children opportunities for expression. Furthermore, both children and teachers were placed in empowering and dynamic roles, so that they became *subjects* or active architects rather than objects or passive recipients.

Focusing on the Institutional Project

Program organizers pursued improvements, not only in educational attainment, but also in living conditions, determinants of health, and the well-being of the children and the community. It was clear to the project team from the very beginning that it was necessary to look at all aspects of the interrelationships between health and education. The overall outcome pursued for the project was an educational one. Thus, it was important to keep the activities of the project consistent with the professional *leitmotif* of teachers and the fundamental goal of the school as an institution.

Through the preparation of the Institutional Education Plan (PPP in Portuguese) (starting from a situation analysis conducted by the whole school community), the school created a framework to analyze the social context in which the school was immersed; from that baseline, the school then developed learning experiences consistent with the framework. The framework also facilitated the identification of resources and tools needed to intervene and to plan for the specific actions aimed at facilitating a change process.

The PPP was at the center of the Alexandre de Gusmão school's process. Its motto was "Transforming children into citizens of a new era," and it committed all school members *to generating an educational environment that goes beyond the school boundaries through participative solutions and the promotion of change agents and new social objectives.* Such participative solutions were constructed in synergy with the objectives of improving quality of life and health and based on three strategic areas: best possible teaching and learning strategies, individual empowerment, and community-based promotion of culture and art.

Permanently Seeking Partnerships

To legitimate and mobilize support and resources for this initiative, it was important to create the Columbia Park Council,[3] inviting the most prominent activists of the community to accompany the school. The project made a significant (for the community) investment in musical instruments and set up the first workshops on drama, guitar, percussion, and folk dances, initially for enrolled students. Rapidly, the interest of people outside of the school grew so much that the workshops and classes opened to anyone from the community. With time, elderly people from the community also became involved in the music classes. The school decided to open doors to people of all ages to participate in the initiative, which in itself sent a message of inclusion and interest in social justice.

Soon the school was physically not big enough to hold all these initiatives. It was again necessary to gather support from other organizations in the community. Two community centers were rented, and soon approximately 500 people of all ages joined a wide spectrum of activities and workshops including classic ballet, guitar, singing, percussion, music history, and drama.

A Supportive Public Policy

The implementation of this project, in one of the most deprived areas of Rio de Janeiro, did not just develop out of the blue. Rather, it developed in the context and with the support of a well-established Health-Promoting Schools initiative led by the Secretary of Health in Rio de Janeiro. The Municipal School Health program was created in 1992. It proposed a "critical approach" that sought to reorganize school-based health services and redefine the meaning of the link between health and education (Silva, 1999).

For a city of six million people – where the health system comprises more than 100 health centers, 25 hospitals, 6 maternities, 80 family health teams, and 742 community health agents - to coordinate with an education system formed by 1,100 schools, 750,000 students, and 35,000 teachers is a huge challenge.

In 2000, a pilot project involving 100 schools sought to develop a model of Health Promoting-Schools that reflected the characteristics and identity of the city. The program emphasized the strengthening of three critical axes: participative management, popular education, and intersectoral action. The project sought to

---

[3] Initially composed of Alexandre de Gusmão Municipal School, Andréa Fontes Peixoto Municipal School, Baptist Curch of Columbia Park, Church Nossa Senhora do Perpétuo Socorro, and Neighbors Association of Ildefonso Falcão Av. Later added were Seson School, Educational Centre *Lúcia Leitão*, Church God's Assembly, Church New Jerusalem, Columbia Neighbors Association, and Church *Os Sabidinhos*.

address some of the coordination needs and opportunities that existed between the health sector and its counterparts in education and social welfare.

The program was indeed an enabling factor for the coordination between schools and health services/facilities and a mobilizer of a collaborative will. For instance, the seminars and subregional workshops regularly organized by the Secretary of Health provided meeting and networking opportunities for representatives of the schools with health and social assistance managers, who were in the position to help and facilitate collaboration. The implementation of the Alexandre de Gusmão's school health project is one example of how to operationalize on the ground a policy that is generated and cultivated from the central level.

Highlights and Lessons Learned

Addressing complexity requires sound leadership and dialogue skills. Implementing the principles of a global school health strategy in a context of such complex conditions, such as those faced by the Alexandre de Gusmão school in Rio de Janeiro, does not happen without contradictions and different points of view between regional managers and people on the ground. Disagreements on the process and clashes of interests and leadership have been common. The role of the school's principal as a leader and facilitator in creating a consensual plan of action has helped to solve conflict and provide strategic orientation each time these contradictions have challenged the process. It was important to protect the process from misunderstandings, conflicts, and the influence of personal and institutional dynamics, sometimes conflictive and shortsighted. Clear and representative rules, based on collective interests and understanding of what was at stake, provided the way to moderate such differences and protect the long-term sustainability of the project.

Dialogue has also been a key tool of the process. This included not only an openminded and interactive approach to teaching and learning, but also a permanent exercise to expand the network of collaboration and find new partners for the strategy. This dialogue was essential in order to legitimate the strategy in the community and with governmental authorities. This dialogue often took place in a context of diverse ideas and philosophical or ideological backgrounds. Once again, Morin's premise was verified: "What is progressive is not an idea but the dialogue of ideas" (Morin & Coppay, 1983).

There are many ways to become a Health Promoting School. The ABC & Art approach does not necessarily follow the "conventional" HPS model. The process has involved working with all four of the most typical components of the HPS strategy (health education with emphasis on life skills development, coordination with health services, healthy school environment, and healthy school policy). But the Rio de Janeiro model has not addressed all components simultaneously; for example, the early stages of the project gave priority to putting health services in place. Rio has also promoted exploration and experimentation of complementary dimensions of an HPS, especially active participation of children and community involvement.

The approach is enlightening in relation to the controversy between "comprehensive" and focused approaches to health promotion in schools. What this experience illustrates is that comprehensiveness is a necessary response to complexity, while focus is also important to address most basic needs and create conditions to reach specific goals.

Empowerment is about learning. Empowering children and families has been at the center of this experience. However, empowerment does not consist of simply "giving away" power but of facilitating a process that requires the attention of subjective and social variables. The "power" to change reality must be discovered through various individual and collective learning.

Health promotion in schools does not necessarily fit into a "log frame." The itinerary followed by the project was not at all a "linear" route. From the perspective of the most active participants, it meant that planning was not strictly a "logical framework" model, but a continuous exercise of appraising emerging needs and opportunities. This process required the ability to deal with the unexpected, to be ready to change, and to respond with creativity and imagination, at times spontaneously, to a challenging institutional and social environment.

References

Freire, P. Retrieved from http://www.paulofreire.org/Capa/WebHome

Instituto Brasileiro de Geografia e Estatística (IGBE) [Brazilian Institute on Geography and Statistics]. (2000). *Brazilian human development index 2000*. Retrieved March 2008, from http://www.ibge.gov.br/

Meresman, S. (2007). *Health and education in the labyrinth*. Technical paper prepared for the Pan American Health Organization and the Education Development Center, Inc.

Morin, E., & Coppay, F. (1983). Beyond determinism: The dialogue of order and disorder. *Substance, 12*(3), 22–35.

Pantoja, A. Unpublished documents and reports.

Silva, C. (1999). *Programa de Saúde Escolar numa Perspectiva Crítica* (3ª edição). Rio de Janeiro, Brazil: Secretaria Municipal de Saúde.

Chapter 10
Canada: The Evolution of Healthy Schools in Ontario, Canada: Top-Down and Bottom-Up

Carol MacDougall and Yvette Laforêt-Fliesser

Contextual Introduction

The stories from the urban, highly multicultural city of Toronto (population 2.5 million) and the mixed urban and rural area of Middlesex-London (population 400,000) paint a perfect picture of the reality of Canada's 20-year involvement with the Comprehensive School Health movement. These two centers are in Ontario, one of the ten provinces and three territories spreading east to west across the northern border of North America. Each province has its own education and health ministries, so there is a great deal of variation in how each jurisdiction manages its programs and services. In addition, the province of Ontario includes 72 district school boards (plus 33 school authorities for geographically isolated or hospital school boards) and 36 public health units that direct the work of local education staff and public health staff, respectively. Public health units receive both provincial and municipal funding, so they address provincial mandates as well as locally identified health needs.

The Canadian Association for School Health (CASH) was established in 1988 following a national conference that identified Comprehensive School Health (CSH) as the most effective strategy to address the country's health and social issues at that time, such as AIDS, drug abuse, and child abuse. Over the next few years, each province and territory established its own "Association for School Health." A consensus statement on "Comprehensive School Health," initially released in 1991, was revised in 2007 and has been endorsed by 37 national organizations (Canadian Association for School Health, 2007). It includes four key components: teaching and learning, health and other support services, supportive social environment, and healthy physical environment. Policies and partnerships at all levels involving all key stakeholders are embedded within these components. The combined advocacy efforts of the CASH and other national

C. MacDougall(✉)
School Program, Perth District Health Unit, Stratford, ON, Canada

C. Vince Whitman and C.E. Aldinger (eds.),   143
Case Studies in Global School Health Promotion: From Research to Practice,
DOI: 10.1007/978-0-387-92269-0_10, © Springer Science + Business Media, LLC 2009

organizations have successfully moved "Healthy Schools" onto the federal agenda. In 2005, a Pan-Canadian Joint Consortium for School Health (JCSH) was established, comprising senior officials (deputy ministers, assistant deputy ministers) of the Ministries of Health and Education. Each participating province/territory (11 of 13) has established a School Health Coordinator position. The goal of the JCSH is to act as a catalyst and strengthen the capacities of health, education, and other systems and agencies in school health promotion (Joint Consortium for School Health, 2008).

Ontario's "Coalition of Ontario Agencies for School Health" (COASH), based in Toronto, functioned from 1989 to 2000 with very limited resources. In the wake of unprecedented cuts to the education system in the nineties, it merged in 2000 with the Ontario Public Health Association's School Health Working Group and the Centre for Health Promotion's Healthy Schools Interest Group to form the currently flourishing Ontario Healthy Schools Coalition (OHSC). At present, the OHSC has over 210 members representing 38 organizations (public health units, school boards, hospitals, mental health agencies, universities, and a range of organizations related to health, education, parents, and students) and interested individuals. It holds four teleconferences per year, each with 60–80 participants from across the province, as well as one annual face-to-face forum. The goals of the OHSC are to raise awareness of the benefits from and need for Healthy Schools, to build the knowledge base and capacity for implementation of a Healthy Schools approach, to influence policy development and the provision of adequate public funding for Healthy Schools, and to provide a forum to share Healthy Schools initiatives and best practices across health, education, and related sectors (Ontario Healthy Schools Coalition, 2008).

The combined advocacy efforts of the OHSC and other organizations have been fruitful. In 2003, the Policy and Program Branch of the Ministry of Education dedicated staff to Healthy Schools, and several policies have been announced under the Healthy Schools umbrella. In particular, the "Foundations for a Healthy School" framework based on the four components of CSH has been produced and is widely supported (Ontario Ministry of Education, 2006).

Overview of the School Health Programs

Overview of the Toronto "Health Action Team" Initiative

With the 1998 amalgamation of six municipalities to form the City of Toronto, there was acute awareness of the importance of coordinators as entry points to large organizations. Significant effort had been expended to build strong working relationships between school board Health and Physical Education Coordinators and the Toronto Public Health (TPH) Planning and Policy School Health Consultant, four regional School Health Services Coordinators, and other TPH staff and managers. In 2003, an opportunity arose that proved critical to moving Healthy Schools forward in Toronto. The Toronto Heart Health Partnership was accepting proposals involving strong community partnerships to address heart health risk factors. The TPH Planning and Policy School Health Consultant supported the Toronto Catholic District School Board (TCDSB) Health and Physical Education Coordinator in applying, while another TPH School Health Services Coordinator supported the Toronto District School Board application. Both applications were successful; however, this case study will focus on the TCDSB project. The TCDSB is one of four school boards TPH works with; it serves 95,000 students in 201 schools (170 elementary and 31 secondary). The TCDSB received a grant of Cdn $60,000 for April 1, 2004 to December 31, 2005, as well as two grants of Cdn $56,000 for subsequent years. This successful proposal-writing process was important because a solid partnership was a prerequisite for applying; this was an automatic incentive or mechanism for cross-sector collaboration. In addition, the funding that was obtained assisted greatly in securing internal administrative and management support within the two organizations and leveraging additional financial and human resources.

The TCDSB project involved establishing Health Action Teams for Physical Activity Action Planning in elementary and secondary schools. Health Action Teams comprise representatives of school administration, teachers, students, parents, public health, and other relevant community partners such as recreation (Toronto Catholic District School Board, 2008a). These Health Action Teams work together to conduct a baseline assessment and then plan, implement, evaluate, and celebrate physical activity initiatives over the funding period. Principals of each school submit these plans as part of the local school action planning requirements of all TCDSB schools. Issues have broadened since the first year to include nutrition, bullying, substance misuse, tobacco, and others. Each school receives Cdn $500 once its plan is submitted.

The TCDSB project also set up a central school board-public health unit coordinating committee for the Health Action Team initiative, comprising the board Health and Physical Education Coordinator, his resource staff, a frontline teacher whenever possible, the TPH Planning and Policy School Health Consultant, one of the four TPH School Health Coordinators, and a TPH Physical Activity program staff member. This central committee developed tools consistent with the CSH approach and components, secured resources, and planned events, such as principal presentations to encourage sign-up, fall kickoff events, mid-year networking and in-servicing, and end-of-year celebrations for Health Action Teams. Concurrently, the school board was establishing Professional Learning Centres for a range of subject areas. The Health and Physical Education Coordinator was able to advocate for Healthy Active Living and Learning (HALL) Centres in one school in each of the four quadrants of the city, to promote ongoing professional development in Health and Physical Education for staff (Toronto Catholic District School Board, 2008b). These centers became the sites for the majority of Health Action Team events, with students at the school frequently demonstrating their leadership skills.

Healthy Schools in Middlesex-London: 14 Years and Counting!

Interest in CSH began in 1992, following an extensive review of literature as well as an environmental scan of Canadian efforts with this health promotion strategy. An implementation plan for CSH in London and Middlesex County schools was endorsed by the public and Catholic directors of the local Boards of Education. The directors recommended a grassroots approach whereby each school would develop its own plan for becoming a "healthy school"; this was consistent with the "community school" movement that was practiced in this jurisdiction at that time. Information sessions for school principals were provided by health unit staff. It was expected that the school community would take ownership for planning activities and projects that responded to the health and social needs and priorities of the school. The health unit was expected to provide leadership and resources to initiate the approach in schools. Public Health Nurses (PHNs) assist a Healthy School Committee to establish a shared vision, see the link between health and learning, and seize opportunities to actively engage the community in finding solutions to health-related issues of the school or community.

The process was piloted in seven schools during the first year. One tool that was developed was the *Healthy School Profile*. It maps out the actual capacities and needs of school communities according to the four components of CSH. All materials that were developed by the public health unit were tested, evaluated, and revised with the expert input of principals and teaching staff. School principals identified the profile as the key event that mobilizes the school community to identify and act on a variety of health and social issues (Mitchell, Laforêt-Fliesser, & Camiletti, 1997). Using interviews, focus groups, and survey methods, the PHN gathers information from school staff, students, parents, and key members of the school community. Only aggregate data are included in the written report that is prepared by the PHN, to protect the anonymity of individual responses (Laforêt-Fliesser & Mitchell, 2002). While issues such as physical inactivity continue to receive considerable attention in the profile, other popular issues such as school yard and traffic safety, quality of hot lunches or cafeteria food, cleanliness of washrooms and access to hand-washing facilities, safe routes to school, and encouraging healthy, caring relationships (i.e., antibullying initiatives) are also addressed in a Healthy School Committee's action plan. In addition to the profile, schools are encouraged to use a Healthy Schools suggestion box in which school members can inform the Healthy School Committee of any emergent issues. More recently, schools have opted to have a "town hall" meeting to identify health and social issues and to create a vision for the school. High school students are more likely to use a focus group method to solicit opinions from their peers and school staff.

Because Middlesex-London was one of the first public health units in Canada to adopt CSH as a philosophy and framework for school-based health promotion, staff and managers have consulted widely on planning and implementation approaches. They have also shared lessons learned and practical tips at numerous conferences and workshops for health and education professionals and in publications. Parents, students, and school staff have been active contributors to these knowledge-exchange efforts.

Toronto Achievements and Impact

In Toronto, as a result of the strong leadership by the school board, and because the initiative assisted schools in meeting the immediate need to implement the provincially mandated Daily Physical Activity (DPA) policy, there was significant uptake by schools. In Year 1 (04/05), 70 schools signed up; Year 2 (05/06), 98 schools; Year 3 (06/07), 126 schools; and Year 4 (07/08), 135 schools (118 elementary and 17 secondary). Currently, the total reach is approximately 54,000 students. A wide range of creative activities were implemented, such as Grade 8 student leaders and teacher advisors choreographing a dance/exercise routine that these students regularly lead for a gym full of younger students, performing skits involving a respected student playing a hero who eventually "gets" the health message, designing a rubber chicken team sport, and hosting Family Fun Nights and multicultural dances. End-of-year process evaluations in 2006 provided very positive findings, for example:

* 88.5% agree/strongly agree that the students are more physically active during the school day (slight dip from 93% in 2005, but this was anticipated to some degree).
* 90.5% agree/strongly agree that there are more leadership opportunities for our students.
* 81.9% agree/strongly agree that the school spirit/climate has improved.
* 91.5% agree/strongly agree that this Health Action Team initiative has been a positive experience for our school.
* 88.6% agree/strongly agree that their school is becoming a healthier school community.

Anthony Petitti,
personal communication, March 7, 2008.

There has also been a gradual increase in the involvement of PHNs on Health Action Teams, with 43 schools currently involving their public health nurses. And in 2006 the school board revised their system priorities to include specific reference to "health" – "Safe, Inclusive and Healthy Learning Environment: To enhance the quality of the working and learning experience through improving schools and workplaces so that they contribute to positive health and respectful relationships" (Toronto Catholic District School Board, 2006).

Middlesex-London Achievements and Impact

As noted earlier, the health unit was to provide the leadership and resources for the initial implementation of Healthy Schools. From 1995 to 2000, about 25 of 150 elementary schools and 4 of 18 secondary schools were engaged. Regular reports to board of education administration and school trustees provided updates on the many success stories during this period. School-board amalgamations and educational reforms during the late nineties had a negative impact on sustaining Healthy School Committees in some schools. The retirement or transfer of many supportive school principals often resulted in the disbanding of the Healthy School Committees despite the successful outcomes for the school. By January 2001, only seven elementary schools and three high schools had sustained their Healthy School Committee.

A restructuring of the public health unit at this time established two teams focused on school-based health promotion: an elementary school team and a team focusing on youth health and secondary schools. Public health management reaffirmed the benefits of Healthy Schools and that PHNs would continue to practice within a CSH framework for school-based health promotion. Meetings with the superintendents of education through the School Health Education Council confirmed the public and Catholic boards' endorsement of this approach; however, they wondered how principals might react, given the multitude of demands and new mandates emanating from the Ministry of Education at that time, such as safe schools and school improvement and effectiveness. Information sessions with school administrators linked the benefits of CSH with school effectiveness, student performance, and safe school environments. Public health staff joined the board Safe School Advisory Committee to identify opportunities for working on initiatives that would promote a safe and healthy school environment. The board of education consultants for physical and health education replaced senior administrators on a joint education and public health school action team. Increasing the capacity and competence of PHNs, parents and students were a priority during this period of "reenergizing" the Healthy Schools movement in our jurisdiction. Numerous presentations and workshops were held, and the Healthy School Profile was revised in collaboration with school principals and staff. In the fall of 2002, the first Annual Healthy School Workshop for high school students and staff was offered to increase uptake in secondary schools. A Guide to Healthy Schools was developed, distributed to school principals, and posted on the health unit Web site for easy access (Middlesex-London Health Unit, 2004).

Within a 6-year period, 42 elementary and 13 secondary schools have established a Healthy School Committee or a similar committee such as a Safe and Healthy School Committee or Wellness Council. Two schools have had a committee in place since 1994 with another 20 committees operating for at least 3–5 years. We have witnessed a gradual increase in principal and superintendent engagement with and endorsement of the Healthy Schools approach as they acknowledge the value of health and health promotion and their link to the academic success of students. Since 2001, financial support from the public health unit (grants of up to Cdn $100 per school) and provincial "heart health/healthy living" and "tobacco-free living" grants of up to Cdn $1,000 have contributed to an increased number of schools participating in Healthy School initiatives.

Surveys of principals (Oliva, Mouritzen, BucklandFoster, Laforêt-Fliesser, & Madden, 2004), parents and staff (Steel, BucklandFoster Laforêt-Fliesser, & Madden,

2004), and high school students (Vandenheuvel, Laforêt-Fliesser, Steel, Bainbridge, & Hofstetter, 2005) have reported the following: an improvement in students' ability to discuss issues and to problem-solve, a high degree of agreement among students that working together can make a difference in resolving issues, and an increased likelihood for students to speak out and take action on identified health and social issues as a result of their membership on Healthy School Committees. Principals, parents, and staff placed a high value on this approach and reported an increased awareness of strengths and issues in the school, public health services, and community resources. Evaluations also reported a high level of participation and ownership of the Healthy Schools process by the school community. Principals and staff agreed that the committee's work contributed to the school improvement/school success plan, increased links between school and community services, and increased use of health unit services and programs.

Specific Aspects of Implementation

Champions and Leaders at All Levels

In the Toronto experience, the central school board-public health unit coordinating committee was, and still is, key. Strong collaboration occurs for the planning of the kickoff, mid-year, and end-of-year events, as well as for the development of needed resources – principal sign-up letters, baseline survey, event flyers, PowerPoint presentations, letters to parents, school health assessment tool, planning template with example, minutes form, CSH handout, resources list, end-of-year activity reporting form/evaluation report, and tip sheet for Health Action Team sustainability. The planning template helps the schools to name their priority health issue and to state activities in each of the four CSH component areas (curriculum, services, supportive social environment, and healthy physical environment) to ensure comprehensiveness and lasting impact.

The school board Health and Physical Education Coordinator champion and his team are a critical strength. They were able to ensure that at every step of the way, there was a clear connection between Healthy Schools and other aspects of the core business of education, such as safe schools, student engagement, connectedness to school, student leadership opportunities, behavioral issues, antibullying programs, student focus/time on task/attentiveness, attendance, and academic achievement. The Coordinator was also able to advocate to higher levels in the school boards to formalize their commitment to health in their mission statement. With such clear direction from their organization, it is no wonder that many local school-level principal, teacher, parent, and student champions emerged.

Within the public health unit, the school health consultant, coordinators, and managers championed partnerships with both school boards externally and championed the CSH concept internally. CSH was endorsed in 2000 as the framework for the delivery of school health services in the newly amalgamated city, and reaffirmed in a visioning process in 2003/2004. Coordinating personnel have worked hard with a range of public health practitioners to clarify roles, and this continues as an ongoing challenge.

In Middlesex-London, the positive, consistent working relationship between the PHN and the school's administration and members lays the foundation for initiating and sustaining the committee. Furthermore, school principals have indicated that the support and leadership of the PHN is necessary for up to 2 years, until members of the Healthy School Committee gain the confidence and skills they need to lead and sustain the process (Mitchell & Laforêt-Fliesser, 2003). Parent, student, and school staff champions have emerged in several schools over the years. PHNs have successfully engaged school-based champions to chair this committee, including secondary school students as co-chairs. We have also learned that a critical mass of students on a committee is essential to mitigate the power imbalance that can occur when adults and children are members of a committee together. PHNs and principals have been mindful of encouraging meaningful student and parent participation. As staff and principals have moved to other schools, they have championed the initiative in their new schools. Students who graduate from elementary school often continue their involvement on a committee throughout high school.

For us, the identification of a school board champion, such as the superintendent or learning coordinator, has varied over a 13-year period and has created challenges in keeping Healthy Schools on the agenda of school boards. The recent adoption of a Healthy Schools Framework by the provincial Ministry of Education has certainly generated greater interest, and we are moving toward a school board steering committee and possibly a public health school liaison position in the near future. In the fall of 2006, one local board acknowledged the success of several of its schools committed to Healthy Schools and, as a result, embarked on the creation of a board-wide policy that expects all principals to work with parents, students, and community partners to build safe and healthy school environments. This policy work was done in collaboration with public health staff. Other local boards of education are now giving serious consideration to supporting Healthy Schools.

Team Training and Ongoing Coaching/Learning Community

In Toronto, the concurrent establishment by the school board of four regional HALL Centres in September 2004 – each with Cdn $50,000 of funding from the school board budget – is a major strength. The HALL Centres are dedicated to providing teachers with excellent professional development opportunities in Health and Physical Education curriculum delivery and to becoming model schools for healthy, active living and learning.

Public health representatives are included on the Central Steering Committee as well as steering committees of each of the four centers. In 2007, the number of HALL centers increased to 5. In addition to offering teacher in-services on Health and Physical Education, these professional learning centers host the annual Health Action Team regional events (kickoff, mid-year in-service, end-of-year celebration) and profile local success stories. Principals, teachers, parents, and students learn from each other's experiences.

Within public health, there was, originally, one central Planning and Policy School Health Consultant. It was soon recognized that this central coordination, internally within the health unit and externally with school board partners, was crucial, so four School Health Coordinators (now called Consultants) were put in place, linked to the School and Youth Teams of liaison nurses working with schools. A large part of the coordinators' role has involved in-servicing frontline PHN and health promotion staff. Training for public health staff has focused on explanation of the CSH model and commonalities with other models such as Health-Promoting Schools (Europe, Australia, and elsewhere), FRESH (Focusing Resources on Effective School Health), Coordinated School Health Program (United States), Quality School Health (Canadian Association for Health, Physical Education, Recreation and Dance), and Living Schools (Ontario Physical and Health Education Association). The common elements particularly emphasized have been *partnerships* (in particular, promoting student involvement in decision making), coordinating *structures* (such as Health Action Teams or other relevant committees at all levels), and the planning *process* (committing to a shared vision of a healthy school, assessing strengths and needs, prioritizing issues, creating a plan that includes action within the four components of CSH, and implementing the activities, evaluating, and celebrating successes). The training has also focused on clarification of the respective roles of school liaison nurses who link with clusters of about 25 schools each versus roles of specific program staff, such as physical activity, nutrition, tobacco, substance abuse, injury prevention, sexual health, heart health, and cancer prevention staff. A great deal of emphasis has also been placed on clarifying the role of public health staff in fostering school readiness to engage in Healthy Schools work and in supporting Health Action Teams already committed to this work. It has been a role adjustment to change from traditionally being an "expert" to being a "consultant" – from "doing" to "supporting others to do" – from delivering "programs" to contributing to a "process" as an equal member of a team. Topic-specific content is still supplied upon request, but the biggest struggle has been with the liaison role to Health Action Teams.

During 1993–1994, PHNs at the Middlesex-London Health Unit received training on how to facilitate the engagement of school communities in becoming a healthy school. PHNs were reminded that their abilities to listen, assess, enable, and build trusting relationships were core nursing skills that would lay the foundation for facilitating the planning, implementation, and evaluation of this collaborative approach. They were expected to act as a catalyst and facilitator of the process. Over time, various tools and resources were developed to assist the school with implementation, specifically the Healthy School Profile (Mitchell et al., 1997), the Healthy School Committee, a resource kit, and evaluation tools. New activities such as completing the Healthy School Profile, analyzing the data, and mobilizing a school community required additional in-service training and support. Advocacy, negotiation, and mediation skills were also enhanced through training and supervision. Health unit staff also provided workshops to educate and inform school principals and vice principals about the process.

Since 2002, the Healthy Schools Workshop for Secondary School Students has been successful in attracting youth and teachers interested in becoming champions in their schools and in training youth to identify health issues and plan activities in their schools. This strategy has encouraged the sharing of success stories among peer leaders and has created a network of support among youth who are promoting Healthy Schools (Vandenheuvel et al., 2005).

Stakeholder Ownership and Participation

The Health Action Team initiative in Toronto is primarily "owned" by the education sector (school board), with public health in a supportive role. This has been key to sustaining the initiative over time. As principle stakeholder, central education staff have convened coordinating meetings; maintained a focus on the concrete needs of students, teachers, and principals in the field; streamlined requirements to avoid overburdening school staff; and developed user-friendly, concise tools and resources, all the while incorporating insights and input from public health. The school board staff and Professional Learning Centres' staff are "insiders" to the school system, so they were able to secure buy-in both from local school stakeholders and higher level board leaders. At the start, primarily principals and lead teachers for the Health Action Teams attended launch and in-service events. It has been an evolution for these adults to recognize the need to involve students in leadership roles and in decision making on Health Action Teams. The most successful schools have been given opportunities to profile their student-led successes to encourage other schools to pursue this approach. Most recently, a close partnership has developed between the school board Health and Physical Education coordinator and the Student Leadership coordinator, and workshops have been held where secondary students have done leadership development with elementary students.

In Middlesex-London, we learned very quickly that the Healthy School Committee is an important "vehicle" or "clearinghouse" for discussing a variety of health and social issues in the school. Given that each school was to determine its participation in this initiative, an effective committee comprised of students, parents, teachers, community members, and the school principal or vice-principal was key. This committee continues to operate collaboratively with other formal structures in the schools, such as the School Council, the Student Parliament, or other standing committees. Parents can talk to other parents and not leave all of the responsibility to the school's administration and teaching staff. What has amazed many principals is the variety of issues that are discussed at the committee meetings. One principal stated: "For me, it's almost an open agenda... there's very little that I don't feel is appropriate to be on the agenda of a Healthy School

Committee... because a healthy school is everything..." (Laforêt-Fliesser & Mitchell, 2002, p. 14). Process evaluations during the initial years of implementation clearly indicated that the formation of a Healthy School Committee was at the heart of a successful Healthy School.

The PHNs' approach is grounded in principles of health promotion whereby the PHNs enable school communities to identify health and social issues that are important to them. The community "names the concern or issue" and develops its own action plan. Community development and building capacity are at the heart of public health's work within schools. The PHN links the school to various community resources and facilitates the process by providing structure and facilitative leadership. Surveys of principals, staff, and parents have strongly endorsed the PHN as facilitator and resource provider and stressed the importance of sustaining this level of support. Eighty-eight percent of staff and parents reported that the process had increased their knowledge of strengths and health and social issues in their school communities. A high level of participation was noted among committee members, and 70% indicated that their school community was taking ownership for the initiative. Students have commented favorably on the functioning of the Healthy School Committee, with 88% reporting that the committee worked well together and 83% that the student voice was heard at the table. Almost all students (98%) reported that the committee made realistic plans in acting on health issues. All stakeholders reported that competing demands for time and limited resources negatively impacted the consistent participation of committee members. This has been particularly true for teachers and administrators who have been experiencing additional workloads related to the implementation of several educational reforms.

Lessons Learned and Recommendations

A great many lessons have been learned in Toronto, in Middlesex-London, and in Ontario as a whole. It is wonderful to be given the opportunity through this case study to reflect on these.

- *Both top-down and bottom-up strategies work.* In comparing the Toronto experience of school board leadership that rallied school level support for Healthy Schools, with the Middlesex-London experience of local school successes that led to board-level support, it is clear that either top-down or bottom-up approaches can work. This is very encouraging because there are many differences across jurisdictions, so it gives hope that one can initiate healthy schools work at either higher or lower levels, or perhaps even a combination of the two. Moreover, in Ontario, we have a combination of top-down Ministry of Education directives around Healthy Schools developed through consultation, as well as bottom-up successes that are making a difference and drawing attention from higher levels.

- *Emphasizing connections between Healthy Schools and the core business of education is important.* School boards and school administration have priority areas of focus within their mandate; to secure acceptance of Healthy Schools, it is critical to show the connections between Healthy Schools and the core business of education. In the Toronto experience, schools were being asked to submit a school improvement plan, so including a plan to implement Ministry-required DPA was reasonable. Establishing Health Action Teams to develop DPA plans contributed to this requirement. Twenty minutes of DPA contributed to less bullying on the school grounds and improved classroom behavior and student attentiveness. Having older students learn to be peer activity leaders for younger students at recess was consistent with a board focus on developing student leadership skills and promoting student engagement in their school. These connections were emphasized with principals and teachers at every opportunity. Subsequently, expansion to other topics could occur, as other priorities rose to the top, such as the school nutrition environment.
- *Relationships are key.* In both the Toronto and Middlesex-London experiences, positive working relationships were essential to advancing Healthy Schools work. In Toronto, the school board-level connection with public health was the main driver of board-wide work. In Middlesex-London, the frontline PHN connection with principals was foundational to local school successes.
- *Focusing on the concrete element of a Health Action Team/Healthy School Committee is pivotal.* It has been the experience of both Toronto and Middle-sex-London that, by itself, the term and concept of CSH is often daunting, vague, and intimidating to many school stakeholders. Our major successes occurred when we focused on the concrete coordinating structure of a Health Action Team or Healthy School Committee. People can grasp the visual of representatives of administration, school staff, parents, students, and community partners such as public health at one table, working together to make the school more supportive of health and learning. We have found the term "Healthy School" to be more user-friendly than "Comprehensive School Health." In fact, our provincial Ministry of Education has launched a Healthy Schools Recognition Program, and our OHSC has endorsed the "Healthy Schools" term. It is important also to note that, in reality, not all Healthy School committees include representatives of all stakeholder groups. Often, it is primarily students and a teacher advisor, particularly in secondary schools. In some instances parents cannot attend meetings held during the day, but are accessible for support in other ways. Flexibility is the key.
- *Funding is a necessary incentive.* For many jurisdictions in Ontario, it has been the Heart Health Partnership funding that has enabled us to get Healthy Schools up and running in a meaningful way. These grants are contingent on strong partnerships across sectors, so they propel health and education to work together. The funding for Toronto enabled the central coordinating committee to provide interested schools with seed funding to help them with meeting costs and with carrying out local plans. Without this incentive, schools would be very unlikely to invest significant time or resources in comprehensive Healthy Schools work.

Moreover, obtaining this significant grant brought credibility to the project and enabled both the school board and public health unit to mobilize additional internal resources and staff for training/coaching/ongoing learning and centralized planning of events.

- *Local successes contribute to policy formulation.* Policy support (within the school boards and at the provincial level) actually occurred *after* the local-level successes. It is interesting to note that policy statements were not necessary in order to achieve local commitment. Rather local-level successes actually convinced higher levels to formulate policy. At some point, it is ideal to have supportive Healthy Schools policy statements at the international, national, provincial, school board, public health unit, and local school levels. Once policy support occurs, it does increase the profile and importance of any issue.

- *Champions and leaders are important at all levels.* Champions internal to the education system and health system at all levels were crucial (in local schools, school board, public health unit, provincial education ministry and health promotion ministry, and at the national level). This has been discussed more fully in previous pages. It is valuable to note that public health roles include both board level support and school level support. The Toronto experience has found it ideal to have dedicated staff at both levels.

- *Capacity building – team training and ongoing coaching/learning community – is important.* One must not underestimate the need for resources to in-service all stakeholders on the Healthy School concept, structures, and process. This significant investment is necessary to ensure common understanding and commitment. The schools that took on the role of Professional Learning Centres in Toronto were key to building grassroots support as they were local sites where Health Action Team kickoff, networking, and celebration events were held. In addition, not only principals, teachers, parents, and students, but public health staff as well, require a significant amount of in-servicing or preparation in order to feel confident in their new roles with Healthy School Committees/Health Action Teams. Sharing success stories was found to be very valuable.

- *Stakeholder ownership and participation are crucial.* This also has been discussed at length, but is important to highlight in these concluding remarks. Because the school board champion was the primary lead for the Health Action Team initiative and was an "insider" in the school system, the uptake by schools was much greater than ever expected. In addition, all materials were specifically designed with the time limitations of teaching staff in mind, so they were well received.

- *Youth involvement matters.* It is important to emphasize from the beginning that schools should involve youth on their Healthy School committees. Planning in-services that build youth leadership skills can greatly enhance local Healthy Schools efforts.

- *Healthy Schools work is evolutionary.* It is clear from 4 years in Toronto and 14 years in Middlesex-London that working toward Healthy Schools requires long-term commitment and vision. Simple aspects are grasped at first; across time, schools gradually incorporate more elements to become more comprehensive in their approach. This was seen in the Toronto experience where teachers and principals were often the initial participants and they gradually engaged more students and PHNs as the concept of working in partnership was better understood.

- *Advocacy is necessary at all levels.* Finally, the Canadian experience makes it clear that advocacy at all levels has been necessary to get us to where we now are, and will still be necessary to secure support to move us further along the road to full implementation. Advocacy should not be perceived as negative or as a threat, but rather as a reality check between what is and what should be.

Acknowledgments The authors wish to acknowledge the support they received from Toronto Public Health (Liz Janzen and Vincenza Pietropaolo), Toronto Catholic District School Board (Anthony Petitti), and Middlesex-London Health Unit (Irene BucklandFoster) in preparing this case study. The authors would like to thank them and all the school and health unit staff, parents, and students who make Healthy Schools happen. This case study is dedicated to the memory of Andy Anderson, PhD, Canadian visionary leader for Healthy Schools, who passed away in 2007.

References

Canadian Association for School Health. (2007). *Comprehensive school health: Canadian consensus statement (revised)*. Retrieved March 6, 2008 from http://www.safehealthyschools.org/CSH_Consensus_Statement2007.pdf

Joint Consortium for School Health. (2008). Retrieved March 6, 2008 from http://www.jcsh-cces.ca

Laforêt-Fliesser, Y. & Mitchell, I. (2002). Healthy school communities: Collaborative approaches that work. *Physical and Health Education Journal, 68*(2), 12–18.

Middlesex-London Health Unit. (2004). *A guide to Healthy Schools*. Retrieved March 6, 2008 from www.healthunit.com.

Mitchell, I. & Laforêt-Fliesser, Y. (2003). Promoting healthy school communities. *Canadian Nurse, 99*(8), 21–24.

Mitchell, I., Laforêt-Fliesser, Y. & Camiletti, Y. (1997). The use of the healthy school profile in the Middlesex-London, Ontario schools. *Journal of School Health, 67*(4), 154–156.

Oliva, N., Mouritzen, M., BucklandFoster, I., Laforêt-Fliesser, Y., & Madden, J. (2004, May). *Healthy school committees: Perceptions of principals in participating schools*. Paper presented at Transforming Health Care Through Nursing Research: Making it Happen, Canadian Nursing Research Conference, London, ON.

Ontario Healthy Schools Coalition. (2002, revised 2008). *Terms of reference*. Retrieved March 6, 2008 from www.opha.on.ca/ohsc

Ontario Ministry of Education. (2006). *Foundations for a healthy school*. Retrieved March 6, 2008 from http://www.edu.gov.on.ca/eng/healthyschools/foundations.html

Steel, S., BucklandFoster, I., Laforêt-Fliesser, Y., & Madden, J. (2004, November). *Healthy school committees: Teachers and parents tell us how they work!* Paper presented at 55th Annual OPHA Conference: Public Health: The Best Health Investment, Toronto, ON.

Toronto Catholic District School Board. (2006). *System priority: Nurturing our Catholic community*. Retrieved March 7, 2008 from http://www.cateam.ca/

Toronto Catholic District School Board. (2008a). *Health Action Teams*. Retrieved March 6, 2008 from http://www.tcdsb.org/physicaleducation/hat.htm

Toronto Catholic District School Board. (2008b). *Healthy Active Living and Learning Centres*. Retrieved March 6, 2008 from http://www.tcdsb.org/physicaleducation/plcs.htm

Vandenheuvel, N., Laforêt-Fliesser, Y., Steel, S., Bainbridge, J., & Hofstetter, A. (2005, November). *Healthy schools, healthy youth: Building capacity for healthy living.* Paper presented at Joint Conference of the Ontario Public Health Association and the Association of Local Public Health Agencies, Toronto, ON.

Chapter 11
Nicaragua: The Social "Treasure" of Participation

Sergio Meresman and Anyoli Sanabria

> *Unite, shine, support each other, so many separated wills*
> Ruben Darío, Nicaraguan poet

Contextual Introduction

Basic Data

- 36 out of 100 school age children do not attend school.
- Of each 100 Nicaraguan children that start primary school 41 drop out.
- There are more than 7,000 schools in Nicaragua, the majority rural.
- Only 20% of primary schools have access to proper water and sanitation.
- Only 23% of the teachers are professionals.
- Under-5 mortality is 38 per 1,000 live births, and chronic malnutrition is 16%.
- Teen pregnancy accounts for 20% of all pregnancies.

Nicaragua is one of the poorest countries in Latin America. Of its 5.5 million people, 46.2% live in poverty and 15% in extreme poverty. In rural areas, these conditions worsen: two out of three Nicaraguans are poor (Government of Nicaragua, 2001). The autonomous communities of the Caribbean coast are the poorest municipalities.

S. Meresman(✉)
CLAEH (Latin American Centre for Humane Economy), UNER (University of Entre Rios), Montevideo, Uruguay

C. Vince Whitman and C.E. Aldinger (eds.),
Case Studies in Global School Health Promotion: From Research to Practice,
DOI: 10.1007/978-0-387-92269-0_11, © Springer Science + Business Media, LLC 2009

159

The country's annual income per person is $US3,100 (2007). Social expenditure accounts for 3.8% in education and 3.7% in health, half of what other countries with similar poverty levels invest (Alliance for Childhood Investment, 2007).

Nicaragua has progressed in strengthening its democratic institutions and culture, but social conditions – determined by endemic poverty combined with recurrent political crisis, partisan public policy administration, and corruption – profoundly erode the trust between citizens and governments and foster a permanent institutional fragility (Alliance for Childhood Investment, 2007).

Meeting the Millennium Development Goals is a huge challenge for Nicaragua, particularly for the health and education sectors, which are faced with serious structural limitations that severely obstruct the rights of children and adolescents. Among the most noticeably marginalized groups are those living below poverty lines, the rural populations, the indigenous, and those disabled or with special education needs.

Preschool formal education covers 52.1% of children, while primary education has a gross rate of 87.6% (2006). Approximately, 36% of children and adolescents are not part of the education system. The quality of education is largely unsatisfactory, showing a completion rate of barely 59% in primary school. More than 70% of girls and boys in grades 3 and 6 do not achieve the minimum learning standards, according to tests conducted in 2006.

Bilingual education, which is essential in a country that hosts a large indigenous community, has an even lower coverage, and 13.4% of the children and adolescents ages 5–17 are engaged in child labor (2005). Although boys and girls have fairly equal access to education, disparity persists in terms of the treatment boys and girls receive in school and at home; for instance, girls get assigned traditional roles such as cleaning the classrooms.

Lack of training and professional development opportunities for teachers, limited professional acknowledgment, low salaries, frequent turnover, and the fact that 23% of employed teachers are uncertified (empiric) practitioners also affects quality (Nicaraguan Ministry of Education, 2006). Also, educational materials and support resources for teachers are insufficient.

Many schools face severe problems in infrastructure, water, and sanitation. They have no running water, water tanks, or resources to treat water to ensure that it is drinkable. Latrines or bathrooms are not always up to standards. School compounds often do not meet the necessary privacy, safety, hygiene, and accessibility standards.

Schools and communities in Nicaragua, as well as in many other places in Latin America, have learned a lot about how to survive and develop in a context of extreme complexity, crisis, and emergency. Often they have to carry on operations through severe institutional crisis, with scarce resources, and under precarious political and institutional conditions. So far as complexity and adversity can be tackled only with comprehensive responses, the Friendly and Healthy Schools project has found in complicated Nicaragua a nest for innovation and creativity.

Overview of the School Health Program

The Institutional Fabric

Nicaragua has shown progress in the development of a legal education and health promotion framework. The framework acknowledges the role of schools in transforming families and communities through the promotion of life skills and good practices that influence lifestyles and behaviors. However, limited ability to translate the legal framework into integrated and collaborative health and education practices has often frustrated the effort to operationalize transforming practices at the school and community level.

For this reason, several national institutions – with almost unanimous support from the United Nations Agencies – agreed on the Friendly and Healthy Schools (FHS) initiative. This was an attempt to put into practice an institutional consensus that prioritized the improvement of quality education in Nicaragua and to address a number of critical child development factors through inter-sectoral, multiinstitutional, and children's rights-oriented action.

The construction of the multiinstitutional alliance started in June 2001, when the Ministry of Education signed an agreement with the Ministry of Health and the National Water and Sanitation Company to promote FHS, with support from UNICEF and the Pan American Health Organization (PAHO/WHO). The initiative was officially launched in 2002. To test the proposed approach in different contexts, it began by involving 17 schools from diverse geographic areas and social backgrounds.

The participating agencies – the national Ministry of Education (MINED), Ministry of Health (MINSA), National Water and Sanitation Enterprise (ENACAL), and the international United Nations Children's Fund (UNICEF) and Pan-American Health Organization (PAHO) – formed a Steering Committee to be responsible for overseeing the implementation process at municipal, regional, and national levels. Other agencies such as the Ministry of Natural Resources and Environment, the National School Feeding Program, and Handicap International collaborated in specific activities or components. At the municipal level, local NGOs, government, and private sector groups also joined the efforts.

At the beginning, it was vital to agree that MINED coordinate the steering committee, as the institution that had competency in implementing activities in schools. Other agencies accepted and acknowledged this leadership and acted in a supportive manner.

Building on Previous Experiences

FHS was not about launching new policies but about how to implement what was already on the education agenda through an innovative and coordinated strategy, avoiding duplication, dispersion, and negative competition among the different stakeholders and ongoing programs. The rationale of the initiative emphasized the fact that some previous experiences had not succeeded or were unsustainable because they were imposed on schools without a real understanding of the needs and the institutional cultures of the schools. Most of the earlier experiences were extracurricular initiatives, often innovative and valuable, but never able to take root in the teachers' practice or the education policy. FHS used a nonorthodox approach to integrate various well-tested experiences of different agencies and programs.

The FHS initiative recaptured three regional programs that had been previously implemented in Nicaragua and provided useful background: the New School (Escuela Nueva), in relation to quality education; Healthy School/Health-Promoting School, in relation to health; and Friendly School, in relation to children's rights and responsibilities. The interagency collaboration and agreements were based on the FRESH (World Bank et al., 2002) framework and supported by all the UN agencies. Its very name shows the determination of the agencies to combine good practices into a model for changing schools and improving education.

Scope and Outreach

FHS were at first predominantly introduced for primary multigrade schools (where one teacher is responsible for all grades) in rural areas. The intention was for these initial experiences to be a showcase to educators and education authorities that schools are effective mobilizers and catalyzers of multisectoral collaboration and that they can achieve improvements through comprehensive approaches. Progressively, the initiative involved also preschool, community centers, and some schools that offered secondary education.

Currently, the initiative is being expanded to the autonomous Caribbean coast, while adapting some of the resources and guidelines into the Miskito and Mayagna cultures and languages. The proposed goal for 2006 was 200 schools. In 2008, the initiative includes all 387 schools in eight departments (provinces) and 42 municipalities.

Some schools started to offer short residency programs to teachers interested in learning about the model. Some others, particularly rural schools, started to act as reference centers for others in their own area, while many nongovernmental organizations and private schools that learned about FHS decided to adopt or support the model.

Revisiting Conceptual Frameworks from a Practice-Oriented Perspective

FHS was inspired by the need to provide Nicaraguan children with the skills they need to address their own lives and the challenges of their changing country and region, which are embarking on a process of social and economic development.

It took almost 2 years for all the institutions and stakeholders involved to come to an agreement on a conceptual framework for the initiative. This process of technical dialogue and consensus building was simultaneous to the implementation of showcase projects, which provided feedback into the process.

The strategy developed into a comprehensive model that takes into account all the diverse factors that determine the ability to learn. The vision was set for "a quality school that is child-centered, involves parents, ensures inclusion, respects equal rights for boys and girls, is flexible and responds to individual needs, promotes health and highlights the moral status, and professionalism of teachers" (Nicaraguan Ministry of Education, 2005).

The main principles of the new initiative were (1) children's rights are indivisible, hence multisectoral approaches are necessary; (2) children should be at the center of the initiative; (3) the schools' institutional project and life skills education should be the main avenues; (4) provide equity and quality education for all; (5) health promotion is key to quality education; and (6) promote leadership and capacity building of the education sector, community, and children's participation.

Taking Ideas into Implementation

A Friendly and Healthy School is defined as "one in which children and adolescents build, practice, and develop knowledge and life skills in a setting that is healthy, safe, protective and respectful of the diversity, where children and adults (teachers, parents and community members) can participate and make decisions" (Nicaraguan Ministry of Education, 2005).

The Friendly and Healthy School comprises five components.

1. *Quality, friendly, and successful learning.* This calls for developing systemic and methodological conditions for teachers to facilitate a learning process that is guided by high quality standards and is friendly at the same time. It requires a permanent effort to provide training opportunities and supportive teaching resources to teachers and school personnel.
2. *Appropriate, safe, and friendly conditions in the school environment.* The physical conditions of the school should be consistent with the educational model. An FHS should provide safe and hygienic classrooms and green areas with sport compounds. It also pursues accessibility measures to ensure that children with special needs are not excluded.
3. *Water, sanitation, and hygiene.* The FHS should provide safe water, an appropiate sanitation system, and a strategy for garbage management. It also teaches children and the community about the importance of hygiene.
4. *Health and nutrition education.* This includes the implementation of policies related to good health and nutrition-related habits, vaccination, oral health, nutrition education, and a school feeding program.

5. *Children's rights and responsibilities.* This works to develop citizenship-related competence such as participatory skills and understanding of democratic and collective decision-making processes. It provides regular opportunities for children and their families to apply these skills in school management.

Proposed Implementation Cycle for HFS

Each participating school and community set up a project team composed of the school principal, community leaders, representatives of the student government and school council, teachers, parents, and children. Figure 1 shows a scheme of the implementation cycle.

The implementation cycle is not linear; only for didactic purposes can it be represented as an itinerary where each stage smoothly follows another. The actual implementation process follows a complicated path characterized by backward and forward maneuvers, strategies, articulations, and decisions that require specific competences to get through each phase.

Specific Aspects of Implementation

Many aspects of the FHS implementation process are seen as innovative by the institutions involved. This does not necessarily mean that the ideas are completely new. The perceived difference in this experience is related to the ability of the organizations leading the initiative to succeed in the implementation and to demonstrate that the model was feasible and effective in improving education in Nicaragua.

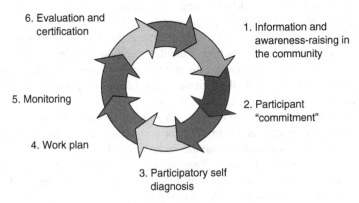

Fig. 1 HFS implementation cycle

Several factors were identified as the most successful aspects in the FHS implementation:

- *A clear and shared vision:* It took time and patience for the various stakeholders to agree on the main conceptual elements for a shared vision. It was also important to build trust and find a clear and shared vision of the difference that implementing this model will make in the life of children and schools.
- *Strong consensus on the conceptual framework and approach:* The highly participative process involved collecting input from the different agencies on the FHS conceptual framework and approach; it also built a strong team spirit among the officials and members of the multiinstitutional technical team. Further, it led to a clear understanding about the need for collaboration and complementation among the different agencies.
- *Integrated approach:* The effectiveness and feasibility of complementing focused interventions with an integrated health promotion approach has been another important lesson of the Nicaraguan experience. Including all relevant actors throughout the process of identifying needs and entry points, planning, training, and technical assistance was key to provide consistent advice to schools. This will be further examined in our final conclusions.
- *Multidisciplinary and multiinstitutional technical team:* A formal agreement among the main institutions supporting the initiative speeded decision-making and sometimes avoided bureaucratic stalemates. Shared preparation of annual plans, reports, and studies among UNICEF and PAHO particularly helped the process of creating multiinstitutional concensus.
- *Ownership and participation throughout the planning, training, and implementation:* Making simple guidelines widely available has been reported as a tangible help to participation of local organizations and communities across the different stages of the process. Children's participation was highly encouraged in concordance with the children's rights approach promoted by the United Nations agencies and the momentum created internationally in favor of healthy and safe environments for children.

Achievements and Impact

In 2005, an independent agency carried out an external evaluation of FHS (Gonzalez et al., 2006). Results were encouraging about the impact of the model on improving the lives of school children. It is interesting to look at some of the results, which showed promising evidence of the success of the FHS model in organizing and carrying out new school-community dynamics and increasingly achieving more participation of the community. The most significant indicators were:

- Increased ownership by the Ministry of Education, which opened up the possibility to influencing the general education policy

- Improved interinstitutional coordination
- Strategic and multiinstitutional technical and political support for the initiative
- Improved school enrollment and retention in the participating schools
- Improved teaching practices in participating schools (e.g., the active, hands-on methodologies introduced for health promotion were increasingly applied to other curricula)
- Increased participation by parents and community

The external evaluation also elaborated a number of recommendations, of which these were the most significant:

- Mainstreaming the concept and methodologies of the FHS initiative as a quality model for all Nicaraguan schools, as well as within the national health policy. The recommended goal is to have quality indicators met by 2015 by all Nicaraguan schools.
- Linking FHS with the process of decentralization and the transferal of schools to the municipal level.
- Strengthening participatory opportunities for children and families (e.g., setting up school managerial councils, providing a seat for children on school boards).
- Strengthening principal, teacher, and health personnel training on children's rights, life skills, and other specific topics highlighted by the initiative.
- Responding to the need to harmonize school infrastructure, water, and sanitation with FHS standards.
- Validating and adapting the initiative to the bilingual and multicultural context of the Autonomous (Miskito and Mayagna) Regions.
- Expanding the initiative by certifying 50 additional schools as FHS in the following 2 years.
- Using the "United Nations Agencies collaboration" experience as a good practice showcase to be implemented in other areas and sectors.

Conclusions and Insights

Main Factors Contributing to Success

Consistent institutional leadership and public support: We have identified in earlier work (Meresman, 2007) the value of consistent advocacy and leadership at the national level as a feasibility factor in implementing initiatives such as FHS. It is the kind of support that makes good practices and collaboration at local level sustainable, by ensuring the appropriate technical and financial resources. It also avoids the reliance of good projects on mere voluntarism or personal leadership, as we have seen in many cases. By the same token, the absence of such national support is a major barrier to developing good collaboration practices on the ground.

Strategic technical and political support for the initiative: A multisectoral and multiinstitutional initiative mobilized complementary resources that supported the needs of schools in terms of implementation at the same time that they enabled a positive political and institutional environment to move forward.

These different views are also contributors to the complexity and diversity of objectives at stake. Rigid institutional agendas, individualism, and striving to impose one's own ideas are hindering factors. Dialogue, communication, and conflict-resolution skills are the competences most needed to build trust among participants and take strategies forward.

Creation of an inclusive, multisectoral network for coordination and collaborative management: Participating institutions signed a written agreement, establishing each sector's commitment, and responsibilities and acknowledging the institutional leadership of the Ministry of Education. The initiative sustained an inclusive approach to mobilizing resources and coordinating actions in support of children and communities. This network originated at national level and exists in each province where there are FHS.

The usefulness of an inter-agency task force is another lesson learned through this project. In addition to UNICEF, PAHO/WHO, UNESCO, and the World Food Program, organizations working on specific education and school health-related areas (such as the World Bank and Inter American Development Bank) and organizations working on specific school health-related areas (such as CARE, Plan International, SNV, USAID, Save the Children, and Handicap International) collaborated with the initiative. The dispersion of resources and competitive relationships between international agencies in promoting slightly different approaches to the link between health and education (Health-Promoting Schools of PAHO and WHO, Child-Friendly Schools of UNICEF, FRESH of the World Bank and UNESCO) are often mentioned as a barriers to good practices on the ground to progress accordingly. However, this experience has proven their enormous potential of complementing technical and financial resources as well as delivering a consistent message to local authorities.

A sound technical framework: Using self-diagnosis and situation-analysis tools, schools were able to generate baseline information and know-how to apply to participatory planning and involve the community. There was room for each school to analyze its reality and find its own way to set up quality, and there was a sound technical agreement on the basic indicators and components.

Progressive scale-up, based on contagious *interest:* The development of FHS was not fast. It grew out of the progressively increasing interest of communities and teachers as the program's reputation among Nicaraguan schools disseminated and grew. The certification of the first five schools as healthy and friendly on the basis of their ability to respond to the needs identified in the situation analysis and the priorities agreed with the community was an important incentive to other schools. Since 2006, the initiative has already been numerically significant, reaching 387 schools and 35,000 children.

Dissemination of technical papers and resources: HFS documents were widely disseminated. Implementation guidelines were widely introduced to education, health, and local development practitioners.

Ongoing monitoring and technical assistance: Good inter-institutional coordination resulted in better capacity to provide ongoing monitoring and technical assistance. Interinstitutional teams were set up to ensure permanent coordination and follow-up of the initiative at all levels – national, regional, municipal, school, and community.

Emphasis on the capacity of schools and communities to address their own needs and wishes: The FHS framework put into practice a model that required a process of self-analysis led by each school and community. This guided participants through an empowering experience, via the identification and mobilization of existing and potential local capacities.

Complementation between focused interventions and comprehensive *approaches:* The Nicaraguan experience shows that focused and comprehensive approaches are not necessarily diametrically opposed, as has often been felt within the school health professional community. From tackling a specific emerging health problem (e.g., the need to provide water and sanitation), complementary actions were triggered at the classroom (health and hygiene education) and community level (mobilizing support of families) to generate a holistic program that was prepared to address the actual causes of the problem and was more likely to succeed in the long run.

Openness and capacity for social participation: Participation does not emerge naturally as a consequence of a health or education promotion process. It requires a planned strategy to facilitate the distribution of different roles and building capacities for participation. The provision of opportunities for meaningful participation and managerial decision-making by parents is still challenging to most school principals.

Unfinished Business and Challenges

Improve tools for evaluation and systematization: Although the numeric goal established by the Steering Committee has been largely met, a significant challenge remains – the very slow progress in developing and applying tools for evaluating the process and for collecting and systematizing lessons. Also, the initiative lacks a way to certify a school as FHS or credit its progress.

Harmonize school infrastructure and water and sanitation with FHS standards: Physical infrastructure does not meet standards in Nicaragua. The strategy has made significant progress in establishing a legal and administrative framework to ensure that schools set goals in this field, but there is still much room for improvement.

Acknowledgments The authors had support from Education Development Center, Inc., and UNICEF, Nicaragua.

References

Alliance for Childhood Investment. (2007). *Social investment study* [in Spanish, Alianza por la inversión en la Niñez, *Estudio de inversión social*]. Retrieved March 2008, from http://www. unicef.org/lac/flash/DW/nicaragua_09.html

Figueroa, A.R. (2007). *Round Table: Inter-agency Collaboration for the development of Health Promoting Schools* (in Spanish, *Mesa redonda: Cooperación interagencial para el desarrollo de las Escuelas Promotoras de la Salud*). Retrieved March 2008, from http://www.ops-oms. org/Spanish/AD/SDE/HS/EPS_RED_MESA.pdf

Gonzalez, D,. et al. (2006). *Mid term evaluation of the friendly and healthy schools initiative in Nicaragua* [in Spanish, *Evaluacion de medio término iniciatativa Escuelas Amigas y Saludables de Nicaragua*]. Managua, Nicaragua: Juarez & Associates.

Government of Nicaragua. (2001). *Strengthened strategy for economic growth and poverty reduction* [in Spanish: Gobierno de Nicaragua, *Estrategia reforzada de crecimiento económico y reducción de pobreza*]. Retrieved March 2008, from http://idbdocs.iadb.org/wsdocs/getdocument.aspx?docnum = 619872

Meresman, S. (2005). Mainstreaming health promotion into education policies, the Uruguayan experience. *Promotion & Education*, 12(3), 178–179.

Meresman, S (2007). *Health and education in the labyrinth* [in Spanish, *Escuelas Promotoras de Salud, el laberinto de la implementación*]. (Technical paper prepared for the Pan American Health Organization and the Education Development Center, soon to be published).

Nicaraguan Ministry of Education. (2005). *Friendly and healthy schools initiative manual for teachers* [In Spanish, *Manual del docente, Iniciativa Escuelas Amigas y Saludables*]. MINED, MINSA, ENACAL, UNICEF and OPS. Managua: Author.

Nicaraguan Ministry of Education. (2006). *National statistics* [in Spanish, *Ministerio de Educación de Nicaragua: Estadisiticas Educativas*]. Retrieved March 2008 from http://www.oei.es/ quipu/nicaragua/educ_basica_media2006.pdf

Sanabria, A. (2002). *The friendly and healthy schools in Nicaragua: An inter-agency initiative* [In Spanish, *Escuelas Amigas y Saludables en Nicaragua: Una iniciativa inter/agencial*]. (Minutes of the 3rd Meeting of the Latin American Network of Health Promoting Schools) Retrieved March 2008 from http://www.amro.who.int/Spanish/AD/SDE/HS/EPS_RED_ MESA.pdf

World Bank et al. (2002). *Focusing resources on effective school health: A joint initiative by the World Bank, PAHO-WHO, UNICEF and UNESCO*. Retrieved March 2008, from http://www. freshschools.org/Pages/default.aspx

World Health Organization, Mortality Country Fact Sheet (2006) Retrieved in August 2008 from http://www.who.int/whosis/mort/profiles/mort_amro_nic_nicaragua.pdf

Chapter 12
USA: The Michigan Journey Toward Coordinated School Health

Laurie Bechhofer, Barbara Flis, Kyle Guerrant, and Kimberly Kovalchick

Contextual Introduction

Schools have a wealth of potential for ensuring the future well-being of young people. You can't educate a child who isn't healthy, and you can't keep a child healthy who isn't educated.

M. Joycelyn Elders, MD

Schools provide an incredible opportunity to improve the current and future health and well-being of young people. A captive audience of young people in our nation's schools awaits health knowledge and guidance from trusted adults. Schools are the best places to promote healthy lifestyles and to provide the primary and secondary prevention needed to avoid and detect diseases that are the predictors of future health. The construct of school systems is conducive to a holistic or coordinated approach to school health.

In Michigan, as in other states, health in the school setting is a challenge as schools undergo continued pressure to focus on learning and greater academic achievement. While schools often see the need, it does not always equate to making health a core mission. Yet, optimism for a healthier future is not based on desire or hope, but on more than two decades of collaborative work among Michigan's school health champions. They speak with conviction that the future health status of Michigan's children is positive. However, no one would say that he or she is completely satisfied with school health in Michigan. The concept of continuous improvement and being "a work in progress" is deeply embedded and has contributed to many school health successes.

K. Guerrant(✉)
Coordinated School Health and Safety Programs Unit, Grants Coordination and School Support, Michigan Department of Education, Lansing, MI, USA

C. Vince Whitman and C.E. Aldinger (eds.),
Case Studies in Global School Health Promotion: From Research to Practice,
DOI: 10.1007/978-0-387-92269-0_12, © Springer Science + Business Media, LLC 2009

This case study follows Michigan's development of school health from its early stages to the important work of building an infrastructure and the events and innovations that became powerful forces for change. The case concludes with insights and lessons learned.

About the USA

The USA is a democratic nation comprising 50 states and Washington, D.C., a federal district. It also includes several territories located in the Caribbean and Pacific. The USA has the third largest land mass in the world, after Russia and Canada, with 3.79 million sq miles. Only China and India have larger populations than the USAs' 300 million people. While vast regions of the country are sparsely populated, the majority of the people (83%) live in urban centers. Immigration from other countries has made the USA one of the world's most ethnically diverse nations. The USA is structured as a representative democracy, with federal, state, and local levels of government. Its economy is the largest in the world. Although many in the USA live in prosperity, a significant number of people still live without adequate nutrition, housing, education, employment, and health care.

Unlike the nationally regulated and financed education systems of many other industrialized societies, public education in the USA is primarily the responsibility of the states and individual school districts. The US educational system reaches more than 55 million students from kindergarten to grade 12, and over 17 million students in colleges and universities, many of them foreign-born. The vast majority of students attend tax-supported public schools. Approximately 10% of the total elementary and secondary enrollment in the USA in 2003–2004 was in private schools (Broughman & Swaim, 2006). In most public and private schools, education is divided into three levels: elementary school, junior high school (or middle school), and senior high school. In almost all schools at these levels, children are divided by age groups into grades. The ages for compulsory education vary by state, beginning at ages 5–8 and ending at ages 14–18. Locally elected school boards, with jurisdiction over school districts, typically make decisions pertaining to curricula, funding, teaching, and other policies. Educational standards and standardized testing decisions are usually made by state governments. The *No Child Left Behind Act of 2001* placed a greater focus on accountability, with the goal that every child achieve proficiency according to state-defined standards by 2013–2014. Approximately one-third of US students – those from low-income families – receive free or reduced-price breakfast and/or lunch every day, paid for by the federal government.

The Great Lakes State: About Michigan

Known as the "Great Lakes State," Michigan has more freshwater shoreline than any other state. It is the tenth largest state in the USA and is geographically, economically, socially, and ethnically diverse. The primary industries of Michigan are tourism, agriculture, and manufacturing (Michigan in Brief, 2008). Automotive manufacturing has been Michigan's hallmark for growth and prosperity. Auto industry declines have led to a financial downturn. Wages in Michigan declined by 0.5% in 2007. The unemployment rate in June 2008 was 8.5%, the highest in the nation (U.S. Congress Joint Economics Committee, 2008). In the fall of 2007, Michigan ranked highest in unemployment among all the states in the nation, with 7.4% of the labor force currently unemployed (U.S. Department of Labor, Bureau of Labor Statistics, 2007). Approximately 38% of Michigan students are currently eligible for the federal free or reduced-price lunch program (State of Michigan, Center for Educational Performance and Information, 2007).

Michigan has over 1.7 million students (U.S. Department of Education, National Center for Educational Statistics [NCES], 2005–2006) and is ranked fifth in the nation for total number of public school districts (U.S. Department of Education, NCES, 2005–2006). Michigan's high school graduation rate is 86% and the dropout rate is 4% (State of Michigan, Center for Educational Performance and Information, 2005–2006). Health risk behaviors of Michigan high school youth parallel those of the U.S. youth overall. Less than half of Michigan students (44%) got the recommended amount of physical activity in a week; only 17% of Michigan high school students ate the recommended daily servings of fruits and vegetables each week; and 42% of Michigan high school youth reported ever having sexual intercourse (Michigan Department of Education, 2008). As with other health and education indicators, there are still disparities related to gender, race/ethnicity, socioeconomic status, and educational achievement that put some students at greater risk. It is a challenge to reach all students while also focusing on those with higher needs. The education system gives broad decision-making responsibility to states. The states in turn provide leadership, guidance, and resources, but they defer to local schools to customize programs to fit their needs. This structure affords local schools the opportunity to design and adopt programs for students with higher needs.

Overview of the School Health Program

School Health in the USA

As far back as the nineteenth century, when the USA first constructed a system of formal education, its primary focus was on educational goals and methods. Health-promoting schools came about as a reaction to pressing health needs. For example, in the mid-1900s, to prevent malnutrition and to provide an outlet for farm surpluses, the U.S. Congress passed the National School Lunch Act, which provided a nutritious lunch program for all students in schools throughout the nation. It established a basic meal pattern requirement and required schools to serve lunches free or at a reduced price to children in need. The Office of Safe and Drug-Free Schools was created as the US government's vehicle for reducing violence in schools and use of drugs, alcohol, and tobacco. And as research began to link academic achievement more closely to mental, environmental, and physical health, financial assistance for activities that promote the health and well-being of students was provided under the America's Schools Act of 1994. One outcome of the America's Schools Act was the Carol M. White Physical Education Program Grants to initiate, expand, and improve physical education programs for students. In 1987, the Centers for Disease Control and Prevention (CDC) Division of Adolescent and School Health (DASH) began providing funds and technical assistance to state, territory, and large-city education agencies to help schools conduct effective HIV-prevention education. The effort expanded in 1992, with additional funding for states to build the capacity of schools to support a coordinated school health approach for addressing risk factors for chronic disease, in particular, physical inactivity, unhealthy eating, and tobacco use.

Early Developments of School Health in Michigan

Michigan has had a commitment to health education and physical education for over 40 years. The Michigan Department of Education (MDE) has sustained full-time consultant positions to lead health education since 1967 and physical education since 1973. Since 1974, the departments of education and public health have shared human and fiscal resources to collaborate on school-health-related initiatives.

In the mid-1980s, many forces worked to develop a statewide model health education curriculum. The nation was focused on substance abuse prevention, and schools were barraged with materials from the public and private sectors. In response to parent and school concerns, Michigan used available resources to expand a pilot curriculum to address Comprehensive School Health Education (CSHE). The resulting model health education curriculum, with lessons in a clear scope and sequence for students in each grade K-6, addressed ten topic areas. A rarity for its time, the curriculum included family and community involvement worksheets and homework assignments that engaged parents and other trusted adults.

The process used to develop the model curriculum was as important as the product itself. A network of 115 professional and volunteer groups – representing agencies (e.g., health department, American Cancer Society), content areas (e.g., HIV education, violence prevention, physical fitness), and disciplines (e.g., nursing, school social work) – came together to develop a "road map." The partners became champions as CSHE emerged as the primary curriculum for health education in Michigan. This collaborative ownership, with the combination of state and local-match funding and the infusion of federal funding, increased the adoption and implementation of the curriculum in a majority of school districts and schools within a few years from its inception. Collaboration among government and nongovernmental agencies has become a trademark among Michigan school health champions and continues to this day to provide the foundation for coordinated school health programs.

Specific Aspects of Implementation

Building Capacity to Deliver Coordinated School Health

Success of the model health education curriculum depended on its adoption and implementation by school districts. Because Michigan has over 800 school districts and over 1.65 million students, a statewide structure of 25 regional school health coordinators was created to provide an efficient and effective delivery system for school health education. The structure of coordinators, housed in regional education service centers or large urban school districts, has become one of the hallmarks of school health education in Michigan, and still stands strong today. The funding came from an initial Michigan legislature allocation of $1 million in 1984/1985 and increased to $1.2 million in its second year.

In the early years, the coordinators focused on marketing, formation of local advisory committees, instructional material procurement and distribution, and teacher training to implement curricula. Given the number of teachers, Michigan used a train-the-trainer model. As the vision for school health expanded beyond curricula, the coordinators continued to broaden their scope of work. Coordinators serve an important role in closing the gap between state-level agencies and local school districts by being the "eyes and ears" for emerging needs, and leaders for innovation.

The state funding for school health laid the foundation for coordinated school health, while federal Safe and Drug-Free Schools funding, provided by the US Department of Education, accelerated implementation. In 1987, Michigan received additional funding from the CDC/DASH, to develop a statewide HIV and AIDS prevention program. The funding was timely, given the national attention to this emerging epidemic and new Michigan laws that required school districts to teach about HIV and AIDS as part of their communicable disease instruction.

The use of federal funds to support state departments of education was a novel approach at the time. State and local education agencies were a common-sense choice to have an impact on the health of young people, because they spend a considerable amount of time in school. In the USA, the educational system is an institution with its own mission, operating principles, governance structure, and culture. Like any other long-standing institution, schools are not easily influenced by external factors. The most effective school health endeavors are those that work within the educational system in collaboration with key partners to effect change in policies, programs, and practices.

In the late 1980s, the MDE was awarded a 5-year competitive CDC/DASH National Training and Demonstration grant of $250,000 to build the capacity of other states to effectively manage their HIV and AIDS grants. Because the state had a professional development leadership role, the funding enhanced Michigan's expertise as master CSHE trainers.

In the early 1990s, the CDC/DASH increased state funding for school health with Expanded Program dollars to build the infrastructure for a state-level Coordinated School Health Program (CSHP). State departments of education received funds to work in partnership with state departments of health to build the capacity of schools to use a coordinated approach to address physical activity, nutrition, and tobacco use (PANT) and ultimately prevent chronic disease. These funds allowed Michigan to expand the model health education curriculum to address secondary school students, support a needs assessment and gap analysis of current structures and resources in state government that addressed CSHP, and provide guidance for future program planning and decision making. The same collaborative decision-making process used to develop and implement model curriculum and to address emerging issues such as HIV and AIDS has been replicated for fitness, tobacco prevention, physical activity, asthma, and sun safety.

Changing the Way We Do Business: Moving Toward a CSHP Model

The CSHP model makes sense because it is a holistic approach that looks to the entire school environment to have an impact on the health and well-being of the whole child. A seminal article published in the *Journal of School Health* (Allensworth & Kolbe, 1987) defined an eight-component model to impact the health of students. It included health education, physical education, health services, school nutrition services, counseling and psychological services, healthy school environment, health promotion for staff and family, and community involvement. This CSHP model emphasized the importance of each of the components to creating a more coordinated and efficient way of providing programs and services. It also expanded the vision for affecting the health and well-being of students within a school setting from the classroom to the whole school.

Within the realm of HIV and sex education, the family and community involvement component became a key vehicle for increasing implementation of comprehensive prevention education. The MDE developed a brief model parent survey instrument that school districts use to learn what topics parents wanted to be taught at specific grade levels. The survey results helped shape local programs that were aligned with parent and student needs. It also provided schools with documentation needed if decisions were ever challenged.

One of the challenges for "selling" the CSHP concept was to work collaboratively with people from different professional disciplines. Michigan has realized success, but does not claim to have fully arrived at implementing CSHP. Key to arriving at this juncture is being adept at simultaneously maintaining a vision, collaborating with key stakeholders, conducting ongoing assessment, being aware of emerging needs, conducting evaluation, and taking action as opportunities arise. The examples below illustrate the benefits to school health in Michigan of ongoing strategic vision.

The Time Is Right: Capitalizing on Emerging Health and Safety Concerns

The Obesity Epidemic: In the mid-1990s, the nation began to examine the prevalence of obesity, the human and fiscal costs associated with chronic disease, and the importance of primary prevention in addressing the obesity epidemic. National media identified Michigan as one of the heaviest states in the nation, and school leaders sought guidance about the school's role in promoting healthy weight. Excessive weight puts school children at greater risk for a host of health and social-emotional issues that become barriers to learning.

In 2001, the MDE convened a state-level Healthy Weight Advisory Group to examine the school's role in addressing obesity. The resulting consensus paper, *The Role of Michigan Schools in Promoting Health Weight* (Michigan Department of Education, Office of School Excellence, 2001), provided vision and guidance to schools on how to address this issue appropriately. The critical mass of more than 50 state and national leaders shared supportive norms necessary for creating new thinking and practices to address healthy weight in Michigan districts. The process fueled a paradigm shift from a narrow focus on weight loss to a broader model that promoted healthy students of all shapes and sizes. The impact of strengthened partnerships and collective new thinking was monumental in its influence on future health initiatives. Through these strengthened partnerships, shared goals and objectives were created, leading to increases in shared resources (funding and staffing) and similar messaging to achieve a common vision.

High-Risk Youth: In early 2001, the Michigan Department of Education took a bold step and convened a state-level group of stakeholders to examine how to better meet the HIV prevention needs of youth who self-identify as lesbian, gay, bisexual, transgender, or who are questioning their sexual orientation or gender identity (SMY). Several forces came together to move the initiative forward: The field was asking for help; several regional sites had piloted professional development; the CDC/DASH encouraged states to focus their HIV prevention on high-risk populations, and, finally, the American Civil Liberties Union (ACLU) and the Gay, Lesbian & Straight Education Network (GLSEN) Detroit had just published a call to action, *What Schools Need to Know: Gay, Lesbian, Bisexual and Transgender Students and the Law* (ACLU & GLSEN, 2000).

The MDE worked with key partners to spearhead the multitiered statewide initiative with three major components: (1) the Safe Schools for SMY Workgroup, (2) the *A Silent Crisis* resource guide, and (3) the professional development workshops, *A Silent Crisis: Creating Safe Schools for Sexual Minority Youth.* The initiative was based on the CSHP premise that safe and supportive school environments increase academic achievement and reduce risk-taking behaviors and risk for HIV. With representatives from grades K-12 and higher education, parent and youth-serving groups, legal advocacy, and public health organizations, the workgroup provided the foundation for the SMY project. Now in its fourth edition, the resource guide (Michigan Department of Education, 2005) delivers vital resources to educators and youth-serving organizations and has been disseminated to more than 1980 educators in Michigan and the nation. Finally, a total of 26 workshops have been implemented to reach over 880 educators in 175 school districts. Through the SMY initiative, Michigan learned that a strong coalition with passion and commitment can make progress in addressing a tough issue.

Together We Can Do More: Pooling and Leveraging Resources

It was no accident that teamwork became the philosophy and lifeline of Michigan's school health champions. This quote from baseball legend Babe Ruth is the embodiment of Michigan's work: "The way a team plays as a whole determines its success. You may have the greatest bunch of individual stars in the world, but if they don't play together, the club won't be worth a dime."

Michigan Action for Healthy Kids (MAFHK): The alarming trends of obesity and lack of physical activity among young people drew 12 state and other partner agencies together as part of the national Action for Healthy Kids (AFHK) initiative, which is dedicated to improving children's nutrition and physical activity in schools (http://www.actionforhealthykids.org). Members of MAFHK have moved swiftly to diffuse health innovations through local schools. The coalition has held more than a dozen statewide meetings and regional trainings; developed model local wellness, physical education, and healthy food and beverages policies; provided regional and statewide grants to build regional coalitions and assist local schools in their wellness efforts; trained facilitators to assist schools with assessment using the Healthy School Action Tool (HSAT); and, in partnership with the state Surgeon General, honored 190 schools over the last three years for making positive changes. They also created a Healthy Schools Healthy Students Web site (http://www. mihealthtools.org/healthyschools.asp) to register for HSAT, share success stories, conduct a student survey, or apply for the Healthy School Environment Award. Most impressive was the development of the Healthy School Toolkit to assist schools in moving to a CSHP. The toolkit contains data that make the case for healthy eating and physical activity, steps for conducting an assessment, guidance for developing and adopting policy, and ways to communicate success. More than

4,000 toolkits have been distributed and used by teachers and parents across the state.

Through teamwork, MAFHK has accelerated the pace of implementing health initiatives in schools. In 6 short years, it has become the clearinghouse for reliable information, tools, and resources needed to implement a CSHP in schools and earned the status of "school health central." The fact that it is the largest AFHK state coalition, with over 500 members, representing more than 200 Michigan public and private organizations, is a proof that "together we can do more." Michigan has proven that bringing together passionate, well-intended, action-oriented people will build capacity and sustainability, limit controversy, and sustain revenue streams.

Securing Additional Funding

American statesman Barry Goldwater said: "A government that is big enough to give you all you want is big enough to take it all away." Too often, promising programs disappear because funding is reduced or taken away. Michigan has experienced this firsthand. To maintain sustainable programs, state leaders have learned that additional funding is vital. Securing it requires resourceful, creative, and ongoing advocacy efforts. Additional funding creates more staffing positions, allows initiatives to expand, assists in addressing emerging health issues, can be a gateway to accessing more resources, and helps channel funding to districts and communities.

School Meals: In the USA, the US Department of Agriculture (USDA) provides funding and donated foods so that schools can offer nutritious meals to students. School nutrition services are one of the eight components of CSHP. The USDA-funded nutrition consultant provides leadership for nutrition services and works with local school food service directors to also make the school nutrition programs learning labs for healthy eating. Additional USDA funding was granted to support compliance with federal requirements of Public Law 108–265, 2004 (http://www.fns.usda.gov/TN/Healthy/108-265.pdf) to adopt and implement a local wellness policy.

School-Based Health Centers: The addition of school-based health centers to help provide health services (another of the eight components of CSHP) on school property has been critical to improving students' health. Families encountering barriers to accessing health care for their child could conveniently send their child to the center during the school day. In some communities, the health center has become a resource center where the entire family can use services that include case finding, screening, on-site primary health care, behavioral health services, health promotion/disease prevention education, and referral services. In 2004, Michigan was the first in the nation to secure a unique funding structure that allowed for state funds to be put up for federal match. In 2007/2008, this funding structure brought over $6.5 million into Michigan to help implement this component of CSHP.

Mental Health: Mental health in schools is an emerging need that requires additional attention and focus. A mental health grant of more than $375,000 was recently awarded by the federal Office of Safe and Drug-Free Schools for a collaborative project between the MDE, Michigan Department of Community Health (MDCH), Michigan Department of Human Services (MDHS), and the School Community Health Alliance of Michigan (SCHA-MI). Three school-based pilot sites will work directly with their local community mental health offices to increase access to mental health services for their students. The MDE will also partner with MDCH, the MDHS, and the nonprofit SCHA-MI to develop statewide policy to overcome barriers to mental health services for students. In addition, the funds will help build partnerships and system changes at the state and local levels to increase capacity, referral and follow-up procedures, and access to a formalized network of community providers. The hope is to eventually leverage additional resources to create a position within the MDE focused on the mental health component of the CSHP model.

Advocacy and the Power of Parents

For more than two decades, Michigan school health champions have been passionate change agents with a focus on the future. They have learned, however, that if others do not know about the work, it will become stagnant or cease altogether. Educating new legislators and decision makers about the importance of coordinated school health has become a key part of "the way we do business." Anyone can be an advocate - all it takes is dedication to informing, educating, and empowering others.

Michigan is a national leader in recognizing and utilizing the power of parents. The importance of parents has been understood ever since the early days of the model curriculum. In 2001, the $3.7 million that supported the school-based health centers was eliminated with a single executive order. Within days, advocates came together with a unified voice demanding reinstatement. Parents and students who were local school health advisory board members and consumers were so outraged that they protested on the lawn of the State Capitol. The pressure mounted with letters, editorials, and phone calls until the funding was fully restored. Advocacy saved the centers.

The belief in the power of parents has truly been embraced at the state level. Parents are given information and resources about how they can be school health champions on issues such as healthy snacks, the importance of physical activity, and effective school-based sex education. Conversely, school administrators and teachers are encouraged to see parents as crucial advocates and change agents for school health. Parents can be the most powerful voice in education since they are not bound by the same rules and restrictions that govern school employees.

In 2004, changes in sex education laws (http://www.michigan.legislature.gov) gave additional power to parents via district sex education advisory board membership and a complaint process. Parents embraced that power and induced change.

In a suburban school district with more than 15,000 students, a parent took the lead to work with a key administrator to reinstate sex education for all students in the district. In a rural district of 2,000 students, the parent majority on the sex education advisory board went beyond their charge of sex education and convinced the district to hire a new teacher for an added high school health education course. Once again, parents demonstrated their ability to effect change, despite budget challenges and pressure to keep the status quo.

The Power of a Champion: Selling School Health Through Leaders

Michigan is fortunate to have leaders in high-level positions who are passionate about school health and willing to take stands on controversial issues affecting the health and well-being of Michigan school-aged youth. The Healthy School Network (HSN) was funded by the CDC/DASH and led by the National Association of State Boards of Education. HSN reinforced Michigan's State Board of Education's (MSBE) belief in the importance of school health. In the words of the late champion and former MSBE President Beardmore (2002),

> ... [there is a] connection between health and learning and a gradually increasing understanding of the human and financial cost benefit of early intervention at the first sign of learning or health problems. Society cannot afford to wait to address the needs of children and their families.

In 2003, the MSBE adopted the first in a series of landmark policies to support the relationship between health and academic achievement. Topics included CSHP, comprehensive school health education, sex education, healthy food and beverages, physical education, wellness, tobacco-free schools, and bullying. The policies have provided vision and guidance to school districts, and they have shaped subsequent legislation.

History was made when the first-ever state Michigan Surgeon General (MSG) was appointed in 2003. Within a year, the *Michigan Surgeon General's Prescription for a Healthier Michigan* highlighted the importance of primary prevention in protecting families and communities (http://michiganfitness.org/Publications/documents/Rx-HealthierMI.pdf). The MSG became a spokesperson on physical activity, nutrition, and tobacco prevention through the statewide Michigan Steps Up campaign (http://www.michigan.gov/surgeongeneral), which gave credibility to existing CSHP efforts and established a recognition program – the Surgeon General's Healthy School Environment Award (http://www.mihealthtools.org/greatschools) – to highlight and reward the extraordinary efforts of local schools. Because of unwavering commitment to high-need communities, the MSG was instrumental in securing over $5 million from the W.K. Kellogg Foundation to empower youth to become peer leaders for making positive health choices. Once again, a high-level champion yielded impressive results.

Working Smarter: Using Data to Drive Decisions

Data drive decisions at all points in program planning, implementation, and evaluation. With limited resources, leaders need to focus energy on real school and community needs. At the state level, the MDE uses CDC's School Health Profiles (http://www.cdc.gov/healthyyouth/profiles/) and the Youth Risk Behavior Survey (YRBS) to provide a snapshot of the status of school health programs and student health risks in Michigan (http://www.cdc.gov/HealthyYouth/yrbs/index.htm). CDC's Division of Adolescent and School Health provides funding to states to conduct the YRBS and technical assistance for the YRBS and the School Health Profiles surveys. At the local level, districts use the Health Schools Action Tools – HSAT (http://www.mihealthtools.org) – and the Michigan Profile for Healthy Youth – MiPHY (http://www.michigan.gov/miphy).

The HSAT, developed in 2003, combined the best of the School Health Index from the CDC (http://apps.nccd.cdc.gov/shi/default.aspx) and Changing the Scene from the USDA (http://www.fns.usda.gov/TN/Healthy/changing.html). After considerable discussion and consensus building, the HSAT became the single assessment instrument endorsed by the Michigan Departments of Education and Community Health (MDE and MDCH), and a host of other partners in health and education. The mutual endorsement of HSAT provided a streamlined system of assessment for each of the eight component areas of CSHP, together with tools for gap analysis, planning, implementation, and sharing successes. To date, 400 schools have completed HSAT, impacting nearly 220,000 students; 800 additional schools are currently signed-on, with potential impact on approximately 353,000 students.

For many districts, data collection, needs assessment, and evaluation are difficult, avoided, or neglected tasks. In Michigan, the MDE and the MDCH have provided tools and technical assistance to make data collection a standard practice. The MiPHY was developed in 2005 to provide a standardized tool for local student needs assessment. The survey can be taken online by middle and high school students in one class hour; districts can receive results instantaneously. The MiPHY results, along with other school-reported data, help districts make data-driven decisions to improve prevention and health promotion programming and to meet specific needs assessment and reporting requirements of virtually any federal or state grant. In the 2007–2008 school year alone, 173 school buildings in 79 districts and 33 counties used the MiPHY data collection system.

Helping Schools Move Toward a Coordinated School Health Approach

Michigan has developed many resources that districts use to implement comprehensive and coordinated school health approaches. Thus, systems were developed to maximize their use at the district level including the following:

- Information dissemination via Web site, e-mail lists, and communication networks
- Development of a cadre of passionate "experts," spokespeople, and advocates
- Professional development, coaching, and technical assistance
- Financial incentives for districts to build capacity, buy-in, and sustainability
- Sharing of best practices and success stories via conferences, Web sites, and e-lists

For example, in 2004, the US president signed a law requiring all school districts that receive federal funding for school meals to establish a school wellness policy. MDE capitalized on this requirement with development of a model policy, statewide needs assessment, technical assistance for school districts, advocacy trainings for parents, and minigrants for student involvement. The systems developed to increase use of school health resources raised local compliance with the requirements in this multitiered initiative from 66% to well beyond 85%.

With the large number of districts in Michigan, MDE has needed to utilize all of these strategies to facilitate sex education program implementation in districts. Sex education is not mandated and is seen by some as controversial or peripheral to academic achievement, the core mission of schools. Nevertheless, Michigan has moved forward and implemented programs. For example, the regional school health coordinators formed an ad hoc sex education workgroup that has developed resource documents, planned annual professional development opportunities, and provided leadership in the promotion of the new or revised *Michigan Model for Health*® curricula. In addition, the MDE provided minigrants to district sex education advisory boards to review and recommend curricula aligned with research and best practice. Supplemental grant funds were used to support intensive technical assistance with local advisory boards. The technical assistance process provided districts with state-developed tools, but – even more important – it gave them structure, process, and motivation to use those tools to make concrete changes in the way sex education was delivered. The dialogue among various required constituencies on sex education advisory boards (e.g., parents, clergy, students, community health professionals) expanded to other key issues relevant to CSHP. For example, parents advocated for additional parent and community involvement through parent surveys as well as district-wide assessment of bullying and school climate.

Putting It All Together: MICHIANA

Michigan school health champions have made incredible progress. In 2004, enthusiasm was high, and there was optimism that the vision of CSHP would become a reality in all Michigan school districts. The MDE and the MDCH embarked on a joint venture with Indiana State Departments of Education and Health and the American Cancer Society (ACS) and launched the MICHIANA School Health

Leadership Institute. The goal of the five-year initiative was to assist a limited number of school districts in developing sustainable local CSHPs.

Replicating the success of earlier ACS School Health Leadership Institutes, 18 school districts, representing 98,000 students from 190 schools in Indiana and 49,000 students from 107 schools in Michigan, were selected to participate in MICHIANA. During the first three years, district teams of two to seven staff each participated in six semiannual trainings designed to provide team members with knowledge and skills needed to successfully implement and sustain a CSHP. Now, in the fourth year, districts in both states have experienced substantial successes. Michigan's successes include the following:

- Receipt of over $1.6 million in grant funding
- Implementation of five district policies regarding healthy vending machine choices and improved options in the cafeteria
- Passage of 24/7 tobacco-free campus policies
- Formation of eight district-wide CSH councils and 26 CSH building-level teams
- Opening of three school-based health centers
- Increased implementation of *Michigan Model for Health*® in eight districts

As a result of the success of the initial MICHIANA Institute, the ACS has committed to supporting another five-year institute that will reach approximately 20 new school districts. By pooling financial and human resources and maintaining support and commitment to the project, MICHIANA partners were able to have a greater impact in each state than any one partner could have accomplished alone.

Lessons Learned and Conclusion

If you can find a path with no obstacles it probably doesn't lead anywhere.
                                                                    Frank A. Clark

It has been challenging to help school districts change the way they do business and create a healthy school environment that supports learning. School professionals, like any other professionals, are comfortable working in their own silos and spheres of influence. With limited resources and increased accountability, however, schools are looking for creative ways to blend funding sources and increase efficiencies throughout the educational system. The coordinated school health approach encourages key stakeholders including the school board, school administrators, teachers, the food service director, school social workers and counselors, and parents to think about how they can collectively promote a healthier school community.

This chapter has highlighted landmarks in Michigan's journey toward a coordinated approach to school health. Champions have developed a statewide delivery system; expanded the vision of coordinated school health; created model policies, tools, and curricula; pooled and leveraged additional resources; capitalized on leaders and grassroots advocates; and facilitated implementation of CSHP in school districts and schools at the local level.

The school health journey has not always been easy. Leaders have learned important lessons that will continue to guide future efforts. They include the following: build relationships and trust with those at every level – from leaders to grassroots supporters; do not underestimate the "power of one"; work within the rules of systems, but look for opportunities to be flexible and move toward systemic change; meet people where *they* are; do not get stuck on what cannot be done – instead, focus on opportunities to make even the smallest of changes; remember that for every one step forward, there may be two steps backward; look at ways to change and improve how you do business; build capacity in communities by "teaching people to fish" rather than "giving them a fish"; include follow-up, mentoring, and coaching in professional development efforts; and, finally, be proactive rather than reactive – advocate before a crisis erupts.

Every locality has its own cast of characters, sets, and events, but the lessons learned from the Michigan experience are universal. With commitment and perseverance, champions can facilitate change in schools. The vision, however, must continue to be about young people. Success is ultimately measured by the ability to change the culture of schools to promote students' health and learning. Students deserve to learn and thrive in an environment that fosters mental, physical, and emotional well-being.

Acknowledgments Additional thanks to Carolyn Fisher, EdD, CHES, and Nancy Haney, MA, for their thoughtful edits on the chapter

References

Allensworth, D.D., & Kolbe, L.J. (1987). The comprehensive school health program: Exploring an expanded concept.*Journal of School Health, 57*, 409–412.

American Civil Liberties Union of Michigan & the Gay, Lesbian, and Straight Education Network of Detroit (2000). *What schools need to know: Gay, lesbian, bisexual and transgender students and the law. The rights and responsibilities of Michigan school administrators, educators, and school personnel regarding sexual orientation issues and the education of our gay, lesbian, bisexual, and transgender students.* Detroit, MI: Author.

Beardmore, D. (2002). *Keynote "healthy schools network ten year history".* National Association of State Boards of Education Annual Conference. San Diego, CA. Keynote given on October 9, 2002.

Broughman, S.P., & Swaim, N.L. (2006). *Characteristics of private schools in the United States: Results from the 2003–2004 Private School Universe Survey* (NCES 2006-319). U.S. Department of Education. Washington, DC: National Center for Education Statistics.

Michigan Department of Education. (2005). *A silent crisis: Creating safe schools for sexual minority youth.* Central Michigan University, Educational Materials Center. Mt. Pleasant, Michigan: Author.

Michigan Department of Education. (2007). *Local wellness policy implementation grant data report: Status of local wellness policy adoption and implementation among Michigan local education agencies.* Retrieved March 22, 2008, from http://www.michigan.gov/documents/mde/LWPGrantDataFinal_221612_7.pdf

Michigan Department of Education, Coordinated School Health and Safety Programs Unit. (2008). Unpublished data from the 2007 Youth Risk Behavior Survey.

Michigan Department of Education, Office of School Excellence. (2001). *The role of Michigan schools in promoting healthy weight: A consensus paper.* Retrieved March 22, 2008, from http://michigan.gov/documents/healthyweight_13649_7.pdf

Michigan in Brief. (2008). *Michigan facts.* Retrieved March 22, 2008, from www.michigan.gov

Michigan State Board of Education. (2005). *Model local wellness policy.* Retrieved March 22, 2008, from http://www.michigan.gov/documents/Policy_on_Welness_141434_7.pdf

State of Michigan, Center for Educational Performance and Information. (2005–2006). *Michigan graduation/dropout rates.* Retrieved March 22, 2008, from http://www.michigan.gov/cepi

State of Michigan, Center for Educational Performance and Information. (2007). *Free and reduced lunch rates.* Retrieved October 15, 2007, from http://www.michigan.gov/cepi

U.S. Congress Joint Economics Committee. (2008). *State by state reports, July 08: State median wages and unemployment rates.* Retrieved August 13, 2008, from http://jec.senate.gov/index.cfm?FuseAction = Reports.StateByState

U.S. Department of Education, International Affairs Staff. (2005). *Education in the United States: A brief overview.* Washington, DC: Author.

U.S. Department of Education, National Center for Education. (2005–2006). *Common core of data (CCD) survey, local education agency universe survey. Table 2. Number of public schools, by 2007 urban-centric local types and states, 2005–06.* Retrieved August 13, 2008, from http://nces.ed.gov/surveys/ruraled/TablesHTML/06_school_total.asp

U.S. Department of Education, National Center for Education Statistics. (2005–2006). *Public elementary and secondary school student enrollment high school completions, and staff from common core of data: School year 2005–06. Table 1. Public school student membership, by grade and state or jurisdiction: School year 2005–06.* Retrieved August 13, 2008, from http://nces.ed.gov/pubs2007/pesenroll06/tables/table_1.asp

U.S. Department of Labor, Bureau of Labor Statistics. (2007). *Unemployment rates for states.* Retrieved October 29, 2007, from http://www.bls.gov/news.release/pdf/laus.pdf

Chapter 13
Uruguay: Mainstreaming Health Promotion in Education Policies

Sergio Meresman

Contextual Introduction

Uruguay is a middle-income country with a population of 3.4 million; the population growth rate is 0.6%, and per capita income is US $3,790. However, Uruguay enjoys a literacy rate of 98%. Similarly, 98% of the population has access to potable water, a remarkable situation in comparison with Latin America averages.

Uruguay is characterized by an export-oriented agricultural sector and satisfactory levels of social spending. Its formal health and education systems have always been recognized as among the best in the region and are valued as some of the country's most precious assets.

Uruguayans are kind, well-mannered people. They can also be perceived as introverted, especially when compared with other, outgoing Latin American people. Uruguayan schools are typically overcrowded; most classrooms accommodate about 35 or 40 children for each teacher. Uruguayan boys love to play soccer whenever they can, so that is what they usually do in school breaks. Girls are sometimes welcome to join in the matches, or they walk hand-in-hand in small groups, jump hopscotch, or play an old-fashioned game called "rock-paper-scissors."

Education and Health Context

Free and universal access to all levels of education was introduced early in the twentieth century. The country attained universal primary education in the 1960s. Education spending tends toward equity, and 85% of primary schools are public.

S. Meresman
CLAEH (Latin American Centre for Humane Economy), UNER (University of Entre Rios), Montevideo, Uruguay

C. Vince Whitman and C.E. Aldinger (eds.),
Case Studies in Global School Health Promotion: From Research to Practice,
DOI: 10.1007/978-0-387-92269-0_13, © Springer Science + Business Media, LLC 2009

This is important because children in Uruguay tend to be born into lower-income households; the poorest 20% of families have 42% of the country's children.

Uruguay achieved universal education in the 1990s. Primary education coverage has reached 98%. In 2004, preschool coverage reached 90% of 5-year olds and 85% of 4-year olds. Special schools catering to the disadvantaged through extended school days and enriched programs increased from 58 in 1996 to 106 by 2004.

Uruguay's life expectancy at birth is 76 years, a figure currently exceeded by six Latin American countries. The main problems affecting the health status of the Uruguayan population stem from an aging population and the high prevalence of incommunicable diseases.

Uruguay is living through a time of major change. In 2002, Uruguay suffered from the effects of the economic crisis affecting its neighbors, Argentina and Brazil, and the economic situation deteriorated to an extent previously unknown. Poverty worsened between 2002 and 2004; the number of people living below the poverty line reached one-third of the population and 54% of children. More children in need, more complex education needs, and more issues generally related to disadvantaged contexts naturally became part of what school systems had to address and also affected the systems themselves.

In the context of increasing demands on schools, inclusive policies became more and more crucial at all levels. Many new needs emerged, and many social safety-net programs were implemented through the education system (e.g., expanding the number of school meal beneficiaries). Integrating health promotion approaches with essential health and education components and local development resources has become, more and more, a purposeful and decisive approach of schools.

Since 2005, Uruguay has been in the midst of an economic and political transition. The victory of a left-wing coalition in the general elections marked a new phase in the country's political history. Since the aforementioned economic crisis, the country has experienced a steady recovery, although unemployment is still high (around 13%) and poverty is close to 30% for the general population and 40% for children (Uruguayan National Institute of Statistics, 2006).

Overview of the School Health Program

Between 1994 and 2005 Uruguay implemented – with support from the World Bank – a comprehensive strategy to improve its basic education system. The strategy was devoted to expanding preschool education, building institutions (particularly teacher training reform and small grants to support the implementation of quality education projects administered by schools), and introducing a full-time-school model.

Between 2002 and 2004, the program supported the implementation of an Education for Life and Environment component [or *Educación para la vida y el ambiente (EVA)*] as well as Inclusive Education initiatives in more than 250 out of the country's 4,000 primary schools. The EVA project invited schools to identify, through a situation analysis, a specific health-related issue they wanted to change. Schools then received technical assistance and a number of resources to tackle their problem and improve the health and well-being of children and teachers.

All the typical Health-Promoting Schools components (improving school environments, strengthening health education contents and methods, improving the coordination between the school and other health and welfare services in the community) were included as possible strategies of action for schools to choose.

Assistance provided to participating schools included resources that were meant to benefit quality education in general, not just health and inclusion objectives. Technical and financial components included were the following:

- Technical assistance to formulate, implement, and evaluate theme- or problem-based projects identified by the school community
- Specialized technical assistance relating to health and environment issues, as a means to strengthen the project, build capacity among the teachers, and mobilize the school community to promote healthy environments and lifestyles
- Assistance in the development of course syllabi and educational materials for the courses selected by the schools
- School infrastructure renovation and development to create healthier, safer, and friendlier environments
- Participation in a network of exchanges of experiences and material, including a bimonthly electronic newsletter and two annual retreats

Specific Aspects of Implementation

Observations and questions related to the most significant implementation aspects and lessons learned from this project are summarized below.

1. *Mainstreaming health promotion and inclusive approaches into general educational policy.* One of the most remarkable characteristics of implementing Education for Health and Environment (EVA) is that it was inserted as a component into a sector-wide effort to transform education, rather than being a separate initiative. Health promotion concepts and practice were integrated into a general policy-making process that aimed at improving the quality of education and were implemented by the Uruguayan National Administration for Public Education, involving most schools and teachers in the country. This improved the project's actual chances of becoming sustainable and resulted in a significant reinforcement of the Uruguayan National Administration for Public Education's capacity to deliver health and environmental projects as part of the general education policy.

Today, it is more common for schools in Uruguay to have health and environmental education objectives included as part of their institutional improvement project, and the school community (teachers, students, and parents) is aware of the need and ways to improve children's living and development conditions in schools.

This change can be attributed to the schools' responses to the deteriorating economic conditions and to the policies and practices that became institutionalized.

The continuous encouragement to participating teachers to analyze, discuss, document, and exchange their understandings on the processes of implementing Education for Life and Environment has strengthened the culture of monitoring and evaluation amongst teachers and schools.

2. *Autonomy and sustainability.* In operational terms, schools have received technical support and seed money to develop a health promotion program while making a number of tangible changes at the level of the school's physical and educational environment, involving all groups in the school community in a participative manner.

The decentralized use and management of the resources made available by the component was in many cases the first opportunity for a school community to make autonomous decisions (management of resources has traditionally been highly centralized in Uruguay) and to commit to a plan for achieving results on the basis of their own strategies and skills. This in itself was an empowering experience and an institutional strengthening tool that provided schools with a sense of autonomy that was highly appreciated. The fact that schools had to prioritize their problems and focus on a single issue they wanted to address was also a learning and motivational experience.

Having to decide on the action track that was most meaningful in the context of their most relevant needs and their capacity to respond effectively was an opportunity to identify and mobilize the professional expertise available in the community, which again strengthened the feeling of "being able" to improve their situation using their own resources and increased sustainability of the whole implementation process.

3. *Education ownership.* It is very often assumed that Health-Promoting Schools is a health sector initiative. A frequent consequence of this view is the potential alienation of the education sector, leading to limited influence on education policy. EVA stressed from the very beginning the role of the education sector in leading and owning the initiative, placing project development at the heart of education policies and institutions. More than a few meetings were used to explain to colleagues and prominent health institutions that if the initiative was perceived by educators as pursuing health outcomes, or prioritizing the participation of health specialists, it would probably have very little effect on long-term education policies and their institutions. Teachers were always treated as the main stakeholders and the education authorities as the owners rather than as participants in the initiative.

Although our experience was limited to the administration of the EVA and Inclusive Education components, we tried actively to engage and collaborate as much as possible with all other parts of the strategy and the teams involved in the general education project, seeking all possible synergies and programmatic reinforcements. Convinced as we were that collaboration is what will make health promotion sustainable in schools, *all our efforts were directed toward integrating the program into the existing policies of improving teaching and learning and putting it into the hands of those who construct everyday life in the schools.*

4. *Participation*. Implementing participatory approaches to health in schools is often the biggest sticking point. While thousands of great content and technical resources are available in Uruguay and internationally, the actuality of having children participate directly and involving them in shaping health promotion and development projects is a challenge; it happens too rarely.

The EVA initiative stated clearly, in the many workshops and teacher training activities and materials, the need to involve children actively in the process of implementing health promotion activities. A range of specific opportunities for children's involvement in activities of high educational value were discussed, such as the following:

- Producing a situation analysis of school and community through consultation with children and the community
- Mapping issues that affect health and well-being, through problem trees
- Identifying things that could be changed in their school and planning strategies for change

All teachers agreed in principle with the concept of active education and participatory approaches to Health-Promoting Schools. The majority of children were also keen on the idea of getting involved, reacting enthusiastically to any opportunity to express their views, wishes, concerns, and creativity in favor of a healthier school. However, participatory approaches were rarely implemented beyond sporadic or particular opportunities. The demands of daily life in schools tend to be overwhelming for teachers and headmasters, and participation brings additional complexity. When resources (personnel, support, etc.) are limited and can support just the basic daily operation of schools, it is a constant struggle to introduce change and innovation. In our experience, at some point schools and teachers tended to impose *their* priorities and apply "pragmatic criteria" over students' suggestions.

School "health day" activities – in which children sing songs that praise the nutritional value of carrots – are the epitome of this kind of children's participation in school health projects.[1] Many times we disappointedly attended presentations in which children, who had been actively mobilized in the beginning, ended up playing a decorative role.

Similar situations tended to arise when parents were organized to *play their part*. Bringing people "from outside" the school to participate in health promotion activities was initially perceived as an additional resource, but careful coordination with school authorities was required so that they would not perceive themselves to be losing control of the dynamics of the project and feel alienated from it.

Most schools and teachers did not seem prepared to accept genuine participation. Institutional culture is a key factor: Authorities and civil servants are unaccustomed to sharing power. Public policy will have to actively pursue this cultural change, to

---

[1] To further explore the discussion on different uses and misuses of children's participation, see Roger Hart's (Hart, 1997) work.

create conditions for better long-term, real participation by children and families in
health promotion in schools.

Implementation in the Labyrinth of Words and Tools

According to the American College Dictionary, implementation is "a means of
achieving an end, an instrument or an agent." It signifies semantically *to put into
practical effect, carry out*. From its very definition, the word *implementation*
indicates the need to look at a correlation between means and ends. Hence, it puts
us in confrontation not only with what we do (how we act), but also with where
we go.

Choosing implementation as the theme for this collection of case studies implic-
itly points to an area of weakness in our work related to the definition itself. By
concentrating on this aspect, we acknowledge that implementation is a concern
with particular challenges and problems. Addressing implementation within the
initiative of promoting health in schools implies an examination of the gaps
between what we preach (the concepts) and what we practice (what we do, what
we get out of what we do, and, most important, where we go).

It is very important to consider the relationship between concepts and frameworks and what changes take place in schools' daily practice. In Uruguay, the
discourse of Health-Promoting Schools has been around for some time. When EVA
first began in 2001, teachers, health officials, and other key informants – whom we
interviewed for the purpose of outlining the strategy – recognized the Health-
Promoting School concept as "an idea promoted by the Pan American Health
Organization." Many regarded it as a valuable concept and ideal. There was a
degree of recognition, but also a mixture of ignorance and indifference, as to how to
put the concept into practice in their lives – the specific aspects of implementation.
There was also very little practical evidence or experience in implementing such a
concept.

It is necessary to consider this, as some concepts are very useful to project a
vision. However, concepts do not provide the tools and competencies that are
required for implementation. We know the value of symbolic efficacy: Words do
shape reality in many ways; for changes to actually occur, they first need to be
expressed. But words can also bewitch: It is necessary not to mistake words for
facts. Health-Promoting School can be a way for a school to name a vision, to
visualize itself in a way that combines needs, desires, and a work plan to achieve
them. But the concept or term can also be just a brand name, a decorative poster, or
a window dressing, in accordance with what an international organization says
"schools should be" and what children and teachers should and should not do.

When evaluating health promotion means and ends 20 years after the Ottawa
Charter, it is very important to separate the progress made by our discourse and
conceptual framework from the stalemate in which we find ourselves as an initiative
that aims to contribute to improving children's health and education. For instance,

public health has made appreciable and significant progress, adopting and using health promotion concepts in the mainstream public health discourse. The empty half of the cup relates to the scarcity of evidence that such concepts have become an integral part of policy and public health practice.

From the EVA experience in Uruguay, we have learned that there is no need for a program to be the initiative of health organizations and professionals or for a school to be named as "health promoting" by an external/international party for a community or school to embrace the spirit, accomplish the goals of improving the school's environment, promote healthy lifestyles, and develop a process of empowerment and self-determination among the children. There is no need for a strategy to be named a "network of health promoting schools," for example, to create a dynamic of innovation, exchange, and cooperation. In fact, it is only when those who are responsible for what is actually implemented within the school environment all-year-round have the objectives, means, and culture of health promotion that it actually can happen.

We have been asked (and have asked ourselves) many times if health promotion approaches and objectives were relevant in a context such as the one (characterized by the economic and institutional crises) that existed in Uruguay in 2002. We came to believe that health promotion – as a means of empowering people to gain control over the determinants of their living conditions – is even more relevant in a context of increasing hardships. The valid question is, "What kind of health promotion actions should a school prioritize: fostering 'healthy behaviors' in a context that strongly determines the actual choices of children and their families or promoting participatory action as a means to learn, to understand, and to address those determinants and change the options at stake?"

Acknowledgment The author had support from Education Development Center, Inc.

References

Hart, R. (1997). *Children's participation: The theory and practice of involving young citizens in community development and environmental care.* New York: UNICEF; London: Earthscan. (Also available in Chinese, Japanese and Spanish)

Uruguayan National Institute of Statistics. (2006). *Poverty and inequity in Uruguay* (in Spanish: Pobreza y desigualdad en Uruguay). Retrieved March 2008, from http://www.ine.gub.uy/biblioteca/pobreza/Informe%20pobreza%20y%20desigualdad.pdf

Chapter 14
Germany: Anschub.de – "Alliance for Sustainable School Health and Education"

Peter Paulus

Contextual Introduction

Educational and Health Indicators

Germany is a federal republic of 16 states and 82.3 million inhabitants. The general education system includes 9,356,000 pupils, with 668,300 teachers, in 36,300 schools. About 10% of the pupils leave school without completing the lowest level of high school (there are three different levels of high school in Germany). This percentage is much higher in pupils from migrant families. Nearly one-fifth of the population has a migration background and 8.8% are migrants. The unemployment rate is 9.1% (7.1% in the under-25 group) and 18.6% in the migrant population.

Concerning the health status of children and adolescents, the German Health Interview and Examination Survey for Children and Adolescents (www.kiggs.de), which was conducted from 2003 to 2006 and included a population-based sample of 17,641 of ages 0–17, revealed much new information. It made very clear the strong connection between health behavior, on the one hand, and health status and social status, on the other. Related to this, educational research (e.g., 2003 Program for International Student Assessment) has shown that the German educational system is very selective. Pupils from lower-income or migrant families have a much smaller chance of reaching higher levels of education. Inclusive strategies, from either the health or the educational perspective, can support each other and promote positive child and youth development. Following this line of thinking, the linking of health interventions with educational aims and objectives seems to be a very reasonable strategy.

P. Paulus
Institute for Psychology, Center of Applied Sciences of Health (CASH), and MPH Program Prevention and Health Promotion, Leuphana University of Lueneburg, Lueneburg, Germany

C. Vince Whitman and C.E. Aldinger (eds.),
Case Studies in Global School Health Promotion: From Research to Practice,
DOI: 10.1007/978-0-387-92269-0_14, © Springer Science + Business Media, LLC 2009

Brief History and Context for the Case and Date Boundaries

Anschub.de, an alliance for sustainable school health and education in Germany, is planned as a nationwide program in Germany. The core target groups of the program are pupils, teachers, and parents, and also the responsible bodies for schools in the community, in the educational and health ministries, and in the administration. At the moment, Anschub.de covers four out of the 16 German states. It is built up as local or regional school networks. Nine networks are in place with more than 200 schools of different types, including about 70,000 pupils and 5,500 teachers, mostly primary (30%) and lower secondary schools (15%). The networks of schools are supported by local or regional steering groups. The steering group consists of a coordinator and supporting governmental (e.g., Ministries of Education, Ministries of Nutrition and Consumer Protection) and non-governmental organizations (e.g., health insurers, local accident insurance associations, health promotion agencies). At the national level, there is an alliance of more than 40 institutions, most of which are actively involved in school health promotion and education nationally. This alliance supports activities in school health promotion and education from the national level down to the regional or local level. The alliance has a Web site (www.anschub.de).

Anschub.de was established in 2002 by the Bertelsmann-Foundation (Germany) and will run as a program until the end of 2010. In the beginning, more than 60 national institutions, organizations, associations, and prominent researchers were invited to three expert forums. They discussed health problems of school-aged children, health of teachers, school health and educational problems, demands on the school system, and individual schools in Germany. They also discussed strategies from different professional and disciplinary perspectives on how to cope with the problems related to school health and education. Most of those attending formed the above-mentioned alliance and produced a mission statement in 2003. This alliance will be transformed in 2008 into a formal association at the national level: "Anschub.de – Program for the good and healthy school." Negotiations with the potential partners are under way. This will be a reliable structure for future developments of the good and healthy school.

Key Cast of Players/Agencies

The members of the Anschub.de alliance come from different fields: (a) Ministries of Education, Social Affairs and Food, Agriculture, and Consumer Protection; (b) health and accident insurers; (c) teacher training institutes; (d) professional organizations of teachers, psychologists, and architects; (e) drug-abuse prevention agencies; (f) the National Association of Child Guidance Centers; (g) National Sport Youth Association; (h) the National Associations of Pupils and Parents; (i) NGOs for health promotion; and more.

Overview of the School Health Program

Vision and Challenges

Anschub.de is innovative in three ways: *First of all, it has created a national alliance of supporting organizations and experts in school health promotion and education.* This has never been done before in Germany. Over the last 15 years of school health promotion, teachers and schools have been the main target groups. They were invited and trained to develop their schools in the direction of Health-Promoting Schools. Now decision makers from school administration and education or health-related organizations and associations at the state and federal levels, as well as private companies are invited. Accordingly, Anschub.de acquires political power, and the decisions that are made influence and change school health promotion much more than before, because the level of action is different. These are strategic partners in an endeavor to support schools. The idea is that schools cannot develop solely from the bottom up with input from enthusiastic people. Schools also need powerful and long-lasting support from the top down. Formation of this alliance is also driven by the idea that support for schools is not only the obligation of school ministries and administration; it also needs coordinated action from all the organizations that have a (legal) responsibility or that feel a social responsibility to support pupils, teachers, nonteaching staff, and schools in general. Schools thereby experience stronger and wider support for what they are doing, than through ministerial support alone.

The challenge for Anschub.de is to overcome conflicting intentions of partners and to establish a cooperative structure that can produce synergetic effects. The first step was to establish the above-mentioned three forum meetings with the initial group of interested entities. They created a basis of shared understanding of relevant problems in the area of school health promotion. To assess this aspect further, an economic evaluation was undertaken. It revealed for each individual partner of the alliance what it would cost to cooperate in and with Anschub.de, compared to doing the same projects alone. This evaluation was based on the Nash Equilibrium of game theory in economics. It showed that it makes sense to the partners in economic terms to be part of the alliance. This is the first step in the direction of a more rigorous evaluation from an economic perspective. This has never been done before in Germany in the area of school health promotion.

Second, Anschub.de has created a new concept for school health promotion in Germany, the concept of the "good and healthy school." This concept links health interventions in schools directly to the activities that schools must carry out to meet the quality criteria of good schools. Seen in this way, health is an input or throughput factor, not an output or outcome factor. The aim of the good and healthy school is, therefore, the promotion of the educational quality of school through health interventions. In school health education, health is conceptualized as health literacy, which is an output factor. And even health education has to show how it contributes not only to certain health outcomes that are part of a good school, but also to educational outcomes of the school in general. The challenge here is to communicate this new direction of health promotion and education in the health and educational system. Many professional people are still of the opinion that Anschub.de is a type of school health promotion program they already know, that is, making schools, teachers, and pupils healthier.

To communicate the difference, and to attract the interest of all those schools and teachers with the desire to be good schools and teachers, is no small challenge in a world where schools are confronted with excessive advertising, information, and ministerial or administrative demands. Anschub.de has created a communication strategy to overcome those barriers inside and outside the school. One of the key points is to involve pupils more in the process of developing a good and healthy school. Another is to ask teachers and parents what they know about and how they experience Anschub.de. This supplies information on the attitudes, beliefs, and values such persons attach to Anschub.de. Anschub also has created more than ten new modules for heads of schools, for classroom teachers, and for parents to support them in building up a good and healthy school and healthy learning and teaching. And it has produced a fan-fold document and a brochure (both also available in English), which inform the target audiences and the general public about the good and healthy school concept, values, principles, and strategies.

Third, Anschub.de has created a new form of cooperation in school health promotion. Networks of schools supported by a local or regional steering group consisting of strong and influential governmental organizations (GOs) and non-governmental organizations (NGOs) (e.g., parents or pupils associations) as partners are fairly new in Germany. The challenge here is to build up such steering groups and keep them working in a community setting. Anschub.de has developed a set of modules for the training of coordinators of these networks, qualifying them for networking and supporting schools, teams of teachers, parents, pupils, and others involved in the development of their good, healthy schools. Coordinators who are chosen for training should preferably come from positions such as school psychologists, school development specialists, or experienced teachers. Anschub. de tries to use existing structures of school support. Cooperation with regional in-service teacher training institutes has started to integrate modules of the good and healthy school into their formal curriculum.

Specific Aspects of Implementation

Self-Evaluation

The schools in Anschub.de evolve in Deming cycles that are very similar to the typical stages in the process of implementing an evidence-based program. They use an instrument called Self-Evaluation in Schools (SEIS), which encompasses relevant quality dimensions of the good school:

- Fulfillment of educational tasks} (Outcome dimension)
- Learning and teaching process}
- Leadership and management process} (Process dimensions)
- Climate/culture}
- Satisfaction} (Outcome dimension)

These dimensions are further characterized by criteria that give a more detailed picture. Indicators show how these criteria can be identified. Figure 1 represents the quality dimensions of SEIS with its criteria (www.das-macht-schule.de). This concept of school quality is used in several federal states of Germany and in the Anschub.de program as well.

Every 2 or 3 years, in the spring, teachers, parents, and pupils fill out a questionnaire, which is a part of that instrument. In a guided process of triangulation, using discussion on the questionnaire results, the school defines its educational

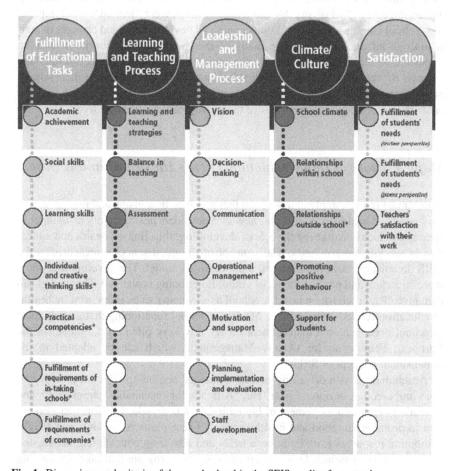

Fig. 1 Dimensions and criteria of the good school in the SEIS-quality framework

problems, assets, and action priorities for the next school year, starting in August. Health interventions are selected that support the school development process or address health education outcomes directly. Schools use the modules as teaching material (e.g., module for drug prevention in primary schools, module for healthy eating) or as training material for teachers (e.g., module for teachers' health) or as support for school management (e.g., module for facility management for head of schools, quality physical activity school program); or they create interventions on their own (e.g., inviting experts from outside the school, rearranging the classroom or schoolyard together with pupils). All these actions are documented by the school and are also used for process and outcome evaluation by an external evaluation agency. Anschub.de has developed its own outcome measures; it also uses other, well-established questionnaires and interview measures.

Evaluation results comparing the development of 43 schools in 2003 and 2007 showed that they carried out several hundred health interventions related to the quality dimensions of the good school. Initially, most of them aimed at "leadership and management," while in 2007 more interventions were directed toward improving "school climate and ethos." Pupils perceived developments and changes in their schools in all dimensions and in many of the more specific criteria. This is an important result, because pupils are the main target group, next to teachers and parents. By recognizing that good health creates an improvement in their school, pupils demonstrate having learned a great deal about the role of health and the contribution of health interventions to the quality of their (school) lives.

Major Factors of Implementation Theory Illustrated in this Case

Anschub.de is an example of a program that is driven by a vision and the big idea of the "good and healthy school." This new idea considers health mainly as an input or throughput factor that keeps the school developing, thus linking health and education in schools more directly. The concept of the good school represented in the SEIS dimensions is, at the moment, a dimensional model. The development into a more structural and process model of school functioning is planned. That model can then give clearer advice on how the school as a system can be influenced by health- or education-related interventions. Models of school functioning that already exist in school organizational management theory rely very often on the model of the European Foundation for Quality Management, which can be adapted to the dimensional concept of SEIS.

Anschub.de is also driven by several elements, beginning with *national guidelines and creation of a movement*. The "Alliance for sustainable school health and education" creates a movement of big national partners who will form an association to promote the good and healthy school. These partners are GOs and NGOs, combining resources from both these fields and also from educational, health, and private sectors. Anschub.de is also an example of a program that takes its starting point from its *adaptation to local concerns* – for instance, it has a local or regional steering group and school health teams. Further, it relies on *data-driven planning and decision making*, for example, through the SEIS self-evaluation tool and external formative evaluation. Self-evaluation on a regular annual basis strengthens the school development process. These are the most relevant and most characteristic elements of Anschub.de. What is missing in Anschub.de is close cooperation within a local or regional school network, which itself is linked to community planning and development.

Conclusion: Reflection for Implementation

Anschub.de has a greater chance of implementing a sustainable movement in school health promotion and education in Germany than any earlier initiatives. The link between the health and education sectors, the strong direction in the promotion of educational quality of schools, the vertical cooperation of single schools (bottom-up) and nationwide operating organizations (top-down) in an alliance, and the cooperation of schools at the local level in a network of schools and partners give Anschub.de an unusual strength. What is needed at the local or regional level is a coordinating person who can bring all these activities together to form a synergetic effect and can link it with other ongoing initiatives at the local or regional level (e.g., community development). Such sizable implementations need time, a vigorous management, and sufficient financial opportunities to have significant impact on school health promotion and education. Eight years for the Anschub. de pilot would seem to be an adequate and suitable time scale.

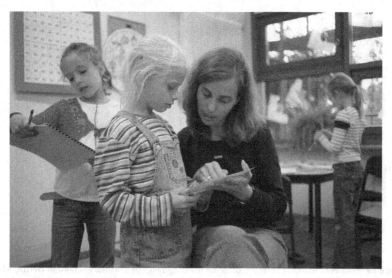

Picture 12 Students working on self-directed learning tasks in a primary school in Berlin, which is part of the Anscub. de – program

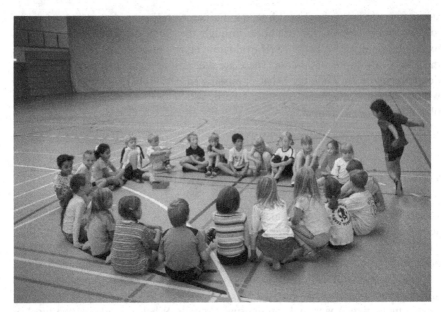

Picture 13 Students working on self–directed leaning tasks in a primary school in Berlin, which is part of the Anschub. de – program

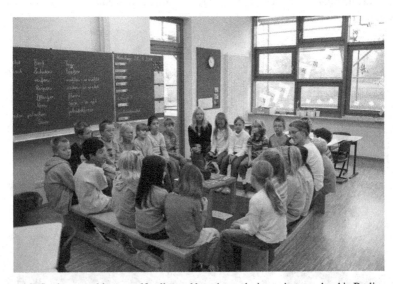

Picture 14 Students working on self – directed learning tasks in a primary school in Berlin, which is part of the Anschub. de – program

References

Bockhorst, R. (2005). Schulen in Bewegung. Gesundheit als Motor für Schulentwicklung. Forum Bildungsqualität, Heft 2, 24–25

Nilshon, I. & Schminder, Ch. (2005). Die gute gesunde Schule gestalten. Stationen auf dem Weg der Schulprogrammentwicklung. Gütersloh: Bertelsmann-Verlag

Paulus, P. Gröschell, M. & Bockhorst, R. (2002). Anschub.de – Allianz für nachhaltige Schulgesundheit und Bildung. Prävention, 25(3), 75–77

Paulus, P. (2003). Schulische Gesundheitsförderung – vom Kopf auf die Füße gestellt. Von der Gesundheitsfördernden Schule zur "guten gesunden Schule". In K. Aregger & U. Lattmann (Hrsg.). Gesundheitsfördernde Schule – eine Utopie? Konzepte, Praxisbeispiele, Perspektiven (S. 93–114). Luzern: Sauerländer

Paulus, P. (2006): Psychische Gesundheit. Rückgrat für die Seele. In Fritz, A.; Klupsch-Sahlmann, R. & Ricken, G. (Hrsg.). Handbuch Kindheit und Schule. Neue Kindheit, neues Lernen, neuer Unterricht (S.138–148). Weinheim: Beltz

Paulus, P. (2007a). Die gute gesunde Schule. Mit Gesundhit gute Schule machen. Gütersloh/ Wuppertal: Bertelsmann/Barmer Ersatzkasse

Paulus, P. (2007b). Schulische Gesundheitsförderung – auf dem Weg zur guten gesunden Schule. In Röhrle, B. (Hrsg.). Prävention und Gesundheitsförderung. Band III. Kinder und Jugendliche (S. 323–345). Tübingen: dgvt-Verlag

Paulus, P, (2007c). 20 Years of health promotion research in and on settings in Europe – the case of school health promotion. Italian Journal of Public Health, 2007, 4(4), 108–114

Paulus, P. (2008). Aktuelle Konzepte schulischer Gesundheitsförderung . Eine neue Perspektive durch Anschub.de – ein Programm für die "gute gesunde Schule" . Moderne Ernährung heute, Heft 2, 1–8

Stern, C. Ebel, Ch., Vaccaro, E. & Vorndran, O. (Hrsg.) (2006). Bessere Qualität in allen Schulen Praxisleitfaden zur Einführung des Selbstevaluationsinstruments SEIS in Schulen. Gütersloh: Bertelsmann-Verlag

Chapter 15
Kosovo: A Health-Promoting Schools Approach to Reduce the Risks of Lead Poisoning and to Establish Cross-Ethnic Collaboration

Ian Young and Ardita Tahirukaj

Contextual Introduction

On 17 February 2008, Kosovo declared itself an independent state. Since then, several countries have recognized its new status, but others, such as Serbia and Russia, have not. This case study describes activities that took place in the years leading up to the declaration of independence, when Kosovo was a United Nation's Administered Province with Provisional Institutes of Self-Government, divided into five administrative regions encompassing 30 municipalities. Kosovo has a population of approximately two million people. The proportion of children of school age and younger is almost one-half of the population, and 37% are under 14 years of age.

The conflict in the Balkans in 1999 and also the gradual deterioration of conditions left Kosovo with severe problems in its infrastructure, local capacity, and relationships among the main ethnic groups. Environmental pollution has left a legacy of severe heavy metal contamination in specific, heavily populated industrial areas.

As a response to the environmental contamination and its impact on human health, WHO, in collaboration with local institutions, worked towards by establishing sustainable structures to implement a comprehensive program of activities that will raise awareness of and decrease exposure to the complex problem of pollution from metal lead and other poisonous heavy metals. Industrial pollution from heavy metal smelting activities is one of the main sources of this pollution. WHO collected and analyzed soil samples in Mitrovica/ë and Zvecan municipalities; over 90% of the samples had lead higher than the safe limits (Dutch List, 1999).

I. Young(✉)
Health Promotion consultant, Edinburgh, Scotland, UK, e-mail: imyoung@blueyonder.co.uk

C. Vince Whitman and C.E. Aldinger (eds.),
Case Studies in Global School Health Promotion: From Research to Practice,
DOI: 10.1007/978-0-387-92269-0_15, © Springer Science + Business Media, LLC 2009

Addressing the lead pollution that affects both the Albanian and Serbian communities is considered to be one of the practical ways to unify the efforts of the two communities in the divided city of Mitrovica/ë. This chapter describes how the Health-Promoting School model has played a strategic role in attempting to address the environmental contamination and, also, a role in rebuilding the damaged human relationships that resulted from a bitter conflict.

The Problem

Mitrovica/ë had the largest metallurgic and mining complex (Trepca) in Europe, which began its activities in 1939 with the extraction of lead, cadmium, and zinc. Many industrial plants existed in the complex: a huge lead smelter, a fertilizer production plant, a refinery, a battery factory, a zinc electrolysis facility, and a sulfuric acid plant. These industries released high concentrations and a wide range of pollutants known to be associated with the health risks of all the population and particularly for children and pregnant mothers.

The complexes were shut down in July 2000; however, lead and other heavy metals (cadmium, nickel, arsenic, and zinc) from the abandoned sites and contaminated soil from the decades of mining and smelting activities have continued to pollute the environment and to pose a health threat to the population.

A survey carried out during and after the closing of the plant in 2000 showed high levels of lead contamination in the blood of children, adults, and pregnant women in the area (Molano & Andrejew, 2000).

In 2002, WHO carried out preliminary assessments of environmental samples, which showed excessive levels of lead and other heavy metals in soil, dust, paint, and some locally grown vegetables. Drinking water appeared to be within acceptable limits.

In 2004, WHO's Risk Assessment to assess exposure pathways and ongoing impact revealed high blood lead levels in children, with those from 2 to 3-years-old causing greatest concern. The "acceptable" level of lead in blood is 10 mcg/dL (US Department of Health and Human Services, 2000). In the areas assessed; 58% of those tested were above this level in Zvecan, 40% in North Mitrovica/ë, and 15% in South Mitrovica/ë.

This is a serious risk to the health and education of children, because the developing brain and nervous system are very vulnerable to damage by lead poisoning. Studies have reported a strong association between high lead levels in children's bodies and lowered IQ, impaired attention, and speech performance (Needleman, 1993).

The threat to the future of the population and the area is also serious because of the effects on the developing fetus as well as on young children. A pregnant woman will pass lead directly to her fetus through the placenta (Groszek, 2002);

this is especially important in a population with a high birth rate, such as Kosovo. Lead can stay in bones for 30 years; during times of increased calcium needs, such as in pregnancy, an increase in the release of lead from the bones can occur.

Because of the consequences of the conflict and a subsequent lack of financial investment, Kosovan schools must address significant physical infrastructure issues. For example, some schools are not completely weatherproofed, and some schools require up to four shifts per 24 h to accommodate all their students.

The above problems are particularly acute in Mitrovica/ë, where the displacement of population has resulted in great pressure on school buildings. However, despite the issues of a poor working environment for many students and teachers and the modest salaries of teaching staff, the schools show a positive and purposeful atmosphere and great energy to improve the situation. This good spirit probably relates to the fact that improvements have occurred and that there is an expectation that Kosovo's political status will be resolved in some way soon. Some new school buildings have been provided, and there is considerable pride in this achievement, although maintenance budgets are limited.

The Response: Building the Health-Promoting School Network

In collaboration with local institutions, WHO is currently implementing a program of activities in the Mitrovica/ë area, with funding from the Dutch and Norwegian governments. Activities aim to raise population awareness of the environmental pollution caused by heavy metals and to decrease exposure. Through local capacity building, local cross-ethnic and inter-sectoral working groups are carrying out health risk assessments, a public awareness campaign, the development of a health strategy (screening, diagnosis, and management protocols), and environmental remediation activities.

The public-awareness working group chose the Health-Promoting School approach as a main tool for raising population awareness on how to live more safely in a contaminated environment. The working group includes officials from different sectors such as health, education, environment, women's associations, the Institute of Public Health, and the Trepca Institute. Both ethnic groups, Albanian and Serbian, are represented on this working group.

This multi-sectoral method of implementation aims to improve the environment of schools through environmental health risk management activities (cleaning and greening activities). Through collaboration, activities also raise awareness in the community and local institutions about environmental problems, their health effects, and methods to decrease exposure. Building the capacity of health and education personnel and providing opportunities for professional development have been shown to be effective strategies in the development of Health-Promoting Schools in other countries (Young & Williams, 1994).

In this short case description, we have chosen to focus on a few major strategies that played a key role in the implementation: A multi-sectoral approach has been used, together with capacity building at the national, municipal, and school levels. For example, at the national level, an Inter-Ministerial Committee on Health-Promoting Schools has been established; it includes representatives from the Ministry of Health; the Ministry of Education, Science, and Technology; the Ministry of Environment; the Institute of Public Health; the Ministry of Youth, UNICEF, International Organization for Migration (IOM); and WHO.

The Ministry of Education, Science, and Technology; the Ministry of Health; the Ministry of Youth, Culture, and Sports; and the Ministry of Environment and Spatial Planning formalized their commitment in a Memorandum of Understanding, stating they would:

- Develop policy and ensure inter-ministerial collaboration in the areas of health education and health promotion
- Promote a healthy school environment, where pupils can acquire new knowledge and skills
- Improve and strengthen the partnerships between the school, parents, and community, with all agencies having a positive role in the welfare of all (See Fig. 1)

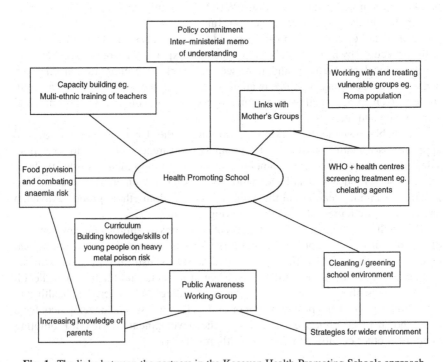

Fig. 1 The links between the partners in the Kosovan Health-Promoting Schools approach

Kosovo has a relatively small, but very active, network of Health-Promoting Schools, which have the support of these four government departments, a national coordinator, and a national coordinating committee that represents all key stakeholders. Kosovo has developed a progressive, flexible school curriculum, which has the potential to provide an excellent framework for health education and promotion in the future. There is a great opportunity to develop a health education curriculum, which meets the purpose of these reforms. Senior staffs in the Ministry of Education recognize that developing this curriculum is important for the future of Kosovo and its young people.

There is also a well-established network of UNICEF, Child Friendly Schools, which offers a whole-school approach to the health and welfare of young people. In addition, a UNICEF lifeskills program offers a curriculum-based initiative with a strong health component. Research surveys have been undertaken in Kosovo relating to specific topics or identified problems, for example, substance use and blood lead levels.

The European Network of Health Promoting Schools (ENHPS) has considerable experience in building sustainability into the program. Kosovo has managed aspects of this very well; the next stage will be to increase the number of schools in the network. The UNICEF Child Friendly Schools initiative has built a larger network of 130 schools; they are now sharing ideas with the ENHPS group and acquiring experience about how to build a sustainable program within schools.

The core values of the new partnership initiative can be summarized as follows:

– Respect for self
– Respect for others (ethnicity, religion, etc.)
– Respect for the environment
– Using a whole-school approach that links with

  • Curriculum
  • Family
  • Community
  • Other specialist agencies, including the health sector

– Respect for life-long learning, which has great potential, given the age distribu
  tion of the population
– Belief that only healthy individuals can fully benefit from education and that
  education can develop life skills and health literacy

Kosovo developed a logframe (logical framework) as the context for planning the Health-Promoting Schools. This is an important step forward in linking the vision of "full physical, psychological, and social well-being for all students of Kosovo" (Tahirukaj, 2007), with strategic objectives and indicators of achievement. However, this logframe will need further development and revision, as some of the indicators of success appear too modest. For example, one objective is that all schools will have potable drinking water and sanitation by 2017. A decade seems much too long a time to wait for a basic public health provision that needs more urgent attention. Kosovo will be looking at new developments within the ENHPS, which has been exploring indicators of effectiveness and provides case studies from a range of European countries (Barnekow et al., 2006).

There has been a considerable investment in professional development and training. For example, WHO organized a four-day, multi-ethnic training seminar for teachers; school directors; and representatives from the Ministry of Health, the Ministry of Education, the Ministry of Environment, the Institute of Public Health, women's associations, and the Trepca Institute. This seminar was of considerable symbolic importance, as it was the first time that representatives of both communities – Kosovo Albanians and Kosovo Serbs - had trained together in any educational sphere since the conflict. The objectives of this training seminar were the following:

- Train teachers, school directors, and key stakeholders in the Health-Promoting Schools approach, with specific reference to issues related to the heavy metal contamination of the environment
- Raise awareness and generate the support of community stakeholders
- Pilot the translation of the training manual, *Promoting the Health of Young People in Europe* (Young & Williams, 1994), and associated training methods

At school level the appointed coordinators and teachers received training that included the following:

- Identifying ways to include environmental health in the school curriculum
- Exploring methods, such as "starting from where children are" (Wetton & McCoy, 1998), regarding their knowledge on environment pollution, and reviewing how the school, children, and their families can contribute to improving the school and community environment
- Helping schools to make links with parents, mothers' groups, and health personnel
- Exploring technical methods, such as nutritional approaches, to reduce the anemia associated with lead poisoning
- Exploring technical methods to reduce exposure in the children's home environment and in the school and its immediate environment
- Increasing community participation in the solution of environmental health problems

As part of the capacity building of local professionals who were working in the public awareness campaign, a study visit to Slovenia and Poland was organized. The purpose of the visit to Slovenia and Poland was to develop links with institutions in these countries that are involved in environmental research, environmental remedial actions, and public awareness programs.

Conclusions

This program is at an early stage but has made considerable progress over the last 4 years. The Health-Promoting School model has proven to be suitable for developing the approach to a highly specific problem, such as children's exposure to an environmental hazard. Schools, for the most part, are excellent vehicles to reach the at-risk target groups of children and pregnant mothers. In addition, the parents, the children's environment, and the health services are accessible through the schools. The educational role of schools makes it possible to inform children and families about the ways to minimize exposure to pollutants in the young people's environment. The whole-school approach can also play a part in minimizing the effects of exposure on the body through multiple strategies. For example, appropriate nutritional advice and food provision in schools can reduce the risks of the anemia associated with lead poisoning. The activities in schools also generate media coverage of the heavy metal pollution, which helps to reach more of the general population.

However, the model of this development is not merely about schools being a convenient venue for public health initiatives. This is not a short-term project, but a sustained attempt to integrate education and health issues for the benefit of young people in Kosovo. The Kosovo HPS strategy has been developed for the years 2007–2017, and the Health-Promoting Schools program is also included in the Kosovo Education Policy/Strategy as well as in the Kosovo Development Plan for 2007–2015. The strategy has been developed by an inter-ministerial committee with the participation of schools and young people. The strategy also integrates related initiatives such as Child Friendly Schools and life skills with violence prevention and mental health promotion under the overarching concept of Health-Promoting Schools.

The government support with a signed agreement between the ministries, the national coordinator, and the coordinating committee is an indicator of the potential for a sustainable development. At a training seminar in Mitrovica/ë, the teachers showed considerable enthusiasm for, and commitment to, the program despite the daily problems they have to overcome. A significant part of the credit for this achievement is due to the WHO Office in Pristina, which has provided leadership, actively promoted this work, and helped to put in place some of the features that build this sustainable approach.

As a result of increased awareness, knowledge, skills, local capacity building, improved environmental health conditions, and increased individual and community empowerment, Kosovo is hoping to deal both with the source of the problem and with minimizing the effects of the existing pollution. Blood lead levels and levels of pollution in the environment will continue to be monitored. In the interim, it is clear that the development of joint training in health-promoting schools is one small but important way in which the two ethnic groups can work together to improve trust and relationships for the future.

Acknowledgments The authors dedicate this paper to all those working in Kosovo to improve the health and environmental problems that affect all people irrespective of their ethnic origins.

The WHO Office in Pristina and Kosovo HPS Inter-Ministerial Advisory Committee acknowledge the valuable and extensive contributions of Ian Young in the development of the HPS Program and training of the officials from health, education, environment sector, school directors, and teachers on HPS approach.

WHO Office in Pristina also thanks Gay Gray, Katerina Sokou, and Lina Kosterova Unkovska, whose expertise contributed to the training of teachers, health, and environment officials.

References

Barnekow, V., Buijs, G., Clift, C., Jensen, B. B., Paulus, P., Rivett, D., & Young, I. (2006). *Health-promoting schools: A resource for developing indicators.* Copenhagen, Denmark: ENHPS, International Planning Committee, WHO Regional Office for Europe.

Groszek, B. (2002). *Guidelines for the prevention and identification of lead poisoning in pregnant and postpartum women.* Pristina, Kosovo: World Health Organization.

Molano, S., & Andrejew, A. (2000). *Report on first phase of public health project on lead pollution in Mitrovica Region.* Mitrovica, Kosovo: UNMIK.

Needleman, H. L. (1993). The current status of childhood low-level lead toxicity. *Neurotoxicology 14*(2–3), 161–166.

New Dutch List [of hazardous chemicals]. (1999). Retrieved in 2002 from http://www.contaminatedland.co.uk/std-guid/dutch-l.htm

Tahirukaj, A. (Ed.) (2007). *Kosovo Health Promoting Schools strategy 2007–2017.* Pristina, Kosovo: World Health Organization.

US Department of Health and Human Services. (2000). *Healthy people 2010.* Washington, DC: US Department of Health and Human Services. Retrieved in 2002 from http://www.health.gov/healthypeople.

Wetton, N., & McCoy, M. (1998). *Confidence to learn.* Edinburgh, Scotland: NHS Health.

Young, I., & Williams, M. (Eds.) (1994). *Promoting the health of young people in Europe: A training manual for teachers and others working with young people.* Copenhagen, Denmark: WHO Regional Office for Europe.

Chapter 16
Poland: The Health-Promoting School National Certificate

Barbara Woynarowska and Maria Sokolowska

Contextual Introduction

Background

Poland is a country in Central Europe, bordered by Germany to the west; the Czech and Slovak Republics to the south; Belarus and Ukraine to the east; and Lithuania, Russia, and the Baltic Sea to the north. It is one of the largest countries in Europe covering 312,685 km². For administration Poland is divided into 16 regions (voivodships), 379 districts (*powiaty*), and 2,478 local government communes (*gminy*). Poland is a member of the Council of Europe (since 1991) and European Union (since 2004).

The period of political transformation to multiparty democracy and a market economy started in 1989. Successful economic reforms have come alongside, with sustained GDP growth rate at over 6%. The unemployment rate decreased in the last years from 19.6% in 2003 to 13.8% in 2006. A serious problem is the youth unemployment rate, which is 29.6% for ages 20–24.

Poland's population at the end of 2006 was above 38 million, of whom about 8 million were under 18 years. About 61% of Poles lived in urban areas. The overwhelming majority of the population is native Poles and Roman Catholic.

School System

Full-time compulsory education lasts 10 years, including education in "grade 0" (the year of preparation for primary education, obligatory for all 6-year-old

B. Woynarowska(✉)
Department of Biomedical Aspects of Development and Education, Faculty of Pedagogy, Warsaw University, Warsaw, Poland

C. Vince Whitman and C.E. Aldinger (eds.),
Case Studies in Global School Health Promotion: From Research to Practice,
DOI: 10.1007/978-0-387-92269-0_16, © Springer Science + Business Media, LLC 2009

Table 1 Structure of school system in Poland and enrollment rate

Type of school	Student age (in years)	Number of grades	Enrollment rate in 2005/2006
Preprimary (kindergarten)	3/4–6/7	4	At ages 3–6 years, 70% in urban and 37% in rural areas
Primary	7/8–12/13	6	98.6
Lower secondary general	13/14–15/16	3	99.7
Basic vocational	16/17–18/19	3	8.6
Upper secondary general	16/17–18/19	3	74.8
Upper secondary technical	16/17–19/20	4	29.6

children) and in the 3-year lower secondary schools (*gimnazja*). Schools can be of two types: public state schools (which offer free education) and nonpublic schools (civic, church, and private, which make up 2–5% of total schools). In 2006/2007, the total number of schools was 29,986, with 5,698,200 students. Table 1 shows the structure of the school system.

School Health Education

In the core curriculum for general education, established in 2002, health education as a cross-curriculum program is obligatory in all types of school. The implementation of this program is not satisfactory, owing to the lack of teacher training in health education and the underestimate of this academic task.

Overview of Health-Promoting School Program in Poland

In Poland the Health-Promoting School (HPS) movement started in January 1992 as a 3-year project, established with the support of WHO Regional Office for Europe in four countries – Czech Republic, Hungary, Poland, and Slovakia. Fifteen voluntary project schools from different regions, towns, and rural areas were selected in a democratic way, using clear, transparent criteria. They were recognized as laboratories or islands of development. It was part of the initial pilot phase of the European Network of Health Promoting Schools (ENHPS), launched by the European Commission, the Council of Europe, and the WHO Regional Office for Europe. Poland joined ENHPS in September 1992.

The HPS project was implemented in the first 5 years of the political, social, and economic transition, when an explosion of enthusiasm of Poles and readiness to introduce changes was observed. Many schools recognized the HPS concept as attractive; its dissemination started very soon and continued for the next 15 years.

Reach

In 2007 regional networks of HPS existed in all 16 voivodships, in more than 1,400 schools of different types, with elementary schools dominant. The program reaches about 650,000 pupils. In addition, more than 200 kindergartens in the country have implemented HPS concept in their activities.

Scope of Implementation

HPS dissemination has gone through four stages:

- *Initial stage* (1992–1995). Experiences of project schools were systematically disseminated in the magazine *Leader*, sent to almost every school in the country. Two manuals were published and disseminated. Regional conferences were organized. Project schools disseminated their experiences among other schools in their neighborhood. The first regional network was created in 1992 around a single project school. At the end of the project in 1995, 23 regional networks had been created across 49 regions (until 1999 Poland was divided into 49 regions), with 350 schools and kindergartens interested in joining the movement.
- *Continuity* (1996–1998). The HPS concept was disseminated in a similar manner. Two national conferences were organized. Regional networks grew to 31, with around 600 schools, in 1998.
- *Reorganization of regional networks* (1999–2004). School restructure (three education levels instead of two) and country administration reform (16 regions instead of 49) were implemented in 1999. Reorganization of the regional networks was necessary. The last regional network in Mazovia voivodship was launched in 2004. The national coordinator was moved from the health sector to the education sector. This was a significant achievement, which "opened the door" for the HPS concept into the education system. A new manual for schools and brochure for local governments were published; a bulletin, *Health Education and Health Promotion at School* (edited twice per year), was established, and papers about HPS experiences are also published in two magazines, *Remedium* and *Leader*.
- *Creation of subnetworks in the frame of national networks.* Since certain regional networks were growing very fast and coordination of work and support of schools from regional level was difficult, the idea was born to create smaller subnetworks in 2004. The most advanced structure exists in Podkarpackie voivodship (southeast part of the country). There are nine district networks with 357 schools and kindergartens. Each of them has a district coordinator, support team, and task team, consisting of representatives of different organizations (e.g., police, health service, sanitary-epidemiological service).

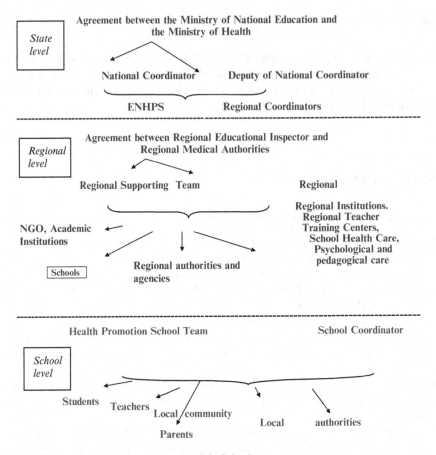

Fig. 1 The health-promoting school network in Poland

The key condition for successful dissemination is the *structure at the national and regional or district level* (shown in Fig. 1) for coordinating and supporting HPS's movement.

The structure functions at either level under certain basic conditions:

- Cooperation between education and health sector as well as with other organizations that have *leading roles in the education sector*, which is the "owner" of schools. The "whole-school approach" cannot be implemented by the health sector. Currently, the national coordinator and all regional and district coordinators are from the education sector.

- Formal agreement between the education and health sectors describing main directions of activities, responsibilities, and forms of support from both sectors. This agreement should be signed at the national level by the Minister of Education and the Minister of Health, and at the regional level by the regional education superintendent (*kurator*) and the head of public health (or similar organization from the health sector).

- Social marketing of HPS concept including systematic publication in magazines for schools, manuals for schools, brochures for local governments, Web site, regional and national conferences addressed to broad audience. National and regional coordinators should be trained in the methods of social marketing.
- Written, clear criteria for membership of regional and district networks.
- Systematic contacts and training for regional coordinators and members of regional supporting teams. Summer schools and other meetings are organized in Poland at least once a year.

There are also certain *barriers* to development of the HPS movement. A growing number of schools in regional networks make coordination and support difficult, mainly at the regional level. People who perform these tasks feel overloaded. Their motivation is based on their enthusiasm; most of them do not get additional pay for this work or resources for management of the networks. Only some of the activities are financed by education authorities, local governments, or sponsors. Many political changes in administration at national and regional levels create many problems for the continuation of formal agreements. Resources are very limited for organization of training, meetings, materials, etc. In some schools with long-term membership in network, decreases of their activities and unfavorable changes in their approach are observed.

Specific Aspects of Implementation of the Health-Promoting School

A reform of the school system was implemented in Poland in 1999. This change also had strong influence on the Health-Promoting School movement, which needed to review its model, first elaborated in early 1990. After several meetings and discussions at schools and in regional support teams, the new model and national standards of HPS were developed in 2006. The model and standards are used as a baseline for planning schools' activities. They provide a basis for developing the indicators and tools for self-evaluation and a national accreditation process for the Health Promoting School National Certificate.

New Model and National Standards of Health-Promoting School

The *model of HPS* developed in Poland is in agreement with the Health-Promoting School approach: (1) It involves students in the process, develops their empowerment and participation. (2) It ensures links between the school, parents, and the community, using a broad and positive concept of health. This model (shown in Fig. 2) is based on Maslow's hierarchy of needs with an open top part of the triangle. It includes three levels:

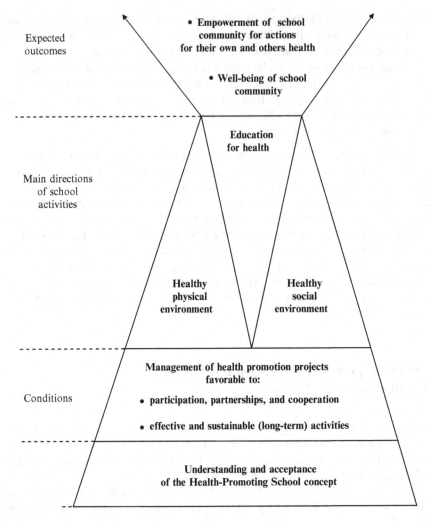

Fig. 2 Model of health-promoting school in Poland

- At the bottom are conditions required for effective activities within a school context.
- The middle part of the model presents the main directions of HPS activities.
- The open top shows expected outcomes (impact): well-being of members of school communities (direct outcome) and empowerment of these members for action for their own health and that of others (direct and long-term outcomes).

For the lower and middle levels of the HPS model, five *national standards* were established: two related to school conditions and three others related to main directions of school activities. A school is assumed to be health-promoting if it:

- Helps the members of the school community to understand and to accept the concept of Health-Promoting School
- Manages health promoting projects in a way favorable to participation, partnership, and cooperation – involving the school community, parents, and local community partners – and to effective and sustainable (long-term) activities
- Implements health education for students and school staff and aims for improving its quality and effectiveness
- Creates a positive school climate that promotes health and development of students and school staff; gives opportunities to achieve success for all and supports their self-esteem; provides conditions for participation, partnerships, and cooperation among school community, parents, and local community
- Creates a physical environment within the school that supports the health and safety of the students and school staff

Indicators and Tools for Self-Evaluation in Health-Promoting Schools

A task force group (specialists from the national level and four regional coordinators) was established in 2005, which worked to elaborate for each aforementioned standard a set of the following:

- Main dimensions (components): the most important components describing the content of the standard
- The indicators for each dimension: characteristics, events, phenomena that can be measured, and signs that identify the achievement of each dimension of a given standard
- Tools: the means of measuring each of the indicators

The examples of dimensions and indicators for the first national standard are presented in Table 2. The authors have presented the tools and procedure of self-evaluation in an earlier work (Woynarowska & Sokolowska, 2006). All indicators and tools were checked in the survey carried out in 24 schools in six national networks (2005–2006). The data were analyzed, leading to modification of indicators and tools. The final version of the indicators and tools, together with a manual for their use and interpretation, was published separately (Woynarowska, Sokolowska, Lutze, & Woynarowska-Soldan,2007).

The Health-Promoting School National Certificate

The idea of establishing the Health-Promoting School National Certificate was born in 2005. It was in response to the needs and expectations of schools belonging

Table 2 Dimensions and indicators for the first national standard: "School helps the members of school community to understand and to accept the concept of Health-Promoting School"

Dimensions	Indicators
Dissemination of the concept of Health-Promoting School and the feeling of knowing this concept among the school community	Informing new teachers, other workers, students and parents about the concept and strategy of Health-Promoting School
	Participation of staff and parents in certain training activities during the past 2–3 years
	Access to publications and other materials concerning the Health-Promoting School
	Feeling among members of school community that their knowledge about Health-Promoting School is satisfactory
Understanding and acceptance of the concept of Health-Promoting School among the members of school community	Acceptance of the Health-Promoting School concept and the rules of its development among teachers
	Knowledge of the basis criteria (characteristics) for Health-Promoting School among teachers
	Understanding what Health-Promoting School means among parents
	Understanding the role of members of the school community in developing the Health-Promoting School

to 16 regional networks of HPS. These schools have regional certificates but perceive a national certificate as a distinction and challenge. The rules of assignment of this certificate were elaborated and broadly discussed with schools and regional HPS coordinators in 2007.

The main goals of establishing the Health-Promoting School National Certificate are the following:

- To recognize and assign value to long-term and systematic school activities according to the conception and standards of Health-Promoting Schools in Poland. This will contribute to the school prestige, be a source of satisfaction for the members of the school community, and motivate their further work.
- To assess how schools that have belonged to a regional network for at least 3 years fulfill the criteria of HPS described in national standards.
- To identify the specific school achievements ("strong sides") as well as examples of good practice. This will help in the national implementation and in the exchange of experiences among schools in different voivodships.
- To make a database about schools and their achievements, which will strengthen the school-support activities at the voivodship and national level, while it will help in the implementation (marketing) of the concept of Health-Promoting School in Poland.

Procedure of Establishing the Certificate

The certificate awarded to schools will be valid for 5 years. A school can get the certificate if it has:

- Been a member of a voivodship network of Health-Promoting Schools or it already has a voivodship certificate for at least 3 years
- Made self-evaluation of its activities in the field according to the five standards
- Made a public presentation of its achievements in the last 3 years, including the results of self-evaluation
- Specified its own specialty ("strong sides") in the field of HPS creating, which it is ready to share with other schools as well as to propose the way of sharing this specialty
- Submitted adequate documentation and received a recommendation from the voivodship coordinator

The certificate is awarded by the local chapter of the Health-Promoting School National Certificate. The members of the chapter are appointed by the head of the Methodological Center of Psycho-Pedagogical Assistance. They are people who work at the Center, honored members, experts in the field of health promotion as well as voivodship coordinators.

First Experience

In 2007, 17 schools from five voivodships applied for the national certificate. Results of the interviews with the school coordinators indicate that:

- The main reasons to apply for the certificate were: (1) the wish to summarize to-date activities, school achievements, and diagnosis of problems that need solving (which was possible on the basis of conducted self-evaluation); (2) fulfillment of the expectations of school community, which is satisfied with its accomplishments; (3) higher prestige for the school in the local community
- The decision to apply for the certificate was made after discussion with various groups of the school community and the voivodship coordinator
- The main benefits are: (1) to conduct self-evaluation, which will bring diagnosis of actual situation in school, identification of "strong sides" and problems that need solving, and activation of school team of health promotion and (2) to experience exchange and cooperation with other schools
- The main difficulties derive from the long and complicated procedure of self-evaluation (many questionnaires, respondents, documents, etc.)

Results of the Analysis of the Documents

Members of the chapter made a serious analysis of documents of the schools that applied for the certificate. In general, the schools overestimated their fulfillment of the criteria of Health-Promoting Schools. While defining their specific achievements ("strong sides") in the process of Health-Promoting School making, schools specified other activities, such as various programs of health education (especially in the field of addiction prevention), other organizations and activities (competitions, parties). On the basis of applied school documentation, one can say that these are active schools in the field of health promotion, but they could not present themselves as Health-Promoting Schools.

It was a difficult task for the chapter. After discussion, the decision was made:

- The schools will not receive the certificate but will gain access to the National Network of Health-Promoting Schools (this level of network has not existed before).
- The headmasters and school coordinators were offered to take part in workshops organized on the national level regarding the concept of Health-Promoting Schools and strategy for its implementation as well as rules for earning the certificate.
- The procedure of awarding the Health-Promoting School National Certificate will be held back for 1 year, in order to work out with voivodship coordinators, school coordinators, and heads of schools a procedure that will show clearly whether a school applying for a certificate has fulfilled the criteria of Health-Promoting Schools.

There was a meeting with voivodship coordinators, to whom the decision of the chapter was presented, where it was agreed that more work is needed for awarding the certificate and that teacher training is needed in schools that belong to the

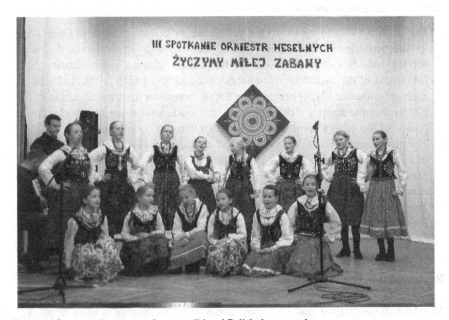

Picture 15   A small group performs traditional Polish dances and songs

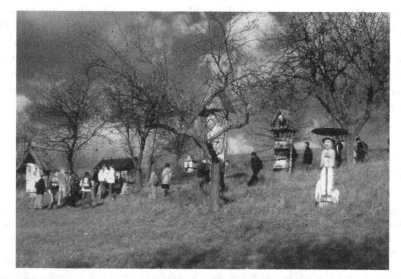

Picture 16 Children get to know and learn the cultural heritage of their region

voivodship network. It was also agreed to organize workshops for school coordinators and headmasters of 17 schools.

These workshops showed that although there is a good knowledge and understanding of the concept of Health-Promoting Schools, teachers have difficulties with presentation of their own activities and achievements in a way that will show their strengths. It was difficult due to complexity of this concept as well as to the multitude and diversity of activities in those schools. The upcoming workshops will team with teachers to create new rules of presentation for schools' special competencies in Health Promoting-School creation and for how to share them with other schools.

Conclusions and Recommendations

1. A movement of Health-Promoting Schools that has been permanent and maintained for 15 years and its infrastructure that supports development at the national and regional level should be acclaimed as successful. This program is the most stable and long-term project concerning health promotion in the country.
2. Working out the national standards, indicators, and methods for measuring these standards was an important phase in the development of the Health-Promoting Schools movement in Poland. These methods made it possible to diagnose and measure school achievements. According to schools, the methods are helpful, but time-consuming as well.
3. Establishing the Health-Promoting School National Certificate corresponds with the school expectations. At the same time, it is a new challenge for schools and it promotes experience exchange with other schools.

4. First experiences with awarding the certificate showed difficulties that teachers have in the presentation of their accomplishments and competencies from the perspective of the Health-Promoting School. It developed from the complexity of Health-Promoting School conception and diversity of activities undertaken by schools from the regional Health-Promoting Schools network. Further work in cooperation with voivodship and school coordinators will aim at supporting schools in the presentation and marketing of their activities.

References

Woynarowska, B., & Sokolowska, M. (2006). A national network for developing and evaluating health-promoting schools in Poland. In V. Barnekow, G. Buijs, S. Clift, B.B. Jensen, P. Paulus, D. Rivett, & I. Young (Eds.), *Health-promoting schools: A resource for developing indicators*. Copenhagen, Denmark: International Planning Committee.

Woynarowska, B., Sokolowska, M., Lutze, I., & Woynarowska-Soldan, M. (2007). Narzedzia do autoewaluacji w szkole promującej zdrowie. *Edukacja Zdrowotna i Promocja Zdrowia w Szkole, 11*, 49–159 (in Polish).

Chapter 17
Scotland: Sustaining the Development of Health-Promoting Schools: The Experience of Scotland in the European Context

Ian Young and Anne Lee

This case study reviews the development of health promotion in Scottish schools and examines the stages of development at the national level over a 20-year period, from the mid-1980s to 2006. The activities over this timeframe have led to the integration of health promotion as an integral and required part of the work of schools within a legislative framework. The case describes the process of change and how the changes initiated in the health sector have now become embedded within government policy and are beginning to be embedded in practice in the education sector.

Contextual Introduction

Population and Health

Scotland is part of the United Kingdom and has a population of 5,078,400, which is growing, because of an increase in the birth rate (in 2007) and because of immigration, particularly from England and Central Europe. Glasgow is Scotland's largest city with a population of 577,000; Edinburgh's population is 448,300. The largest concentrations of social deprivation are associated with the cities. Scotland also has large rural areas, particularly in the north, with very low population densities.

Scotland's health problems have been well documented with high mortality and morbidity statistics in areas such as coronary heart disease, specific cancers, obesity, alcohol-related problems, and mental health. There is a significant link between these problems and socioeconomic status. Although Scotland's health status is showing specific improvements, the overall health profile has continued

I. Young(✉)
Health Promotion Consultant, Edinburgh, Scotland, United Kingdom, e-mail: imyoung@blueyonder.co.uk

C. Vince Whitman and C.E. Aldinger (eds.),
Case Studies in Global School Health Promotion: From Research to Practice,
DOI: 10.1007/978-0-387-92269-0_17, © Springer Science + Business Media, LLC 2009

to lag behind its neighbor, England. In 1991, the standardized mortality rates in Scotland were 12% higher than in England. Health inequalities within Scotland appear to be widening. The gap in male life expectancy between highest and lowest of the 74 parliamentary constituencies in Scotland increased from 7.8 years in 1991 to 13.7 years in 2001 (Whyte & Walsh, 2004). The decline in death rates from common conditions, such as cardiovascular disease, has also been more rapid among the more affluent (Krawczyk, 2004). Thus, despite the overall improvements, the less affluent sections of the Scottish population are falling behind.

The Political Context

The second half of the twentieth century saw a growth of political interest in Scotland, with Scotland eventually having more control over its own affairs through the rebirth of the Scottish Parliament, which was convened in 1999. Certain powers such as defense and foreign affairs are still controlled for all of the United Kingdom by the Westminster Parliament in London, but other powers such as health and education are devolved to the Scottish Executive, and this is significant in the context of this paper.

The Education Context

Scotland has maintained its own distinctive education traditions and system, a right that was established in the Act of Union of 1707. For example, Scotland offers a less centralized and less specialized curriculum at secondary school level than does England. National guidelines are issued, rather than a prescribed national curriculum. Education policy is determined by the Scottish Executive, and the 32 local authorities are responsible for the provision of the education service. Over 95% of young people attend local authority schools, funded by the state, from the ages of 5–16 years. Over 50% of young people remain at school past 16 years. There are high levels of basic literacy in Scotland, and there are national guidelines for health education of ages 5–14.

Overview of Health-Promoting Schools in Scotland and the European Network of Health-Promoting Schools

History

Scotland's commitment to this area of work was formalized in 1993, when it became a member of the European Network of Health-Promoting Schools (ENHPS). The

ENHPS is a partnership among participants in over 40 European countries, with international support from the European Commission, the Council of Europe, and the World Health Organization Regional Office for Europe. With the United Kingdom joining initially in 1993, the Health Education Board for Scotland (HEBS) became the networking agent for Scotland (Crosswaite, Currie, & Young, 1996); separate programs were set up for Wales, Northern Ireland, Scotland, and England.

The Research Context and the Influence of Europe

To strengthen the evidence base for Health-Promoting Schools, links were established with the University of Edinburgh in 1993. This relationship assisted in the evaluation of Health-Promoting School case studies (Inchley, Currie, & Young, 2000). Strong links were built with the Health Behaviours in Scottish Children (HBSC) Study of the Child and Adolescent Health Research Unit (CAHRU) at the University of Edinburgh. The outcomes of the HSBC study (Currie et al., 2004) continue to influence Health-Promoting School policy today in 42 countries with CAHRU playing an international coordinating role.

The HBSC study provides a unique data set on the health of adolescents in Scotland over a 16-year period. The study takes a broad approach to examining young people's health in the context of social factors including family, peers, school and socioeconomic status, and the developmental process of puberty. As an example of the kinds of intelligence supplied, consider the example of gender. Gender and socioeconomic inequalities are evident in many aspects of health behavior and well-being; in general, girls are less positive about their own health and well-being, suffering more frequently from self-reported health complaints, including feeling low. These findings and other relevant trends are presented in Scottish HBSC Briefing Papers (Alexander, Currie, Todd, & Smith, 2004) and in the HBSC international report *Young People's Health in Context* (Currie et al., 2004). This research has played a part in the identification of the specific needs for health promotion among young people in Scotland, leading to specific developments in practice, policy, and legislation.

A major ENHPS Conference on Health-Promoting Schools was held in Thessaloniki, Greece in 1997 (World Health Organization, 1997). At the conference, it was proclaimed that Health-Promoting Schools are an investment in health, education, and democracy. The outcome of that conference was a set of principles that updated the earlier criteria of the Healthy School Report of 1989 (Young & Williams, 1989). The Thessaloniki report defined the values and purposes of Health-Promoting Schools and set out methods that could be used to establish those principles in practice. The new principles put greater stress on equity, democracy, and partnership than the original report; these ideas have been influential in Scotland. The work of Simovska and Jensen in Denmark (Barnekow et al., 2006; Simovska & Jensen, 2003), encouraging the genuine participation of students, has been reflected in research methods (Inchley et al., 2000) and school practice in Scotland (Wetton & McCoy, 1998).

There was also an important follow-up to the Thessaloniki event in 2002 to consider progress made and to take the process forward. It took place at Egmond-an-Zee in the Netherlands (Young, 2002). It included participants from 43 European countries and representatives from many of their national ministries. As a result, the publication of the Egmond Agenda was influential in many European countries in setting out the practical steps that were considered essential in building successful Health-Promoting School programs.

The Egmond Agenda, stating the European experience, suggested that the most successful outcomes arise from programs developed through collaboration between the health and education sectors. The importance of carrying out a national analysis of the health status of young people and of the capacity to promote health in schools was stressed. The report also outlined that for partnerships to achieve lasting success, they must operate in a fair and transparent way at several levels. The experience of the ENHPS in Europe has shown that health-promoting school initiatives are most effective when true partnership is practiced within and between all players in the process. This should include ministries, their institutions, pupils, teachers, NGOs, stakeholders, and interested parties in relevant communities. At the national level, the two most influential partners are generally the Ministries of Health and Education; in the ENHPS, it is deemed that the relevant ministries commit to a formal signed agreement to support the development of health promotion in a member state's schools. The value of this approach will be discussed later. In Scotland, after relatively modest progress in the 1980s and early 1990s, developments accelerated to a level where national legislation has now been set out on health promotion in schools and on nutritional standards in school food (Scottish Executive, 2006).

Specific Features in the Scottish Example

In the mid-1990s there was a supportive base for health promotion in schools in Scotland, but the number of schools that were actively working by the principles set out in the World Health Organization documents was relatively small among Scotland's 2,200 primary schools and 500 secondary schools. However, as mentioned earlier, there was an active research base with both the study on health behavior in school-aged children and a number of case studies on health promotion in schools (Inchley et al., 2000).

Research Base

While there have been few large-scale research programs on the specific impact of health schools on health behaviors, one important longitudinal study

(West, Sweeting, & Leyland, 2004) followed over 2,000 children from age 11 to 15, investigating possible school effects on smoking, drinking, drug use, and healthy diet. The results showed considerable variation in the rates of these health behaviors among 43 secondary schools. After adjusting for prior (age 11) behavior and sociodemographic characteristics, the analyses showed that, with the exception of diet, school-level variation (school effects) remained, meaning that these factors did not account for the differences.

School effects were stronger for smoking and drinking alcohol than for illegal drugs, the effect remaining in a cross-classification analysis of school and neighborhood. Using data from pupils, together with three independent measures, higher levels of smoking, drinking, and drug use were found in schools containing more pupils who were disengaged from education and knew fewer teachers, also in larger schools independently rated as having a poorer ethos. The authors concluded that these results were compatible with the attention given to school ethos in the Health-Promoting School model.

Experimental or comparative studies on school health promotion, such as randomized controlled trials, have not usually been seen as appropriate in complex social settings such as schools for a variety of reasons (St Leger, Kolbe, Lee, McCall, Young, 2007). However, one randomized controlled trial on the impact of an innovative curriculum and associated staff development on sexual health and relationships was undertaken; its positive outcomes have affected both curriculum and subsequent staff development in Scotland (Henderson et al., 2007).

Early Impetus

In addition to this active research agenda, which was broadly supportive of the Health-Promoting School approach in Scotland, there were also supportive colleagues in health promotion posts in the health service and in educational adviser posts in the education service at a regional or area level. The national agency for health promotion at that time had actively supported collaboration between the two sectors by giving preferential funding to initiatives that both sectors agreed to at regional level. However, all of these players could have been viewed as *early innovators* (Rogers, 1962) rather than as mainstream practitioners at that time.

What was generally missing until the second half of the 1990s was unequivocal support and formal commitment from government at a national level. There were, however, new detailed curriculum guidelines developed on health education for the age range 5–14 in Scotland; these were developed by an education committee but with a chair from the national health promotion agency. This was further evidence of effective partnership working. The importance of the wider context of the Health-Promoting School was fully acknowledged for the first time in Scotland in 1999, in an education sector curriculum document. This was evidence of the education sector taking the ideas of the health sector and running with them.

The wellbeing of both pupils and staff is promoted by taking a coherent approach to every aspect of school life. The health promoting school encourages healthy behaviour and, at the same time, recognises that responsibility for improving health does not lie solely with the individual. It is a responsibility shared among all members of the health promoting school community.

Learning and Teaching Scotland, 1999.

Increasing concern about Scotland's health status and the impact of health inequalities produced a formal commitment from government in February 1999, when a major policy white paper on health, *Towards a healthier Scotland*, was published with support from all government ministers in Scotland (Scottish Executive, 1999). This document addressed improving the health of Scots of all ages, including young people.

The government recognises the concept of the health promoting school as important in ensuring not only that health education is integral to the curriculum but also that the school ethos, policies, services and extra-curricular activities foster mental, physical and social well-being and healthy development.

In recognizing this, a ministerial commitment was made to take action and set up a specialist unit for the further development of health promotion in schools (Scottish Health-Promoting Schools Unit). The responsibility for setting it up was given to the national health promotion agency (NHS Health Scotland), the national learning and teaching agency (Learning and Teaching Scotland), and those representing the local government interests (Confederation of Scottish Local Authorities). After much negotiation, this unit was set up within the education service, with support from both the health and education ministries and from the national health promotion agency.

This dedicated resource center, albeit time-limited, was an important first step toward raising the profile of and shifting Health-Promoting Schools to within the education service rather than treating it as an experimental, time-limited *project* initiated by health professionals.

National Implementation

In providing a focus and drive for this work, the government set a formal target in 2003 that all schools should be Health-Promoting Schools by the year 2007; this was another public acknowledgment by government of the extent to which it was starting to take the issue seriously. This target also focused the minds of stakeholders in schools and education authorities on how they would measure and monitor the status of a school in this regard.

With this came a flurry of activity:

- The development of a national framework for Health-Promoting Schools in Scotland, *Being Well – Doing Well*
- The establishment of a Steering Group and National Network
- The production of self-evaluation indicators by the schools' inspectorate

The original steering group for Health-Promoting Schools brought together a range of practitioners at local and regional level, as well as others working more strategically from across health and education to take forward the agenda. This has been further streamlined in favor of the Policy Partners Strategic Group, which brings together the following agencies:

- The Scottish Government's Health and Education Departments
- The national health improvement agency (NHS Health Scotland)
- The education agency (Learning and Teaching Scotland)
- The national sports body (Sport Scotland)
- The schools inspectorate (Her Majesty's Inspectors of Schools)
- The agency representing the interests of local government/authorities (the Convention of Scottish Local Authorities)

The group is responsible for ensuring a coherent and consistent policy approach at national level.

A National Network includes members from each of the 32 local government authorities and each of the 15 health board areas. The members have helped inform and shape national policy and thinking, by drawing on their experience and expertise. They recognized the need for a flexible model to an accreditation process (outlined later). In addition their ownership of and participation in working with this agenda, as regional champions and stakeholders, has been critical to its success. Their ability to think flexibly and link the many initiatives that schools face has reduced the perceived burden of yet another initiative.

The marrying of this top–down and bottom–up approach has proven vital to the successful implementation of the Health-Promoting School approach in Scotland.

The question arises of how to ensure a consistency of approach across Scotland given that there are 32 regional government areas and 15 health board areas, some of whom had already engaged in the development of region-wide systems and approaches, and still ensure local ownership.

Two parallel processes, National Endorsement and Local Accreditation, were necessary to ensure that the target was met. Each local government area had to submit to the National Endorsement Team its local accreditation framework, to show that it met a nationally accepted standard. This ensured a consistency of approach across the country, yet allowed for flexibility. Local Accreditation processes are underway at a local level, gauging the individual school performance. To date, all local authorities/regions have submitted successfully to the national endorsement team; all can say that they have a nationally endorsed scheme in place and that all their schools are on the way to being health-promoting.

Currently the report *Ambitious, Excellent Schools* (Scottish Executive, 2004) is the single most important driver in the education system, arising out of the National Education Debate of 2002. April 2008 will see the mainstreaming of the work of the Health-Promoting Schools unit into Learning and Teaching Scotland's Excellence for All Program, clearly embedding this initiative within the day-to-day business of the education sector.

Evidence of the government's commitment to mainstreaming, however, is in an Act of Parliament in Scotland (Scottish Executive, 2006). The *Schools* (*Health Promotion and Nutrition*) (*Scotland*) *Bill* was introduced in the Scottish Parliament on September 8, 2006 and became a law in summer 2007. This places specific duties on education authorities to build health promotion into their improvement plans and to make clear how they plan to fulfill these duties. The Act also sets out duties on the nutritional standards on the food and drink provided and on the way that free school meals should be provided for those entitled to them. This is a major step forward as Scotland does not have a tradition of bringing about such changes through legislation, usually offering national guidance rather than statutory change in the education system. Such change is taken seriously when it happens, and government inspectors will have a central role in monitoring implementation at education authority and school level.

School inspectors are required to report routinely on wider aspects of school life that influence health, such as the quality of food in the dining areas. Until recently, this was not seen as part of their core work, as curriculum issues were their main focus on quality. Now, given the new Act, the role of the inspectorate will become more visible in *health* as they ensure compliance with the legislation.

Conclusions on the Factors Involved in Stimulating and Sustaining This Change

Working with Complexity

In trying to summarize and conclude, we are mindful of the complexity of the change process; all we can do at this stage is to make tentative suggestions, from our experience, which we *think* are true. We offer these on a tentative basis, as the outcomes could be different in another context or time, given the complexity of the change process.

It is now recognized (Fullan, 1994) that educational reform frequently includes unpredictable shifts and fragmented initiatives. It would be misleading to suggest that progress usually occurs in a simple linear way and in steady increments. Progress is, of course, highly political: Rapid progress is theoretically possible when a strong political will exists; when the political priorities change, the process can stall or go into reverse.

One dimension of the complexity of the change is in the different levels of the system that have to play a part. For example, national government (education, health, and other government departments), area health boards, local education authorities, individual schools, school managers, teachers, parents, and young people. In Scotland change has at some points developed from a top–down approach, while at other times the drive has come from young people, parents, or the exemplary work of specific area health authorities, education authorities, or individual schools.

The Partnership Model: Being Persistent and Being Sensitive to Language, Concepts, and Structures

The original document produced in Scotland to develop indicators of effectiveness of health promotion in schools (HM Inspectorate of Education, 1997) involved a national/local partnership and recognized the importance of health professionals being sensitive to the methods of the education system by utilizing the education system's approach in a parent document *How Good Is Our School?* (HM Inspectorate of Education, 2002, 2004).

In the partnership between education and health, it has become evident that the two sectors have their own distinctive uses of language, which reflect subtle conceptual differences that we need to perceive and acknowledge. For example, educationalists may use the term *curriculum* to cover the whole school experience, whereas health educators may refer only to the learning and teaching in the classroom or the syllabus. The term *health promotion* is not embedded in the mainstream of educational research literature, perhaps because it is not seen as necessary, as education theorists often have a wider conceptual understanding of the term curriculum.

In our work in Scotland and for the World Health Organization in diverse countries in Europe and Asia, one common – if not universal – feature is the relative caution and conservatism of the education sector, so initial reactions to new initiatives are often defensive. This is understandable to a degree, given the scale of change and the failure of many well-intentioned educational initiatives in the past. However, if any joint ownership of Health-Promoting Schools is to be nurtured and sustained, the health sector must try to understand the attitudinal position of the education sector and the beliefs and values that underpin it. It has become evident that partnerships between two sectors such as health and education require time, commitment, and persistence to become effective, requiring processes such as the following:

- The building of trust
- The development of mutual understanding on language, concepts, and values
- Reaching agreement on budget commitments and responsibilities
- Accepting challenges to traditional professional roles

In the ENHPS, it is normal practice to secure a signed agreement by government ministries stating that they will actively work together. This can be important both symbolically and practically, for example, in teachers benefiting from ministry of health expenditure.

In summarizing the historical development of partnership working in Scotland, one sees that in the 1980s and early 1990s early development work in Health-Promoting Schools was initiated by the health sector in what Young (2005b) has termed the *Initial Experimental* phase. This may be followed by a *Strategic Development* phase, in which the education sector starts to perceive the benefits of Health-Promoting Schools in meeting social and educational needs of their schools and communities. A third, *Establishment*, phase may be reached, in which the innovations become embedded in the normal ways of working of the school (Table 1). It is important to note that these phases are not always completely separate or discrete and that the center and regions of one country may be at different stages at any given time. It has been our experience that some countries have reached the early establishment stage when they have had the benefit of up to 20 years of development. Other countries with different levels of health problems and more limited investment or infrastructure in education are often in the first phase of development. While it would be misleading to suggest that progress occurs in a simple linear way and in steady increments, the simplified description in Table 1 may help individual countries to reflect on their current stage of development and to ask the question "How much of this is relevant to our situation?"

Utilizing the Political Will to Improve Health

An important driver that has accelerated the commitment to mainstream health promotion in schools has been the political will to change Scotland's poor health record. There is now a comprehensive policy framework in education, health, environment, and social justice to provide support for tackling health inequalities and improving the health of all. The health promotions in schools' legislation and policies are seen as an integral part of this.

The devolution of political power in matters relating to both health and education and the changing political landscape of proportional representation and coalition government have been positive forces supportive of innovation in Scotland. After the rather slow gestation of Health-Promoting Schools, there has been an acceleration of activity, which has, in our judgment, come from being closer to the seat of political power.

Building Continuity, Capacity, and the Evidence Base

There has been considerable continuity in Scotland in relation to the key partner organizations and many of the key personnel; this has probably been very important in a relatively small country where it may be easier to develop capacity for change. For example, a national health education/promotion agency has been funded by government in the National Health Service for over 35 years, and the education authority structure has changed only once in the last 30 years. Some individuals

Table 1 Phases in the rollout of the Health-Promoting School

Initial experimental phase

Early innovators (mainly from the health sector) raise the issue of health promotion with colleagues in the education sector

The education sector at first tends to perceive health in biomedical terms rather than as a social model, resulting in a deficit of partnership-working between education and health sectors

School Health Services are primarily in a traditional prevention model

Nongovernmental agencies work with individual schools and individual education authorities on specific health issues

Early sporadic or short-term developments occur, which may be driven (and resourced) by political concerns about specific topics such as HIV/AIDS or substance use

Related initiatives such as Community Schools and Eco-Schools are not perceived by education to have anything in common with Health-Promoting Schools because of the prevalence of the biomedical model of health within the education sector

Adoption of some Health-Promoting School terminology by education policy makers. In the early stages this apparent adoption of terminology may not be matched by real changes in practice

Strategic development phase

The education sector starts to perceive the benefits of Health-Promoting Schools in meeting social and educational needs in their schools and communities. Authorities start to build capacity through training and staff development

School health services embrace a wider health promotion role

More strategic approach gradually builds through partnership working at national (government) level and/or education authority/regional level

The health sector funds posts in the education sector

By trial and error and working together, there is a reduction in antagonism between the education and health sectors and a slow, gradual increase in mutual understanding of both sectors. This includes the clarifying of priorities, values, language, and concepts

Some shared posts develop between the education and health sectors, with education contributing resources

More sophisticated research and monitoring of progress is developed as the political profile and the expectations rise

Models are developed to map links between education and health in relation to school health (St Leger and Nutbeam, 2000)

Establishment phase

Policy statements at national level that initially tend to be in the health sector feed into the education sector

Policy statements on specific school initiatives relating to health are increasingly placed in the context of Health-Promoting Schools, for example, curriculum policy statements, food provision policy in schools

The education sector takes on greater responsibility for health promotion in schools and integrates health promotion into mainstream education

At the level of the individual school, health promotion becomes institutionalized, that is, it becomes integral to the schools' core values and normal ways of working

have been involved in this work for over 20 years as practitioners and researchers, both at national level and at area level; this continuity of experience and commitment is probably very important, though difficult to quantify.

There has also been continuity of funding for the HBSC study by the national health promotion agency over the last 20 years. The HBSC team in Scotland has been an effective advocate for addressing health behavior trends in Scotland and has worked actively with the Health-Promoting Schools movement. An example of evidence for the influence of the research agenda is the invitation to the HBSC director onto the partnership group for the Scottish Health-Promoting Schools Unit. There is also a good record of other quality research relating to the health of young people, which also includes qualitative studies where the voices and views of young people have been heard.

The capacity of any education system to adopt innovations will vary in relation to numerous contextual factors. In Scotland the fact that teachers are relatively well qualified, having to go through a registration process, has been helpful. In addition, the salaries and conditions of service of teachers have become more attractive in recent years (Scottish Executive, 2000)

When research (Inchley et al., 2000) has identified a lack of confidence or capacity in the system to respond to innovation in health promotion in schools, action has followed to develop appropriate training resources. For example, *Growing Through Adolescence* was developed in Scotland when teachers made it clear that they required support in dealing with the complex mental health and social health issues concerning young people, body image, self-esteem, dieting, and eating behaviors. It is a training and capacity-building resource designed for trainers working with teachers of children, particularly within the age range 8–14. *Growing Through Adolescence* also serves to bring research data from a number of key resources into an easily accessible format for practitioners, and a European version of this has been developed (Young, 2005b).

To summarize the development in Scotland over 20 years, the main strengths have been in coming to some understanding of:

- The complexity of change and working with it
- The difficulties of partnership-working between the education and health sectors and overcoming them
- Political opportunities and the need to recognize them and work with them
- The importance of good research and its dissemination
- The need to listen to students in relation to their needs
- The need to listen to teachers and to act, for example, in relation to a lack of capacity in the system
- The need to be patient and persistent, as many systemic changes take time.

References

Alexander, L., Currie, C., Todd, J., & Smith, R. (2004). *How are Scotland's young people doing? A cross-national perspective on physical activity, TV viewing, eating habits, body image and oral hygiene.* HBSC Briefing Paper 7. Edinburgh, Scotland: Child and Adolescent Health Research Unit, University of Edinburgh.

Barnekow, V., Buijs, G., Clift, S., Jensen, B. B., Paulus, P., Rivett, D., & Young, I. (2006). *Health Promoting Schools: A resource for developing indicators*. Copenhagen, Denmark: IPC, WHO Regional Office for Europe.

Crosswaite, C., Currie, C., & Young, I. (1996). The European Network of Health Promoting Schools: Development and evaluation in Scotland. *The Health Education Journal, 55*, 450–456.

Currie, C., Roberts, C., Morgan, A., Smith, R., Settertobulte, W., Samdal, O., & Barnekow Rasmussen, V. (2004). Young people's health in context, Health Behaviour in School-Aged Children study. In *International Report from the 2001/2002 Survey, Health Policy for Children and Adolescents No.4*. Copenhagen, Denmark: WHO Regional Office for Europe.

Fullan, M. (1994). *Changing forces: Probing the depths of educational reform*. New York: Taylor and Francis.

Henderson, M., Wight, D., Raab, G., Abraham, C., Parkes, A., Scott, S., & Hart, G. (2007). The impact of a theoretically based sex education programme (SHARE) delivered by teachers on NHS registered conceptions and terminations: final results of cluster randomised trial. *British Medical Journal, 334*, 133–135.

HM Inspectorate of Education. (1999). *The Child at the Centre*. Edinburgh, Scotland: The Stationery Office.

HM Inspectorate of Education. (2002). *How good is our school? Self-evaluation using quality indicators*. Edinburgh, Scotland: The Stationery Office.

HM Inspectorate of Education. (2004). *How good is our school? The Child at the Centre. The Health Promoting School*. Edinburgh, Scotland: The Stationery Office.

HM Inspectorate of Education, Aberdeen City Council, Health Education Board for Scotland (1997). *A route to health promotion: Self-evaluation using performance indicators*. Edinburgh, Scotland: The Stationery Office.

Inchley, J., Currie, C., & Young, I. (2000). Evaluating the health promoting school: A case study approach. *Health Education 5*, 200–206.

Krawczyk, A. (2004). *Monitoring health inequalities*. Edinburgh: Scottish Executive Health Department Analytical Services Division.

Learning and Teaching Scotland. (1999). *Health education 5–14 national guidelines*. Dundee: Learning and Teaching Scotland.

Rogers, E. M. (1962). *Diffusion of Innovations*. New York: Free Press.

Simovska, V. and Jensen, B. (2003) *Young-minds.net/lessons learnt: student participation, action and cross cultural collaboration in a virtual classroom*. Copenhagen: Danish University of Education Press.

St Leger, L. (1999). *The evidence of health promotion effectiveness*. A report for the European Commission by IUHPE, Part Two, 110–122. Brussels and Luxembourg: The European Commission.

St Leger, L., & Nutbeam, D. (2000). A model for mapping linkages between health and education agencies to improve school health. *Journal of School Health, 70*(2), 45–50.

St Leger, L., Kolbe, L., Lee, A., McCall, D., & Young, I. (2007). School health promotion: achievements, challenges and priorities. In D. McQueen and C. Jones (Eds.) *Global perspectives on health promotion effectiveness*. New York: Springer.

Scottish Executive. (1992). HM Inspectors of School Audit Unit, The Health Education Board for Scotland and Aberdeen City Council. *A route to health promotion – Self-evaluation using performance indicators*. Edinburgh, Scotland: The Stationery Office.

Scottish Executive. (1998). *The new community school prospectus*. Edinburgh, Scotland: The Stationery Office.

Scottish Executive. (1999). *Towards a healthier Scotland: A white paper on health*. Edinburgh, Scotland: The Stationery Office.

Scottish Executive. (2000). *A teaching profession for the 21st century*. The McCrone report. Edinburgh, Scotland: The Stationery Office.

Scottish Executive. (2003). *Hungry for success: A whole school approach to school meals in Scotland. The final report of the expert panel on school meals*. Edinburgh, Scotland: The

Stationery Office. Web site: http://www.healthpromotingschools.co.uk/practitioners/eatingfor-health/index.asp

The interim report of H.M. Inspectors of Schools is available from Web site: http://www.hmie.gov.uk/documents/publication/hmiemihs.html

Scottish Executive. (2004). *Ambitious, excellent schools*. Edinburgh, Scotland: The Stationery Office.

Scottish Executive. (2006). Schools (Health Promotion and Nutrition) (Scotland) Parliamentary Bill on Health Promotion in Schools. Retrieved in 2006 from http://www.scottish.parliament.uk/business/bills/68-schoolsHN/

Scottish Health Promoting Schools Unit. (2004). *Being well doing well: A framework for health promoting schools in Scotland*. Edinburgh, Scotland: The Stationery Office.

Tones, K., & Green, J. (2004). *Health promotion: Planning and strategies*. London: Sage.

West, P., Sweeting, H., & Leyland, A. (2004). School effects on health behaviours: Evidence in support of the health promoting school. *Research papers in education, 19*(3), 261–291.

Wetton, N., & McCoy, M. (1998). *Confidence to learn*. Edinburgh, Scotland: NHS Health Scotland.

World Health Organization. (1997). *The Health Promoting School – An investment in education, health and democracy. First Conference of the European Network of Health Promoting Schools, Thessaloniki, Greece*. Copenhagen, Denmark: ENHPS Technical Secretariat, WHO Regional Office for Europe.

Whyte, B., & Walsh, D. (2004). *Scottish constituency profiles*. Retrieved in 2006 from http://www.phis.org.uk/info/sub.asp?p = bbb

Young, I. (Ed.). (2002). The Egmond agenda. In *Education and health in partnership, a European Conference on linking education with the promotion of health in schools*. Woerden, The Netherlands: NIGZ /WHO Regional Office for Europe.

Young, I. (2005a). Health promotion in schools: A historical perspective. *Promotion and education xii*, 3–4.

Young, I. (Ed.). (2005b). *Growing through adolescence*. Copenhagen, Denmark: WHO Regional Office for Europe.

Young, I., & Williams, T. (1989). *The healthy school*. Copenhagen, Denmark: Scottish Health Education Group/WHO Regional Office for Europe.

Chapter 18
Bahrain: National Comprehensive School Health Program, Health-Promoting Schools

Mariam Al Mulla Al Harmas Al Hajeri, Lulwa Abd Al Aziz Al Thukair, and Nayara Sarhan

Contextual Introduction

The Kingdom of Bahrain has a population of 742,562 (2006), living in an area of 720.1 km^2. The population comprises 61.8% Bahraini (459,012) and 38.2% non-Bahraini (283,549).

Some vital statistics (2006)	Socioeconomic indicators
Crude birth/1,000 live birth: 20.2	GDP per capita: US $18,465
Infant mortality rate/1,000 live birth: 7.6	Population growth rate: 2.7
Crude death rate/1,000 population: 3.1	Percentage of population unemployed: 5.5%
Total fertility rate per woman (15–49): 3.0	Average health expenditure per capita: US $392.8
Life expectancy at birth: 74.8 years	Population per doctor: 363
	Population per dentist: 2,435
	Population per nurse: 182

Bahrain is a nation whose foundations are deeply rooted in family values, tribal and community culture and support, with a rich heritage of a high standard of societal health and educational pursuit. Globalization and mass communication have influenced children's lives by opening a world with many new influences, standards, opportunities, and values. Their world is no longer restricted to the environment of family and community. Life choices in this new world are sometimes overwhelming and confusing, so instilling values and knowledgeable

M. Al Mulla Al Harmas Al Hajeri(✉)
Ministry of Health, Manama, Bahrain

C. Vince Whitman and C.E. Aldinger (eds.),
Case Studies in Global School Health Promotion: From Research to Practice,
DOI: 10.1007/978-0-387-92269-0_18, © Springer Science + Business Media, LLC 2009

decision-making skills during the early, formative years is essential. While most young people in Bahrain are doing well, some are at risk of less-than-optimal outcomes. The many factors that place a child at risk have a negative multiplier effect on the youth's health and social outcomes. This potential for adverse outcomes necessitates comprehensive strategies to foster resilience. Vulnerable youth who are provided with a supportive and flexible environment can better access the resources they need to develop their abilities to face life challenges successfully.

Health and Education Indicators

The three leading causes of death in Bahrain are diseases of the circulatory system, neoplasms, and endocrine, nutritional, and metabolic disorders. The three main health problems in youth are obesity and lack of physical activity, unhealthy diet, and smoking (Table 1).

The total number of students in Bahrain is 163,987. There are more female students than male students across all school levels. About three-quarters of students (75.6%) attend government schools (124,010), while about one quarter (24.3%) attend private schools (39,977).

Main health problems in youth:

- Obesity and lack of physical activity
- Unhealthy diet
- Smoking
- Drug abuse
- Sexually transmitted diseases
- Road traffic accidents
- Injury and violence

Table 1 Leading causes of death in Bahrain

Cause of death	Rate per 100,000 population in 2006
Disease of circulatory system	60.5
Neoplasm	34.1
Endocrine, nutritional, and metabolic disorders	46.3
Injuries and poisoning	28.3
Respiratory system	17.1
Infection and parasitic infection	11.4
Genitourinary system	10.9
Digestive system	7.7

Almost all students (99.4% of age 15–17 years) attend secondary level schools, and 98.8% of youth can read and write. Only 350 students, or 0.2%, drop out from school.

The Ministry of Health As One of the Key Players

The Ministry of Health: Our Challenge and Responsibility

The Ministry of Health (MOH) as the custodian and trustee of Bahrain's population health has recognized the importance of the opportunity to work with children and adolescents through their formative years at school, in order to shape and secure the future health and healthy environment of the nation. Ensuring that today's youth grow up in an environment that fosters healthy physical, intellectual, emotional, social, and spiritual development will enable them to become tomorrow's capable parents, caregivers, workers, and citizens.

- The MOH will focus on health education, prevention, and promotion in early childhood and adolescent development, delivered through collaborative school health programs, with high priority on the social and political policy agenda.
- The MOH will sustain and enhance these school programs by policy development and service changes in community-based health services that support the transition from student to young adult and family provider, incorporating the values, practices, and beliefs that promote a healthy lifestyle and future.

Ministry of Health: Strategic Direction

Several high level strategies have been identified for the MOH to meet the needs of youth and their families more effectively. Focusing on these strategic directions will enable the government and communities to contribute to healthy development across the lifespan.

1. *Improve the availability, accessibility, and acceptability of health services* to make them more responsive and supportive to the achievement of students' personal development.

   - All students must have access to a wide range of confidential, youth-friendly health services that are accessible in both urban and rural community settings. Specific programs and services can be created (e.g., establishing outreach programs for vulnerable youth, peer-mentoring programs, parent support groups), expanded (e.g., providing specific benefits not currently offered by the health system), or revised (e.g., removing regulation, rules, and practices that create artificial or unintended barriers to access).

- Services can be provided in locations and ways that are more accessible and friendly to students (e.g., outreach programs, in schools, in malls, through the Internet).
- Finally, improving services in key health issue areas and providing user-friendly information (on topics such as mental health, health promotion, tobacco and substance use, family violence, sexual health, injuries) can also contribute to health and well-being.

2. *Provide supportive environments for students.*

The social and physical environments, as well as the education system, are important determinants of a student's health.

Families, peers, schools, communities, media, and communications, together with the natural and built environments, significantly influence health and the personal health practices of youth. These influences involve multiple sectors such as education, social services, housing, and environment.

3. *Involve students*: Working directly with students to improve their health is a key priority.

- Students have clearly articulated their desire to influence policies and services that are developed to support their safe and successful transition to adulthood. Experts have outlined the benefits to both youth and society when opportunities are provided for students to contribute to policy and program development and service delivery.
- Policy makers and experts must continually consult with students to determine their responsiveness to and acceptance of the directions and strategies.

4. *Collaborate with other sectors.* Many of the determinants of health lie outside the direct mandate of the MOH.

- It is important that the MOH initiates discussion with other sectors, such as education, social services, economic development, recreation, justice, and housing.
- To increase the understanding of how policies and programs of specific sectors affect child and adolescent health and to assist youth by making healthy choices the easy choices, it is necessary to establish a clear role for health in these areas and to develop comprehensive strategies.

5. *Improve the knowledge base for children's and adolescents' health.* To support healthy development, it is essential to have reliable, timely data on all the determinants of health.

- Existing information must be comparable, linked regionally, and made available on a national basis.
- Research, program evaluation, and monitoring are necessary to increase understanding of the conditions that support youth to choose healthy, appropriate risk behaviors over adverse risk behaviors that have a greater probability of lifelong negative health consequences.

- It is necessary to learn which models are the most effective and which approaches work best in specific situations.

Overview of the School Health Program

Impetus and Origin of the School Health Program

The years that children spend in school are an important period for formative development. Students begin to define themselves in relation to their community, culture, and ability to influence the future. They are developing social and civic skills. They are acquiring the capacity to communicate their ideas and feelings effectively. They are refining their ability to resolve conflicts. They are working to make meaningful contributions and to shape how their community or school functions, focusing on local social issues or broad societal issues that will affect their future. They have a passion and an emerging sense of personal power that seeks a voice.

Students in Bahrain's schools are faced with many cultural, economic, health, educational, and social challenges. The healthy attitudes, behaviors, and skills that students learn in comprehensive school health programs, complemented and supported by participation in daily physical education programs throughout their school years, will help them face these challenges.

In Bahrain, all government schools were applying health promotion programs in original ways. For example, all schools had components of health promotion, such as physical education, nutrition, and health education, but these components were not coordinated in an organized way.

The school health promotion project was launched in October 2004 as a program for all government schools in the kingdom of Bahrain. It was gradually expanded.

The first step in planning was advocacy, in order to raise awareness about the concept of Health-Promoting Schools, after building local support. The program was formally announced, and schools were selected for implementation of a pilot scheme. The first group of schools selected (2004–2005) comprised 11 schools in Muharraq governorate. This was later expanded to 50 schools in five governorates (2005–2006).

Scope of Implementation

Model and Vision

Bahrain's Comprehensive School Health (BCSH) initiative requires a model that incorporates a broad spectrum of activities and services offered in the school and surrounding communities. The BCSH model will enable children and youth to:

- Improve their opportunity for enhanced health status
- Develop to their fullest potential
- Establish productive and satisfying relationships in their present and future lives

The attainment of comprehensive goals demands an integrated approach that incorporates specific strategies and elements within three categories:

1. Instruction/curriculum
2. Support programs and social services
3. Healthy physical environments

A common understanding of the comprehensive school health framework among health professionals, educators, teacher educators, social workers, community support groups, students, and families is necessary to achieve health for all.

Bahrain's vision for the School Health program outcome, stated simply, is as follows:

All children and youth living healthy, active lives.

The School Health Program will do the following:

- Provide instruction to develop the knowledge, skills, attitudes, and behaviors related to healthy living
- Support the provision of support services for students and their families
- Create a healthy social and physical environment within the school
- Integrate the concepts of personal health management, health promotion, and education
- Incorporate strategies that are comprehensive, interdisciplinary, and outcome-based
- Be taught by teachers who are competent and qualified in health education and promotion
- Provide sufficient instruction time to elicit behavior change

Mission and Mandate

The mission of the program calls for health and education professionals to work as partners to jointly promote, support, and deliver BCSH in collaboration with the total community (school, home, larger community). In keeping with the mission of the organization to achieve BCSH, professionals will work with key intermediaries that influence students in the school system, through curriculum instruction, support services, and physical environments.

The mandate requires establishment of an "Interdisciplinary Authority" that represents and serves the health professionals and educators who design and implement health education programs and leadership opportunities in the schools. Although educators will join and work very closely with the various government and community agencies (such as community health professionals and centers, national associations, government departments), they will continue to take the lead responsibility for the educational interpretation, implementation, and evaluation of the BCSH program.

Key Strategies

At the MOH level, the School Health Initiative will have six strategic areas of emphasis:

1. Awareness and advocacy
2. Partnerships
3. Resource development and promotion
4. Teacher education (preservice and in-service)
5. Research and evaluation
6. Management, planning, and support

At the School Program level, there are eight key program elements as defined in the WHO model:

1. Health services
2. Health education
3. Healthy school environment
4. Health promotion
5. Nutrition and food safety
6. Physical education and recreation
7. Mental health and social service support
8. Community programs and projects

To implement the program in the selected schools, meetings were held with community leaders to discuss the basic ideas. A small group (team leaders) of interested people from the schools and the community was established. A number of training workshops were conducted for the people concerned in the MOH and the Ministry of Education (MOE) – administrators, teachers, school health nurses, etc. – to explain the scope of the Health-Promoting School program, its importance, methodology of implementation, and evaluation tools. Newsletters and leaflets about the Health-Promoting School program have been produced.

A local planning process was then undertaken for creation of the Health-Promoting School. A school health team was established, and current school health promotion efforts were reviewed. Health problems were assessed, and opportunities for action were determined. After goals had been set and objectives defined, an action plan was developed and mechanisms were put in place to monitor progress. For follow-up and evaluation, the Health-Promoting School coordinators visited the schools to review the implementation of the action plan and discuss the difficulties and opportunities for action (Table 2).

Processes to Implement the Strategies

1. The process started with a circular from the MOE to all 205 schools in the Kingdom of Bahrain to implement health promotion in schools by applying the eight components of school health promotion.

Table 2 Process for creating of the Health-Promoting School

Local planning process for creating Health-Promoting Schools	Training workshops
1. Establishing a school health team	*Workshop 1 (Group 1) June 15–16, 2004*
	What is the Health-Promoting School?
2. Reviewing the current school health promotion effort	How do we develop an action plan (Consultant) (MOE and MOH)
3. Assessing the health problems	*Workshop 2 (Group 1) Jan 15–16, 2005*
4. Finding opportunities for action	Demonstrating progress
5. Setting goals	Collecting information (MOE and MOH)
6. Defining objectives	*Workshop 3 (Group 2) Nov 28–30, 2005*
7. Developing the action plan	Training the trainee (Professor…)
8. Demonstrating progress	What is the Health-Promoting School?
9. Collecting information	How do we develop an action plan?
	Monitoring and evaluation

2. Workshops about the projects were conducted for all the schools' representatives in order to implement school health promotion.

3. All schools were asked to put a short- and a long-term plan in place for implementing the program in their schools.

4. All schools were asked to form committees for health promotion. The head of each committee should be the second person in the school (deputy of the school principal); representative members should include the teacher of physical education, food canteen coordinator, school councilor, and school nurse.

5. Regular meetings of these committees should be conducted with the leaders in the MOE about the plans and implementations.

6. Auditing of the program will be done before, during, and after the implementation, in collaboration with the research committee in the MOE.

7. Each school committee should develop a plan for the next academic year, 2008/2009, which should be submitted before May 2008.

8. The MOE had planned a competition among all the schools; prizes will be announced for the first three winners. The objective of this competition is to empower the project and encourage the schools to implement the school health promotion.

Specific Aspects of Implementation

Policy Directives

The MOH has issued a series of policy directives. These directives reflect a more comprehensive, integrated, responsive, and collaborative partnership approach to population health, delivered through a national health plan that incorporates a shift in program emphasis from acute-care interventions to community-based programs of health promotion and prevention. The MOE has embraced this policy directive and its applicability to challenges in education and to the urgent need for a national comprehensive school health program.

The goal of the Bahrain Comprehensive School Health Programme is to respond effectively to the needs of children and adolescents, based on the population health model and the determinants of the health framework.

The determinants of a health framework require a systematic and comprehensive approach to program and service development. Comprehensive School Health is an approach to school-based health promotion involving a broad spectrum of programs, activities, and services, which take place in schools and in surrounding communities. Such actions are designed not only to affect the health of individual students but also to change the environment in which they live and learn.

Collaboration

The Health-Promoting Schools program in Bahrain is a collaborative effort between the MOH and the MOE. In 2000, a high-level joint committee between the MOH and MOE was formed to put into place a strategic plan for school health in Bahrain: "The Bahrain national school health program." The school health program started in 2002, when the MOH and the MOE reached an agreement to establish a comprehensive school health program for Bahrain.

The MOH collaborates with the MOE in a Joint Committee, as well as with the Gulf Council Committee (GCC) and with the World Health Organization, Eastern Mediterranean Regional Office (WHO/EMRO).

Bahrain has renewed its emphasis on finding ways to link the various sectors that influence the development of children and adolescents. This intersector collaboration is essential because of the following:

- Inter-sectoral action makes possible the joining of forces, knowledge, and the means to understand and solve complex issues whose solutions lie outside the capacity and responsibility of a single sector.
- There are many opportunities to engage health, education, social services, recreation, housing, culture, and justice sectors in joint strategies to achieve shared goals.
- Among the significant potential benefits of collaboration is the enhanced capacity to tackle and resolve complex health and social problems that have proven impossible for individual sectors.
- "Children deserve love and respect for who they are." They are central to Bahrain's investment in its future and must be acknowledged and involved in shaping change and development of the population's health.
- The social services sector is an important partner, particularly in its role to support youth who are experiencing difficulties in family life.

- Each sector has a unique responsibility for initiating discussion, offering its perspective, communicating with its constituents, and providing leadership to engage others in collaborative efforts to better meet the needs of children.
- Most youth spend a significant portion of their time in the school environment. The MOE has a particularly important role to play in the healthy development of children and is a key partner in developing strategies for youth and their families.

Focusing on the determinants of health, *the MOH is well-positioned to act as a catalyst* in the identification of policy, planning, service delivery, and research needs related to child and adolescent health and development.

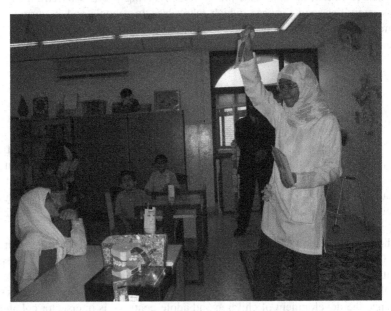

Picture 17 Education for students with special needs about dental hygiene

Conclusions and Insights

Factors that helped in the success of the Health-Promoting School program in Bahrain are as follows:

- Support from WHO and the Gulf Cooperation Council School Health Committee
- Strong commitment and partnership between the health and education sectors
- A well-developed school infrastructure
- The existence of health and safety committees in all schools in Bahrain that support the Health-Promoting School program implementation

Future plans are to expand the program to cover all schools in Bahrain; to develop national standards, guidelines, and evaluation tools for Health-Promoting Schools; to continue the training programs; and to develop a Web site for the national network of Health-Promoting Schools.

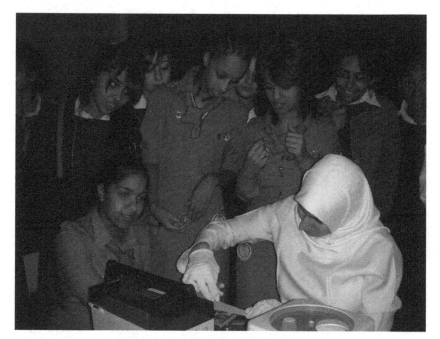

Picture 18 Students checking their blood suger at school during a diabetic health education campaign

The obstacles were as follows:

- The schools were busy with another big project (Future Schools Project), which was strongly supported by people high in the government. The big national project made the school administrators not enthusiastic about the health promotion program.
- The project was a sort of optional recommendation, which made the implementation of the project weak.

The lack of powerful implementation of school health promotion in the majority of the schools led to the trial of another strategy. This strategy was launched in October 2007 as a "modified way of school health promotion." The main objective of the project is to improve school health promotion in all government schools.

Acknowledgments This work was done with support from the Ministry of Health, Ministry of Education (Joint Committee), Gulf Council Committee (GCC), and World Health Organization (WHO) Eastern Mediterranean Regional Office (EMRO).

Chapter 19
Oman: Health-Promoting Schools: Collaboration and Investment

Ali Jaffer Mohamed and Sahar Abdou Helmi

Contextual Introduction

The Sultanate of Oman is located in the southeastern corner of the Arabian Peninsula. Its coastline is almost 1,700 km, from the Strait of Hormuz in the north to the borders of the Republic of Yemen, overlooking three seas: the Arabian Gulf, the Gulf of Oman, and the Arabian Sea in the south. The Sultanate of Oman borders Saudi Arabia and United Arab Emirates in the west, the Republic of Yemen in the south, the Strait of Hormuz in the north, and the Arabian Sea in the east. In addition, several Omani islands are scattered in the Arabian Sea; the most important are Masirah and Al- Halaniyat.

The Sultanate of Oman is divided administratively into 5 regions and 4 governorates with 61 Wilayats. The regions are Al Batina, As Sharqiyah, Ad Dakhiliya, Adh Dhahira, and Al Wusta. The governorates are Muscat, Dhofar, Musandam, and Al Buraimi. The regions of As Sharqiyah and Al Batina have each been further subdivided into two for health and education administration, producing a total of 11 health and educational regions.

The estimated midyear population for 2006 is 2,577,062 (1,883,576 Omani and 693,486 expatriates). The Omani population sex ratio is 102 males per 100 females. It is a young population; about 11.68% and 37.4% of the population are under 5 years and under 15 years, respectively.

The crude birth rate was estimated at 24.17 per 1,000 Omani population during 2006. This shows a drop of 44.9% over the past 15 years (from 43.9 in 1991). It is also accompanied by a decline in the crude death rate, from 7.5 per 1,000 in 1991 to 2.48 per 1,000 population. Life expectancy at birth is 74.29 years. The infant mortality rate and under-5 mortality rate were 10.25 and 11.02, respectively, in 2006 (Department of Health Information and Statistics, 2006).

A. Helmi(✉)
School Health Department, Ministry of Health, Muscat, Oman

C. Vince Whitman and C.E. Aldinger (eds.),
Case Studies in Global School Health Promotion: From Research to Practice,
DOI: 10.1007/978-0-387-92269-0_19, © Springer Science + Business Media, LLC 2009

The economy of Oman has shown a growing trend in recent years. It depends mainly on the income from oil and gas exports, which accounts for over 80.3% of government revenues. The gross domestic product at current prices is RO 13,737.7 million, and the gross national income is RO 13,096.7 million (Oman Ministry of National Economy, 2007).

Education in Oman

Education for all children of school age, with equal opportunity for boys and girls, started in the early 1970s in Oman. It has witnessed a remarkable development in recent years. Basic education – which provides the students not only with information but also with skills – started in the Sultanate 10 years ago.

There is no difference between boys' and girls' enrollment in schools. Girls' net enrollment is even slightly higher (Department of Educational Statistics, 2006).

Enrollment rates show that more than 80% of the population in the age range of 6–18 years are school students; therefore, it is important to promote their health by reaching them in their schools.

Schools in Oman are characterized by high infrastructure standards. All newly constructed basic education schools are well-equipped, with learning resource halls and computer labs. Each school has an open place for physical activity and a school canteen.

In academic year 2006/2007, there were 1,223 schools, including 1,053 governmental schools: 3 of them are special education schools and 170 private schools. The total number of students was 595,736, constituting 23.1% of the population as per the 2006 population estimates. About 95% of the students are in governmental schools. The number of school staff in all schools was 48,365 (42,479 teachers and 5,886 administrators) (Department of Educational Statistics, 2006).

Health in Oman

The Ministry of Health (MOH) is responsible for ensuring the availability of health care to the people of Oman. In the course of implementing its health development plans, the Ministry has developed strategies and objectives (Directorate General of Planning, 2006), which can be summarized broadly as follows:

- Regionalization of health services and decentralization of decision making in specified technical, administrative, and financial affairs
- Emphasizing the role and importance of planning
- Development of education and training in health
- Emphasizing the importance of health system research
- Emphasizing the importance of regional and international relations

Impetus and Origin of the School Health Program

School health activities started in Oman for the first time in 1972, when the basic services were provided through the health institutions. The fourth 5-year health plan (1991–1995) established the school health program with its objectives, strategies, and activities. It provides the preventive aspects of school health in schools, through physicians and nurses, while the curative and rehabilitative aspects are provided in the health institutions.

The main *objectives* of the program (Department of School Health, 1995) are to:

- Raise health awareness of the students and their families, by provision of adequate knowledge of good healthy habits
- Provide comprehensive health services that deal with the physical, mental, and social health needs and problems of this population
- Ensure healthy school environments

Strategies of the School Health Program

The main *strategies* of the school health program (Department of School Health, 2007) are as follows:

- Establishment of *organizational structures* for school health at the central level and in all health regions. At the national level, the school health department, one of the departments of Directorate General of Health Affairs, is responsible for planning, supervising, and evaluating the program. At the regional level, a section was established in the department of health affairs to be responsible for implementation, supervision, and evaluation of the program.
- *Continuous coordination* between the MOH and Ministry of Education (MOE) through various joint committees. A central joint school health committee was formed in 1992, with representatives from MOH, MOE, ministry of municipalities, and Muscat municipality. The MOE established the Department of Guidance and Education to coordinate with the school health department in MOH (see Fig. 1). The school health department also has a collaboration program with regional and international organizations such as the Eastern Mediterranean Regional Office of WHO (WHO/EMRO), UNICEF, and UNESCO.
- Development and *capacity building* of all human resources in school health. Training programs are conducted continually to train school health staff, teachers, and school social workers. The main achievements are as follows:
  - A 4-month in-service training course was conducted in the Oman Institute of Public Health, funded by MOH and WHO/EMRO. It aimed to build capacity of school health nurses. About 101 nurses were trained and certified as trained school health nurses.

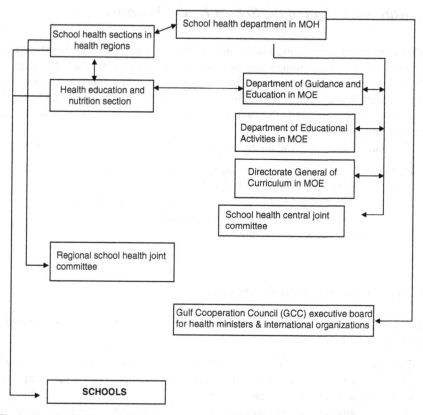

Fig. 1 Organizational structure of the coordination between the school health department in MOH and other concerned departments in the MOE, regional, and international organizations

- – Each school has a health supervisor teacher who is trained in school health. Training programs are conducted continually to train those teachers, especially on first aid and dealing with adolescents' health issues. By the end of 2007, about 1,056 teachers were trained.
- Establishment of a *health information system* in school health programs. Monthly and annual forms are used to monitor and evaluate the process of school health activities. The national data on the main health problems are being published on annual basis through the MOH annual statistical book.
- Conducting *studies and research* that would help to identify the lifestyles of the students. Various studies were conducted to identify the main health behaviors among students.
- *Raising awareness* in the schools and community about the impact of health on the level of educational achievements and educational performance.

Activities of the School Health Program

The school health *activities* that are carried out in all schools are summarized here:

- Conducting a *planned health education* program that targets all school students. This includes distribution of the Omani version of *Facts for Life* (Suliman & Abdulaziz, 2006) as a tool of health education to all students in grades 9 and 11. It aims to provide the readers with some vital health messages and skills that they can apply in their daily lives. A research competition is being carried out among students in grade 11, aimed at encouraging them to read and to look for common health problems in the community.

In addition, MOE is continually updating the curricula, taking into consideration the integration of health messages and skills.

- Providing *comprehensive school health services* to all students in Oman.
  - Each student has a health card. Physical screening is carried out for all students in grades 1, 7, and 10. Students with health problems are referred to primary health care institutions for more management. The school health nurse follows up regularly on chronic cases and cases that need special care.
  - Vision testing is carried out for all students in grades 1, 4, 7, and 10. Appropriate corrective actions are taken for students with defective vision.
  - Oral health screening is carried out for students in grades 1 and 2 aiming for early detection and treatment of dental caries.
  - First aid services are provided in schools.
  - Immunization is provided to all students as per the expanded program of immunization in Oman. All students in grades 1, 6, and 11 get a booster dose of diphtheria and tetanus vaccine, while a booster dose of oral polio vaccine is given to students in grades 1 and 3.

- *Ensuring healthy school environments.* This includes all aspects of a physically healthy environment.
- *Promoting healthy nutrition.* This includes enabling healthy foods in the school canteen and using interactive nutritional education programs.

Assessments

In spite of all the school health activities, the program faced many challenges, especially those emerging from new unhealthy behaviors among students.

These behaviors have been revealed in many surveys and studies conducted in schools:

- Adolescent health survey conducted in 2001 for age range 15–19 years (high school) (Jaffer, Al Ajmi, & Al Wahashi, 2001)
- Global Youth Tobacco Survey conducted in 2003 (Abdulaziz, Al Lawati, & Al Shuaili, 2003)

- School nutrition survey conducted in 2004 (Department of Education and Guidance, 2004)
- Mental health survey conducted in 2004 (Department of Researches, 2004)

All these surveys showed that the students' knowledge, attitudes, and practices are deficient, especially in areas of reproductive health, HIV/AIDS, nutrition, physical activity, tobacco use, accidents, and violence, as well as psychological problems.

We realized that health education alone is not enough to change behaviors and that we needed to focus more on well-organized health promotion programs in schools. These programs should be directed not only to students but also to school staff and families.

There was a consensus that implementing the WHO Health-Promoting Schools (HPS) initiative will help us achieve our aim.

Overview of the HPS Initiative in Oman

Aiming to mobilize and strengthen health promotion and education activities at the local, national, regional, and global levels, the WHO launched the global HPS initiative to improve the health of students, school personnel, families, and other members of the community through schools (WHO, 1999).

Oman, as one of the EMRO countries, started to implement the initial phase of the HPS initiative in 19 schools in the scholastic year 2004/2005:

- Vision: Better health for the school community
- Mission: Working together for HPS

The main *principles* of the initiative in Oman (Department of School Health, 2005) are as follows:

- To link health and education issues and systems
- To provide safe, healthy, and supportive environments
- To promote and empower the health and well-being of both students and staff
- To collaborate with the local community and engage the parents and families in promoting their health
- To integrate with the school's ongoing activities

The main *strategies* of the HPS in Oman (Department of School Health, 2005) are as follows:

- Advocacy aiming to raise awareness of the local community leaders, schools, and families
- Building partnerships with concerned governmental and nongovernmental sectors
- Continuous development of strategies and policies to improve the implementations
- Creation of the national network of schools implementing the HPS as a mechanism for sharing experiences within the schools themselves

In 2004, 19 out of 1,042 schools (1.8%) were selected to implement the initial phase of HPS. Two schools were selected from each health and educational region, except for Al Buraimi, Musandam, and Al Wusta, where only one school was selected.

The selection was based on criteria such as geographical distribution, school level, gender, and previous experience of the school in implementing health programs. Half of the schools were from urban areas, and the other half from rural areas. Nine schools were boys' schools, nine were girls' schools, and one was a mixed school. The team preferred to start with a small number of schools, so that there will be a good opportunity to train them and enable them to learn lessons from each other.

Scope of Implementation

Oman, like all EMRO countries, is following the concept of comprehensive coordinated school health programs, like those modeled in the HPS initiative. The main elements of the initiative (Department of School Health, 2005) are as follows:

- *School health policy:* Schools should follow the MOE national policies that promote health and well-being. Examples of these policies are banning tobacco use, enabling healthy food practices, and providing safe environments.
- *Skills-based health education:* Schools should provide knowledge and skills that support healthy behavior through curricular and extracurricular activities. In Oman, schools have no special health curricula but must follow the curricula produced by the MOE. Thus, the concerned staff in both MOH and MOE worked together to integrate health concepts into the curricula. Individual schools have the freedom to plan and implement extracurricular activities as per their needs.
- *Health services*: These are being introduced in all schools, but HPS can request additional services from neighboring primary health care institutions.
- *School physical environment*: The building, grounds, courtyard, school surroundings, sanitation, water supply, and other elements should ensure a healthy environment.
- *Psychological support*: Schools should help to improve relationships among students themselves and their staff; they should also help students to overcome any psychosocial problems.
- *School nutrition services*: Schools should emphasize changing the poor nutritional habits of students, especially those who fail to eat breakfast or sufficient fruits and vegetables.
- *Physical education*: Schools should promote physical activities, inside and outside.
- *Promotion of health of school staff*: Schools should build the health knowledge, skills, and practices of those who work in the school.
- *Community links*: Schools should make opportunities to link with the families and local community.

Specific Aspects of Implementation

Preparation Phase

To implement HPS in Oman, the concept was discussed in the joint school health committee meeting. A proposal was sent to the decision makers in both the MOH and MOE to get approval and support.

Formation of the HPS Taskforce Groups

To plan, implement, follow up, and evaluate the initiative, teams are formed at the national, regional, and school level.

- *At the national level*: A national taskforce group from MOH, MOE, WHO, and UNICEF was formed to develop a plan of action, develop materials, conduct training, advocate, and assess the initiative.
- *At the regional and governmental level*: Another joint team from MOH and MOE was established in each region and governorate to plan with schools, conduct training, supervise, and assess the initiative on the regional level.
- *At the school level*: A team was created, chaired by the school headmaster or his or her deputy, including the school health nurse, social worker, health supervisor teacher, some teachers, some students, some parents, and persons from the local community. In most schools, the social worker was assigned to coordinate the initiative.

Most schools did their best to convince the local authorities to join the team. For example, Gumah School convinced the Wali (Mayor) to be the chairperson of the team. This, of course, gives schools more support and success in conducting their projects and activities.

Capacity Building of the School Teams

A 5-day training-of-trainers workshop was conducted in November 2004, with the financial and technical support of WHO/EMRO and UNICEF. By the end of the workshop the participants were able to:

- Understand the concept, objectives, and elements of the Health-Promoting School initiative
- Conduct a situation analysis and prioritize the health problems in the school
- Set objectives
- Develop a plan of action

The trainers had conducted other workshops in their regions to train the school teams on the same topics.

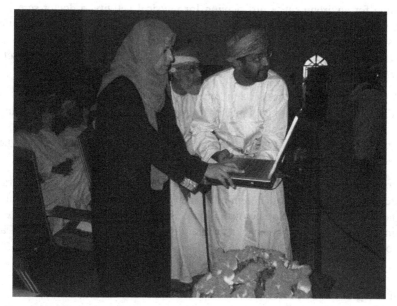

Picture 19 HPS launch

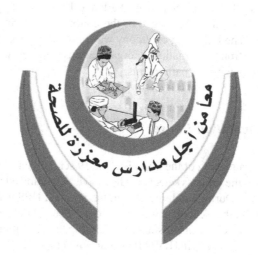

Fig. 2 Logo of HPS

Production of Materials

Production of a logo: A special logo for the initiative was produced with the theme "Together for Health-Promoting Schools." It consists of the crescent as a symbol of health, together with symbols of some of the initiative's elements, such as a school building for environment, a girl playing for physical activity, a doctor screening a student for health services, and a child reading as a symbol of health education. It is surrounded by the colors of Oman's flag.

Production of guideline manuals: The national taskforce has produced a set of three guidelines:

1. A guideline on the process of implementation at different levels
2. A training manual that helps master trainers in the regions to conduct training workshops for school teams
3. An assessment tool that would help the schools monitor their projects and help the external assessors carry out the assessment of the HPS

Production of advocacy materials: To advocate for the initiative and raise awareness of the schools and community, many posters and leaflets were produced on the concept of the HPS. The media were used to advocate for the initiative by writing articles in the newspaper and interviewing members of the national and schools teams on TV and radio.

Launching of the Initiative

The initiative was launched in December 2004 under the auspices of Her Excellency Dr. Muna Salem Al Jardania, Undersecretary of MOE for Education and Curricula, in the presence of the concerned staff in MOH, MOE, WHO, and UNICEF. The launching ceremony was followed by a conference on the initiative. Speakers from international organizations and Arab countries shared their experiences with the participants.

Implementation Phase

After the launching of the initiative, the 19 schools started to implement the plan of action and the projects selected. They have been allowed to continue their activities for 3 years. During implementation, the regional HPS team continued to supervise and retrain the school teams if needed. The schools used interactive learning methods especially in antismoking, antidrug, and nutrition projects. Peer education was used, especially in HIV/AIDS. Various competitions among students were used as tools of health education.

National HPS Network

Aiming to exchange experiences among the schools, the Omani national HPS network was established in different ways:

- *Regular meetings of an HPS Forum*: Two forums were conducted: the first, in November 2006 and the second, in January 2008. In the forums, the schools shared their experiences through presenting and discussing their objectives, activities, and constraints, if any. The main recommendation of the second forum was to expand the initiative to more schools in different Wilayats.
- *Establishment of a Web site* (www.schoolhealthoman.com): This site, with the theme "my health in my school," has helped students and concerned people to discuss and explore their views and knowledge, especially in areas of lifestyle and adolescent and youth issues.
- *Exchange visits between schools*

Assessment Phase

Assessors' guidelines were developed and pretested twice in the field to ensure stability of the tool. The tool has nine modules to measure the achievements of the nine elements of the initiative.

There are three levels of assessment:

1. *Self-assessment*: To be conducted at the school level. This is a continuous process that helps the schools to measure their achievements and update their activities accordingly.
2. *Regional assessment*: To be conducted by the regional teams to determine which schools should get bronze or silver certificates.
3. *National assessment*: To be conducted by the national team to determine which schools have fulfilled the criteria of golden level.

There are three levels of certificates:

1. *Bronze level*: The school can be certified as bronze if it implements the project for 1 year and gets excellent scores in all elements except one or two.
2. *Silver level*: The school can be certified as silver if it implements the project for 2 years and gets excellent scores in all elements except one.
3. *Golden level*: The school can get the golden certificate if it implements the project for 3 years and gets excellent scores in all elements. In addition, the school should support another one to be a Health-Promoting School.

The results of the assessment showed improvement in many elements, such as environment and promotion of staff health and nutrition. In addition, this initiative showed further positive outcomes. First was the strengthened collaboration between the school health department in MOH and the department of guidance and education in MOE with WHO and UNICEF. Second was the development of a sense of responsibility among school members (students and staff), together with increased decision-making skills and initiative-taking.

Conclusions and Insights

Success Factors

Many factors played a role in the success of HPS in Oman. First is the commitment and support of higher authorities in MOH, MOE, and international organizations. Second is a sense of ownership and partnership of health and education sectors, schools, communities, and students. Third is the presence of school health services with objectives and activities. Fourth is the effective role of the Omani community and their participation in health issues. Fifth is the presence of effective parents' councils in all schools.

Constraints

The main constraints are overload by other, similar projects or initiatives; frequent turnover of the team, which necessitates frequent training; limited budget allocated for the schools to implement the activities; and challenges with the assessment, especially if more schools will be invited.

Future Plan

- After approximately four scholastic years of implementation, the time has come to evaluate the initiative. A study is being conducted to measure the impact of the initiative on the knowledge, attitudes, and practices of the school community.
- We will gradually expand the national network to involve many other schools.
- We will review and update the HPS guidelines and criteria every 3 years.

Conclusion

The HPS initiative is an effective approach to promote the health of students, school staff, and subsequently the community. Supportive policies from the higher authorities are one of the success factors. On the other hand, this support may make the schools feel forced to implement the initiative. We suggest that the initiative come initially from the school level and be adapted later by the regional and national level. Proper advocacy is very effective in raising awareness among the schools and helping a school to decide voluntarily to be a Health-Promoting School.

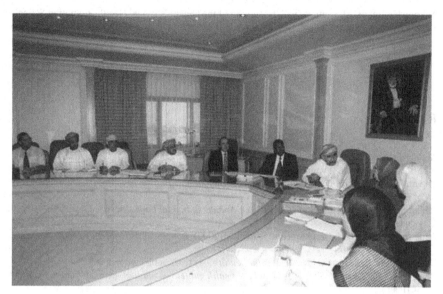

Picture 20 Oman team

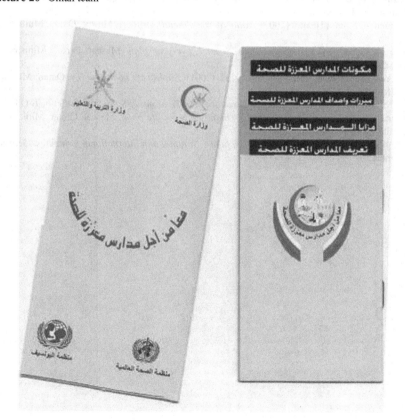

Picture 21 HPS leaflets

Acknowledgment The authors had the support of the Omani National Health-Promoting Schools Taskforce. The authors would like to express their gratitude and thanks to all persons who contributed in the success of the Health-Promoting Schools initiative.

References

Abdulaziz, S.A., Al Lawati, J.A., & Al Shuaili, I.S. (2003). *Global youth tobacco survey*. Oman: Ministry of Health. Available online at http://www.cdc.gov

Department of Education and Guidance. (2004). *School nutrition survey*. Muscat, Oman: Ministry of Education.

Department of Educational Statistics. (2006). *Annual statistical book*. Muscat, Oman: Ministry of Education.

Department of Health Information and Statistics. (2006). *Annual statistical report*. Muscat, Oman: Ministry of Health.

Department of Researches. (2004). *Mental health survey*. Unpublished report.

Department of School Health. (1995). *School health guidelines manual*. Muscat, Oman: Ministry of Health.

Department of School Health. (2005). *Health promoting schools guidelines*. Muscat, Oman: Ministry of Education.

Department of School Health. (2007). *National school health strategy*. Muscat, Oman: Ministry of Health.

Directorate General of Planning. (2006). *Seventh five-year plan*. Muscat, Oman: Ministry of Health.

Jaffer, Y.A., Al Ajmi, F., & Al Wahashi, K.H. (2001). *Adolescent health survey*. Oman: Ministry of Health.

Oman Ministry of National Economy. (November 2007). *Monthly Statistical Bulletin, 18*(11).

Suliman, A.J., & Abdulaziz, S.A. (2006). *Omani facts for life book*. Muscat, Oman: Ministry of Health, Ministry of Education.

WHO. (1999). *Improving health through schools: National and international strategies*. Geneva: Author.

Chapter 20
United Arab Emirates: Health-Promoting Schools: Strategies for Policy Change

Mariam Al Matroushi

Contextual Introduction

The United Arab Emirates (UAE) is a federation of seven emirates: Abu Dhabi, Dubai, Sharjah, Ajman, Umm al-Qaiwain, Ras al-Khaimah, and Fujairah. Abu Dhabi is the largest of the seven emirates, with an area equivalent to 86.7% of the total area of the country excluding the islands. The population of the UAE, estimated to be 4 million people in 2005, is characterized by the presence of a large number of expatriates, who have significantly influenced the social and cultural norms of the country. Excessive mobility has also had an impact on norms and values. The population is also characterized by a high fertility rate, low infant mortality rate (7.7 per 1,000 live births in 2005), and under-5 mortality or child mortality rate (9.9 per 1,000 live births in 2005). Although life expectancy has already exceeded 74 years, the population of the UAE is still relatively young, with 25.3% of the population under 15 years and 90.4% of the total population under 45.

The per capita income exceeded Dh 61,000 in 2005 and is considered to be one of the highest in the world. The high income has facilitated rapid socioeconomic development, as well as the establishment of a modern infrastructure of health and educational services. This rapid change has also affected the disease patterns as a result of changing lifestyle. Cardiovascular diseases, cancer, diabetes, and other chronic diseases have emerged as the leading causes of morbidity and mortality. The ever-rising cost of health care has led to a revision of prospective health strategies, placing a greater focus on risk management and disease burden reduction, as recommended by WHO (Ministry of Health, 2006). All of these factors have been taken into consideration when developing and revising the school health program.

M. Al Matroushi
School Health Program Coordinator, Ministry of Health, Abu Dhabi, UAE

C. Vince Whitman and C.E. Aldinger (eds.),
Case Studies in Global School Health Promotion: From Research to Practice,
DOI: 10.1007/978-0-387-92269-0_20, © Springer Science + Business Media, LLC 2009

Overview of the UAE School Health Program

The school health program in the UAE was established in 1968, and federal administrative oversight for school health was formed in 1977. A year later, in 1978, the federal administrators appointed school health directors in each of the nine medical districts. The mission of the program was to promote, protect, and improve the health of students in UAE, through a comprehensive and coordinated school health program. The components of the program have been developed to ensure that students' physical, emotional, and social health and well-being are maintained in a state that would enable them to achieve maximum benefit from their education.

Strategic Plans

Strategic plans for the UAE school health program have therefore focused on creating a school environment conducive to optimum education and training of students. The main objectives of the plan are to:

- Protect the health of students through positive promotional, preventive, and curative health activities
- Encourage students, parents, and staff to develop knowledge, attitudes, and skills that will help them maintain and improve health, prevent disease, and reduce health-related risk behavior
- Provide a safe, healthy, and supportive school environment that fosters health and learning
- Encourage staff to become positive role models for students by maintaining healthy behavior
- Improve school canteens and provide dietary education to encourage students to adopt lifelong healthy dietary behavior
- Increase the fitness level and promote lifelong safe physical activity among school children
- Improve students' mental, emotional, and social health through health awareness and training programs, as well as by early case detection and provision of early care
- Encourage community participation in the planning, implementation, and evaluation of the school health program (UAE School Health Department [UAE SHD], 2003)

School Health Program Policy

The school health program policy of the UAE focuses on the following:

- Promoting the health of students and of staff in all UAE schools, through the provision of high quality, comprehensive, and equitable services

- Maximizing the benefits of such services and improving their standard though continuous monitoring and evaluation and the rational use of research and development
- Improving health awareness of students and staff and encouraging them to participate in raising the awareness of their families and local communities
- Maintaining active partnerships among all concerned sectors responsible for health and education toward promoting the health and well-being of students
- Strengthening and fostering the cooperation between the schools and their local communities (UAE SHD, 2003)

Financial and Human Resources

The budget for school health programs is from the Ministry of Health and other health authorities. In 2004–2005, there were 512 nurses and 106 doctors distributed among the different medical districts, responsible for implementing the school health program in 745 governmental schools (for 287,098 students) and ten referral school health clinics in the medical districts for students who had special health needs. School health nurses visited 87.2% of the schools during 2–5 days per week. The same staff also supervised the implementation of the program in 480 private schools (for 343,535 students). Of the private schools, 72% had contracts with private doctors or clinics, and 67% had a resident school nurse (UAE SHD, 2005).

The Components and Implementation of School Health Program

The coordinated school health program has been implemented with eight components including school health education, school health services, healthy school environment, physical education, school nutrition services, health promotion of school staff, school counseling and social services, and family and community involvement (UAE SHD, 2003, 2006).

School Health Service

The school health program includes the following:

- Comprehensive screening:
  - Complete medical examination of students in grades 1, 5, and 9.
  - Medical fitness examination for college, university, and institute students, on admission.
- Follow-up of positive cases:
  - Positive cases diagnosed during the check-up are followed up for further investigation, diagnosis, and treatment. They are referred to consultants and specialists in hospitals as needed, to receive proper and free treatment.

– Chronic cases are also followed up according to their individual care plan.

• Vaccinations according to the national immunization program, include the following:

  – Tetanus and diphtheria (TD), oral poliovirus vaccine (OPV), and measles, mumps, rubella (MMR) for grade 1 students.
  – Hepatitis B vaccine (HBV) for students who have not been vaccinated.
  – Rubella to female students in grade 9.
  – TD and OPV are also given to students in grade 11.

The school nurses and doctors check the vaccination history and vaccination card retention to make sure that all previous vaccinations have been completed, so that there will be no need for an accelerated schedule.

• Control of communicable diseases: This depends on early detection, investigation, notification, isolation, and treatment. Students diagnosed or reported from other health care facilities with a communicable disease are not allowed inside school unless the school health doctor or another doctor allows them to do so after the infectious period, to avoid causing an outbreak.
• School dental services: This preventive program for dental health includes screening of students in grades 1, 2, 6, and 7, with application of temporary filling or fissure sealant as needed to maintain oral health. School health also provides limited curative dental service. Dental health awareness and dental hygiene education are also delivered, especially to students in preparatory schools, including kindergarten and first grade.
• First aid and emergency care: School nurses or other trained personnel provide this as needed. Usually students are referred for curative services to the nearest primary health care center or, in some regions, to the central school health clinic.

School Environment

The school environment includes classrooms, halls, school grounds, playgrounds, water tanks, water filters, and coolers. Supervision is intended to ensure the safety, cleanliness, light, and ventilation of the school environment. The school administration solves school environmental problems according to type and intensity, based on the recommendation of the school health team and a report issued semiannually by the central school health department. The educational or school health medical staff monitor the school's social environment and implement interventions when necessary.

Health Education

The health education curriculum in UAE governmental schools is integrated into different relevant subjects, mainly biological sciences. School health staff are responsible for health awareness of students, teachers, and parents through different activities such as lectures, celebration of health-related occasions, and direct student–physician consultations. The health educational materials include video tapes, films, posters, and pamphlets. All the nursing staff are involved in conducting and/or coordinating health education activities once in a week in all schools according to a list of priority topics. Such activities are coordinated with the Ministry of Education and other relevant institutions, such as civil defense or the Red Cross, according to the topic. In 2007, the annual plan included 17 health educational topics to be discussed as a priority, in addition to 11 celebrated occasions.

School Nutrition Program

Supervision of school canteens and cafeterias is undertaken to ensure that all types of food offered in these facilities, together with their methods of preparation, transportation, and storage, meet required standards. All canteen workers must possess a certificate of food handler.

School health staff provide nutrition education. Their activity complements school nutrition education included in the integrated health curriculum in relevant subjects.

Physical Education

The school health program encourages practicing lifelong physical activity inside and outside the school. Physical educators from the Ministry of Education implement the physical activity program in the form of curricular and extracurricular activities. Students who practice competitive physical activities undergo a physical fitness medical examination. This examination is coordinated by the Ministry of Education's physical educators and school health staff. School health staff are also involved, among other things, in training teachers and students in first aid and emergency care, as well as in giving first aid. These same staff provide required medical care during physical activities, excursions, and extracurricular activities as needed.

Psychosocial and Mental Health Services

A screening questionnaire was developed in collaboration with UAE university staff to screen for common psychosocial problems of school-age children. A work plan was developed and seven confirmatory questionnaires were used. Suspected cases are referred for appropriate treatment; a specialist provides follow-up care.

Health Promotion for Staff

Health promotion for staff aims to improve their status through activities such as health assessment. Educational staff are also continuously involved in health education activities to encourage them to pursue healthy lifestyles. The objective of this approach is to improve the health status of the staff to become positive role models for students and to increase their personal commitment to the school health program. Limited school health services are provided to school staff, especially during the time of students' final examination, trips, and special occasions.

Parent/Community Involvement

Parents must be involved in students' health care issues. School health staff attend parent-teacher meetings to communicate directly with parents and to identify students' needs accordingly. Health awareness activities are also organized to promote the health of the family as a whole, as well as of the community at large.

Revision of the School Health Program

The program is regulated by ministerial and administrative decrees issued whenever necessary to ensure that activities in all medical districts are undertaken adequately and to consolidate achievements and overcome obstacles.

Regular Recording and Reporting

Guided by indicators for continuing evaluation, the school health program has been revised regularly to ensure that it attains the required outcomes. An annual work plan is implemented. The plan has clear objectives and indicators for precise evaluation for each component of the program. The information is collected from the districts and tabulated using statistical forms. The results from the analysis of these tables are published in the annual report for the school health program. The results are also announced in a meeting at the beginning of each academic year. The meeting is usually attended by influential people, including the Minister of Health and higher officials from the Ministry of Health and the Ministry of Education.

Research and Surveys

Many surveys are conducted regularly to evaluate the outcomes of the program. The Ministry of Health and the Ministry of Education in UAE have already participated in some of the global surveys, such as the Global Youth Tobacco Surveys in 2002 and 2005 and the Global School Health Survey in 2005.

Challenges

Implementation of the school health program in the UAE has faced many challenges, including the following:

- The continually growing number of students and schools, which demanded more service and staff.
- The uneven distribution of manpower, especially in remote areas where school nurses have not been allocated to schools or have visited schools only once in a week. Vaccination, medical examination, and health education have thus been provided by mobile teams with the cooperation of local primary care centers.
- The shortage of qualified teachers, weakness in active parent and community participation, and scarce school health services.
- Underappreciation and underestimation of the work of school health staff by the concerned authorities.

At the beginning of 2005, Abu Dhabi Emirate started to deliver all school health services through primary health care centers, while school nurses were allocated to some schools inside the cities.

The similarity between the two school health programs – the UAE school health program and the Health-Promoting School – is that both have been developed in the UAE to promote the health of students and school communities. The HPS initiative is applied in the UAE to complement and promote the school health program (Table 1).

Implementing the Health-Promoting Schools Initiative

In response to the WHO initiative on Health-Promoting Schools (HPS), the HPS program in the UAE was established officially in 2000 (Fig. 1). From the beginning, the HPS program in the UAE has recognized the concept of health promotion, which focuses on actions to improve peoples' control over factors that influence their health. Action for health promotion in that context evolves around coordinated activities in a specific setting, such as schools, to create support for health throughout that setting. As this concept involves and requires the combined input of many agencies and sectors, an important aspect of health promotion lies in building partnerships and alliances among these agencies. Efforts in that respect focused on incorporating the Health-Promoting Schools concept into the ongoing school health program in several ways.

Generating Support

The concept of HPS has been carefully explained to senior policy makers in the Ministries of Health and Education, a step that was considered crucial to generating the necessary support for the program in the future.

Table 1 School health program and health-promoting schools in UAE

	UAE School Health Program	Health-Promoting Schools
Scope	Wider coverage of national program covers all government schools and most private schools in UAE	Limited to the selected 46 schools, based on criteria such as willingness, commitment to promoting health and location
Components	8 school health program components • School health services • Nutrition services • Healthy school environment • Health promotion for staff • Family/community involvement • Health education • Physical education • Counseling, psychological, and social services	5 strategies for health promotion mentioned in the Ottawa Charter • Health policies • Environment (physical and psychosocial) • Personal skills • Health services • Community participation
Responsibility	Mainly school health staff in coordination with MOE, educational zone, and schools	Teams within schools with involvement of students, staff, and community. The school community is the main actor
Planning	Planning is imposed in the central school health department (centripetal)	Planning starts at the school community level (centrifugal)
Students and community involvement	Participation of students and parents is limited in service provision	Participation of students and parents and schools in service provision is marked. They are the main players
Setting priorities	Programs target health priorities from health officials' points of view	Program projects special school, community point of view
Continuity of the program	School health program is implemented and sustained through regulations	Program depends largely on the willingness of school community
Empowerment	Limited to school health department	Empowerment of the school community, students, and staff
Budget	MOH budget main is constant provider	Budgets are provided by schools and community resources that are unlimited but not constant
Health problems	Target most of the common health problems, needs, and concern of the students and schools	Target certain, limited health problems that are considered as priorities in the schools

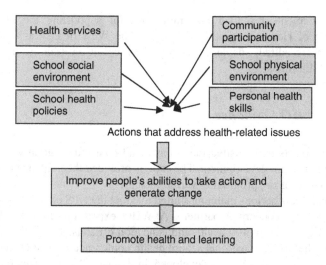

Fig. 1 Interaction between the components of HPS

Capacity Building

To accomplish capacity building for Health-Promoting Schools, the school health program has resorted to international experience on development of the HPS and training of trainers. This international consultation has been followed by the development of training materials and a training program that included the following:

- Training for schools on approach to and development of the HPS concept.
- Training for the trainers and local supervisors on the overall approach, advances, monitoring, and evaluation of the HPS. Trainers also participated in meetings and conferences in the UAE and abroad.

The packages of training material are designed specifically to support workshops for the development of the HPS in the UAE; these training materials were developed by the UAE HPS Coordinating Committee, in collaboration with WHO. Dr. Rose Marie Erben, a consultant from Australia, located within the WHO's Regional Office in the Western Pacific Region, conducted a training workshop to train trainers on the development of Health-Promoting Schools. The training materials used in the workshops were developed after referring to the experiences and workshops conducted in Viet Nam, Mongolia, and Vanuatu. The documents of the training package include the following:

- A manual for facilitators
- Participants' workbook
- National guidelines for the development of Health-Promoting Schools, a framework for action

These documents provided the framework for supporting the growth and development of Health-Promoting Schools in the Western Pacific Region. The documents were edited, adapted, and published to suit the training needs of the United Arab Emirates.

Ensuring WHO Guidance

Four WHO experts have visited the country and contributed greatly to our HPS network and program development. The experts provided the guidance required for the development of the program at various stages.

In the year 2000, serious planning started to adopt the HPS concept by spreading awareness among concerned partners. A WHO expert mission introduced the concept of HPS to about 400 health and education officials. The topic was further discussed in the first international school health conference in Abu Dhabi in 2002.

The first plan for HPS was developed in January 2003 during the visit of Dr. David Rivett from WHO/EURO and the European HPS Network. In December 2003, during a short-term consultancy by WHO consultant Dr. Rose Marie Erben from Australia, a workshop took place to train trainers on the development of Health-Promoting Schools. The workshop was based on a publication of the WHO regional office for the Western Pacific. Later, several other training workshops (4–6 per year) were conducted to train staff from the selected schools on the development of HPS.

Using the outcome of the training workshops, schools started forming teams, analyzing their local situation, identifying the main health problems, prioritizing, and developing an intervention plan by adopting the WHO framework and plan of action. In April 2004, the first annual meeting for Health-Promoting Schools took place to review the school projects.

Plans for implementation were shared for feedback and guidance. The official launching of the program took place in December 2004 with the participation of two Australian experts in this field (Professor Louise Rowling, former president of the Australian HPS Association, and Dr. Bernie Marshall, president of the Australian HPS Association). They visited the HP schools, met the officials and concerned partners, and commented on how to strengthen our efforts.

Agreement Between Ministry of Health and Ministry of Education

The signing of an agreement by the Ministries of Health and Education in December 2003 marked the beginning of their partnership. The health and sports department of the Ministry of Education coordinates Health-Promoting Schools with the school health department in the Ministry of Health, and personnel from these two departments form the working core team for the network.

Higher Coordinating Committee

A higher coordinating committee for the school health program was formed earlier in 2002, following a recommendation from the first UAE school health conference. Steps were undertaken to implement the January 2003 plan, developed in connection with the visit of Dr. David Rivett, a consultant from WHO/EURO and the European Network of Health-Promoting Schools. These steps started by signing the agreement between the health and education officials in December 2003, establishing the higher committee for HPS. The committee consisted of members from the Ministry of Health (MOH), Abu Dhabi General Health Authority, Dubai Health Authority, the Ministry of Education (MOE), and other governmental sectors. These sectors included the General Secretariat of Municipalities, the Ministry of Information and Culture, and the Parents' Council. Members of this committee were the members of the higher committee of the school health program. On the recommendation of Dr. Rose Marie Erben, members from the General Women's Union and the Red Crescent Authority were added to the committee. The committee was very efficient because it included decision makers such as the Assistant Under-Secretary for Preventive Medicine from the MOH (chairman), the Assistant Under-Secretary for Activities and Student Welfare from the Ministry of Health, and the Deputy Director of the General Secretariat of Municipalities.

The responsibility of the committee was to review and approve the HPS strategy and work plans and to provide the required support for the implementation, supervision, and evaluation of the plans. The committee met at least three to four times annually. However, a coordinating team communicated more frequently and when necessary. The coordinating team is formed mainly from the school health department in the MOH and other health authorities as well as the department of sports and health programs in the MOE. A training team from the MOH and the MOE was involved whenever necessary.

Local teams at regional level were also formed from different health and educational departments for the supervision and support of HPS in the region. The support, supervision, and commitment of these teams varied from one region to the other. Therefore, a central team from the MOH and the MOE was appointed to visit the schools with the local regional teams to ensure that the support was provided and to monitor and evaluate the programs and projects in those schools.

Appointment of a National Coordinator

A national coordinator was appointed, for a 2-year period, from the school health department at the MOH.

Formation of a Core Technical Team of Trainers

Since the first training-of-trainers workshop conducted by Dr. Rose Marie Erben about the development of Health-Promoting schools, a number of candidates were selected from both MOH and MOE to train the schools that joined. Follow-up meetings with selected trainers helped form a core team of 12 members. Those members were trained further and helped conduct workshops for the first 18 schools selected to join the initiative. Further training opportunities were offered for this team as possible. Based on expert recommendations, the health staff was trained about health promotion concepts, forming partnerships, and other issues while teachers and MOE staff were trained about health-related issues. As there were a few changes in the organizational structure of the ministry and also changes in working team, we had to replace a few trainers and train more staff.

Establishment of Criteria for the Selection of Piloting Health-Promoting Schools

The establishment of criteria for selecting pilot schools depends on a variety of factors including geographical characteristics and previous commitment to other projects.

Monitoring and Evaluation of a HPS Program

The Health-Promoting School project in the UAE has, ever since, been followed up and evaluated by local teams from the same area and a central team from the MOH and MOE. Monitoring and evaluation was undertaken through school visits, meetings, and documentation of the outcomes. Health-related school activities were assessed by process and outcome evaluation. A baseline study for the evaluation, conducted in 18 of the selected schools, provided baseline data that helped schools in their situation analysis.

On the one hand, the process evaluation focused on certain aspects, such as the level of awareness about the HPS concepts and the health concepts. The process of evaluation also looked for documentation of the directives for the formation of the teams, the minutes for the meeting, and studies conducted for situational analysis. Furthermore, the process reviewed the framework of the work plans that were guided by health promotion strategies in the Ottawa Charter. This content was provided during the training workshops.

On the other hand, the outcome of evaluation focused on comparing the program results to the baseline data and the set objectives of the project or the program. The national program was continuously evaluated by higher committee and external experts and consultation during that time. Their opinions and experience contributed greatly to the improvement of the network.

The HPS schools inside UAE were encouraged to communicate continuously with each other and with HPS schools outside the UAE. The schools were also encouraged to spread awareness about the HPS approach to other schools. One way of measuring schools' contribution to sharing was by their presentations and participation at annual meetings. Most schools participated in the annual meeting, where they were given the chance to present their projects, plans, and achievements orally or through poster sessions.

In 2004 the National Network of HPS was launched, and the first annual meeting for Health-Promoting Schools took place to share experiences and review the project. The UAE HPS network started with 18 schools in 2004. By 2006, the UAE had 30 HPS and another 16 schools registered to join the program. More than 17,000 students have therefore benefited from the project in 46 schools. In several meetings between the representatives of the Gulf Council Committee (GCC) and WHO/Eastern Mediterranean Regional Office (EMRO), suggestions emerged as to how to evolve and grow the HPS program. The establishment of national and regional HPS networks is anticipated in the near future. Workshops are still conducted annually to train more school health and education staff.

Health-Promoting Schools in Remote Areas

Introduction of the Concept

Knowing HPS concepts helped people in UAE to understand that health is created where people live, learn, work, and play, and that they create it themselves in their daily interactions with each other and with their environment. People there started encouraging and calling for action from others living in that area to begin strengthening the health potential of their own everyday settings. They started to understand that health is an option they can make for themselves and not a matter of services delivered by others.

Preparatory Phase

Program coordinators in the MOE and in health services have announced their support for the comprehensive HPS approach, which was envisioned as a suitable alternative to ensure that the school health program components and services are adequately delivered to students, staff, and schools.

The selection of the schools was based on geographical distribution, educational levels, and commitment to previous programs. Resources for the Health-Promoting School projects were provided not from the center, but through the mobilization of community members and local institutions. The network support focused on honoring the distinguished schools. However, the MOE allocated Dh 100,000 that could be used for schools' projects.

Approaches Used for Implementation

Schools have developed many approaches to strengthen the program and to increase community participation. These approaches included the following:

- Making the parents and community leaders aware and informed about the HPS project while calling for and welcoming community and parents' participation
- Holding regular staff–parents meetings
- Involving parents and community leaders in the planning, implementation, and evaluation of the HPS through the supporting local committees
- Involving the students actively in the project, which encouraged them to volunteer for different activities
- Establishing and strengthening links with the media – including local radio and television stations, newspapers, and magazines – to cover school health-related activities
- Publishing and distributing widely a newsletter and health education materials
- Networking and cooperating with other schools, as well as with governmental and nongovernmental institutions and organizations
- Encouraging the establishment of Web pages by some schools
- Contacting and involving influential people and companies to support HPS activities

Practical Steps

The commitment of the MOE, the MOH, and municipalities took the lead in those areas, but generally it was the local coordinating teams that conducted the training workshops, gathered information through a baseline study, and planned and delivered activities in the local schools. This local participation was an important step in sustaining the activities of the HPS projects.

Outcome

The approach adopted by the UAE to encourage the community had significant success, especially with regard to the following:

- It changed community attitudes and the way of looking at the HPS, from a pure educational institution for the children and young people, to an institution for changing the community lifestyles and living conditions.
- The students and staff received positive encouragement from the community to express themselves by trying to change the living conditions and lifestyles in the surrounding environment.

- The greater commitment and dedication of the local communities has motivated local governmental service institutions to take further action.
- The many lessons learned from this experience have the potential to be put to good use in developing future strategies for HPS in the UAE.

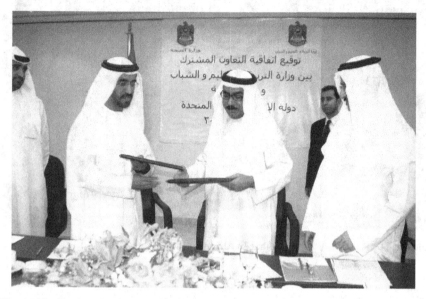

Picture 22   Signing of an agreement by the Under Secretaries of Ministry of Health and Ministry of Education

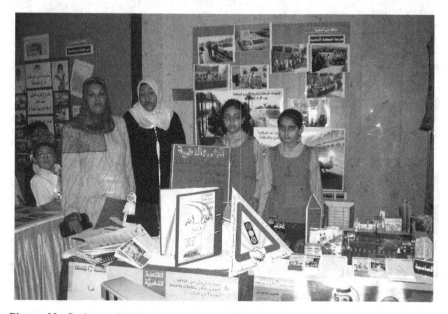

Picture 23   Project on health and school safety, Al Saada school

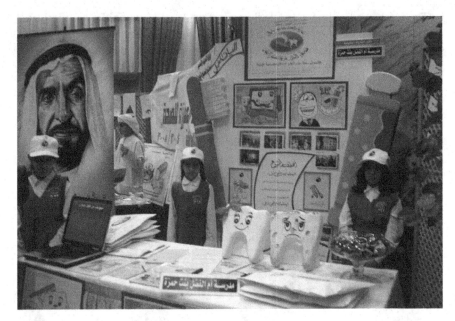

Picture 24 Project on Dental Health, Um Al Fadel School

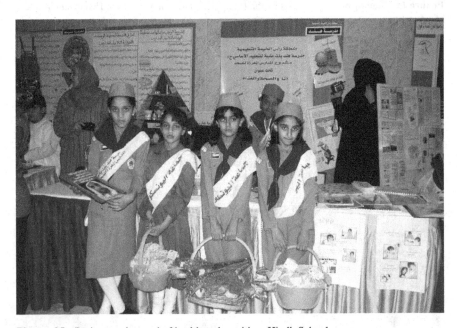

Picture 25 Project on the need of health and nutrition, Hindh School

Acknowledgment The author would like to acknowledge the support from Dr. Abdul Moneim Noor, Advisor in Preventive Medicine, Ministry of Health, UAE.

References

HPS Project in UAE. (2005a). *Workshop for the development of HPS a manual for facilitators.* Abu Dhabi, United Arab Emirates, Ministry of Health.

HPS Project in UAE. (2005b). *Workshop for the development of HPS a participants workbook.* Abu Dhabi, United Arab Emirates, Ministry of Health.

HPS Project in UAE. (2005c). *National guidelines for the development of HPS.* Abu Dhabi, United Arab Emirates, Ministry of Health.

Ministry of Health. (2006). *Preventive medicine sector annual report.* United Arab Emirates. Abu Dhabi, United Arab Emirates, Ministry of Health.

UAE School Health Department. (2003). *Strategic plan.* Abu Dhabi, United Arab Emirates, Ministry of Health.

UAE School Health Department. (2005). *Annual report for the academic year 2004–2005.* Abu Dhabi, United Arab Emirates, Ministry of Health.

UAE School Health Department. (2006). *Work plan for the academic year 2006–2007.* Abu Dhabi, United Arab Emirates, Ministry of Health.

UAE School Health Department. (2007). *Annual report for the academic year 2006–2007.* Abu Dhabi, United Arab Emirates, Ministry of Health.

Chapter 21
China: Implementing Health-Promoting Schools in Zhejiang Province, China

Carmen Aldinger

Contextual Introduction

Brief Introduction to the Country and Province

China is the world's most populated country, with over 1.3 billion inhabitants. China was one of the earliest centers of human civilization and has a history of thousands of years. The People's Republic of China was established in 1949 and is led by the Communist Party of China.

This case study was conducted in Zhejiang Province on the southeastern coast of China, home to more than 47 million people. Eleven cities or prefectures, including the capital, Hangzhou – home of 6 million people and with its famous West Lake – are under the direct jurisdiction of the province. Zhejiang Province has 53 ethnic minority groups, who speak a range of dialects.

Being one of the smallest provinces of China, Zhejiang is also one of the most prosperous. An atmosphere of rapid economic and social development provided the backdrop for the Health-Promoting Schools (HPS) project in Zhejiang. Universal 9-year compulsory education has been established; illiteracy among young people and adults has been mostly eliminated in 1997. In 2002, 84% of junior high school graduates went on to senior high school. Zhejiang officials have a long-term vision for the implementation of an impressive array of economic and social reforms, designed to result in an improved standard of living, a high degree of opening up to the outside world, and a favorable investment climate.

C. Aldinger
Health and Human Development Programs, Education Development Center, Newton, MA, USA

C. Vince Whitman and C.E. Aldinger (eds.),
Case Studies in Global School Health Promotion: From Research to Practice,
DOI: 10.1007/978-0-387-92269-0_21, © Springer Science + Business Media, LLC 2009

Origin of Health-Promoting Schools in Zhejiang Province

In response to the World Health Organization's (WHO) Global School Health Initiative, launched in 1995, and with endorsement of the national Ministries of Health and Education, some of China's health and education agencies began implementing the HPS concept in selected schools. In 1996, an HPS pilot project was established that successfully reduced parasitic helminth infections in rural schools (Xu et al., 2000). This was followed in 1998 and 2000 by two HPS projects in Zhejiang Province that successfully addressed tobacco use prevention and nutrition, respectively (Ma et al., 2002; Xia et al., 2004). A third project in Zhejiang Province used materials from UNICEF to address school-based injury prevention.

Based on the positive experiences of the pilot projects, officials of Zhejiang Province decided to systematically scale up the HPS project over the entire province, partially in an effort to achieve the government-mandated "quality education" that focuses not only on academic achievement but on the whole child.

Overview of the School Health Program

With joint endorsement of the Provincial Departments of Education and Health, Zhejiang Province, under the leadership of the provincial Health Education Institute, launched an effort in 2003 to expand the development of HPS to all 11 prefectures of the province. The program started with a training workshop in the capital of Hangzhou in October 2003 for headmasters and teacher representatives of schools, health educators from the CDC, and education officers of the prefectures.

The participating 51 schools – representing 93,000 students and their families, and 6,800 school personnel – included all levels from primary through junior and senior high to vocational schools, located in rural and urban areas throughout the province. The first phase of scaling up of HPS lasted through November 2005 and was accompanied by extensive quantitative and qualitative evaluation. This case study reports on the qualitative evaluation conducted during this time frame. (In April 2006, 125 new schools joined the effort to become HPS in Zhejiang Province.)

This qualitative case study about the implementation of HPS in Zhejiang Province included nine schools with a total population of about 15,200 students from the above cohort. The sample of 191 participants who took part in group interviews included 26 school administrators (19 male, 7 female), 56 teachers and school staff (21 male, 35 female), 64 students (25 male, 34 female, 5 data missing), and 45 parents (14 male, 31 female).

The remainder of this paper reports findings from this case study.

Scope of Implementation of HPS Components

Schools implemented comprehensive interventions that addressed all of the components of a Health-Promoting School and used the full organizational potential of the schools. Thus, unlike the studies by Lynagh, Schofield, and Sanson-Fisher (1997) and Stewart-Brown (2006), which showed that none of the programs incorporated all five components of the Ottawa Charter in the HPS approach, this study showed that the visited schools in Zhejiang Province addressed virtually all of the components of the Ottawa Charter at school level (policy, supportive environment, community action, personal skills, health services).

Examples of interventions for each component of HPS included the following:

- *School health policy.* Schools became smoke-free, established many health-related regulations such as safety and hygiene regulations, and developed a set of rules for each school department. Some schools posted their school health policy on school walls or display boards, and some issued a handbook for student behavior.
- *Physical school environment.* Schools improved their facilities, such as dining room, dormitories, sports facilities; established multimedia classrooms; and improved sanitation facilities, meeting WHO and national standards. Schools reduced littering and established green, clean, and beautiful school environments.
- *Psychosocial school environment.* Participants had harmonious relationships; teachers and students became like friends. Students were treated equally, and students established support groups with children of various abilities.
- *Health education.* Schools integrated teaching about health into regular teaching; some had special health education classes, and invited professionals to give lectures. Schools conducted drawing and writing competitions with health-related topics.
- *Health services.* Schools or nearby hospitals offered annual medical check-ups for students and staff, as well as prevention and treatment for common diseases. Schools had doctors on duty.
- *Nutrition services.* Schools offered nutritious meals and more food variety. Some schools had balanced fixed plates. Kitchen staff received training and advice from nutritionists.
- *Counseling/mental health.* Schools offered psychological consultation by specially trained teachers and in special, nicely decorated consultation rooms. Some schools had hotlines, special mailboxes, and consultations for teachers.
- *Physical exercise.* Schools established morning exercises and participated in sport matches such as football, basketball, and volleyball. Some schools improved their sports facilities.
- *Health promotion for staff.* Schools encouraged staff to quit smoking. Staff engaged in more exercise and walking and were offered psychological consulting.
- *Outreach to families and communities.* Schools sent letters to parents. Teachers visited and called parents' homes, and offered "parents school." Parent-child communication increased. Students did publicity in the community.

Summary of Achievements and Impact

Following about 1.5 years of HPS interventions, participants reported changes in their attitudes such as paying more attention to health, attaining better "psychological quality" and confidence, forming friendships between teachers and students, and feeling more relaxed. Participants also reported that they were increasing their knowledge of many health issues such as nutrition, hygiene, safety and security, tobacco, injury prevention, and psychology. They were also developing a broader concept of health and increasing their understanding of the HPS concept. Participants further reported that they were actively participating in the project, increasing physical activity, improving sanitary habits, reducing or quitting smoking, changing various bad habits, eating more nutritiously, sustaining fewer injuries, and improving parent-child communication.

A summary of the self-reported changes in attitudes, knowledge and concepts, and behaviors follows.

(a) Attitude changes:

- *Paying more attention to health.* Participants realized the importance of health and paid more attention to health.
- *Attaining better "psychological quality" and confidence.* Students, and some staff, improved their psychological qualities, including their ability to handle difficulties, and increased their confidence.
- *Forming friendships between teachers and students.* Teachers became like friends of students.
- *Feeling more relaxed.* Parents, and some students and administrators, felt more relaxed.

(b) Knowledge and conceptual changes:

- *Increasing knowledge about health issues.* Participants increased their knowledge about health, nutrition, hygiene, safety and security, the harm of tobacco, how to avoid injuries, and psychology.
- *Developing a broader concept of health.* Participants realized that health is a broader concept that includes physical, mental, and social health.
- *Gaining a better understanding about the HPS concept.* Participants expressed a very comprehensive understanding of the components and concept of a Health-Promoting School.

(c) Behavior changes:

- *Actively participating in the project.* Students and parents actively participated in the project, spread health knowledge, and formed good habits.
- *Increasing physical activity.* Some participants increased their physical activity.
- *Improving sanitary habits.* Students decreased littering and improved their hygiene habits, such as hand washing and brushing teeth.

- *Reducing or quitting smoking.* Many teachers, fathers, and grandfathers reduced or quit smoking.
- *Changing various bad habits.* Many participants changed their bad habits, such as sanitary and other living habits, and persuaded others to change their bad habits, too.
- *Eating more nutritiously.* Students and their families changed to a more balanced diet, less fried food, more vegetables.
- *Increasing safety behavior.* Students wore yellow safety caps and walked together; they did not take bicycles or vehicles without certificates to school; parents and teachers wore safety helmets.
- *Sustaining fewer injuries.* Injuries in two schools dropped by about 40%.
- *Improving parent-child communication.* Children had better communication with their parents; parents communicated more with their child.

Specific Aspects of Implementation

Schools went through a detailed process – preimplementation, implementation, and monitoring and evaluation – to become Health-Promoting Schools. Table 1 provides a summary of these steps.

This paper highlights several aspects of implementation: paying attention to external forces, gaining leadership support, obtaining administrative and management support, and adapting to local concerns and training.

Attention to External Forces

The most important external factors that influenced the process of implementing HPS in Zhejiang Province, China, included the one-child policy and the educational system.

One-child policy. China's one-child policy, introduced in 1979 and underpinned by a system of rewards and penalties, allows one child for urban residents and, with some restrictions, two children for rural residents (Hesketh, Li, & Zhu, 2005). The effects of this policy played a role in implementing the HPS project in two aspects.

First, because the government permits parents to have only one child, parents have an intense desire for that child to succeed and prosper and often have very high academic expectations for their child. Parents transfer these high expectations to their child, often creating serious pressure for the child to do very well in school. School administrators, teachers, students, and parents in this study all seemed to agree that students are under much pressure to succeed in school. The pressure extends beyond the children to their teachers, as families expect teachers to enable students to succeed.

Table 1 Summary of the processes of implementing HPS in Zhejiang Province, China

Preimplementation activities

Gaining leadership support
  Getting leaders to "pay attention" or give priority to HPS project
  Obtaining financial support
Being motivated
  Anticipating fame and prizes
  Supporting the government-mandated quality education for students' "all-around
  development" and to moving the society forward
Learning the HPS concept
  School administrators and teachers learning from CDC, training workshop, materials
  Students learning from headmaster, teachers, school publicity
  Parents learning from students
Choosing an entry point
  Perceiving that a specific health issue is important to address
  Conducting observations, referring to government and school surveys
  Already having a "good foundation" in addressing certain health issues
Setting up a special HPS Committee
  Designating principal as the leader in charge of the committee
  Including teachers and school staff, according to their regular area of work
  Including students, parents, community members, and others in some committees
  Committee making rules and regulations and ensuring project implementation
Developing a work plan
  Integrating HPS into school's "regular work" and actual conditions
  Planning activities for each month
Setting up policies and systems
  Improving existing rules and policies
  Developing and publicizing specific HPS regulations, rules, and systems
  Setting up regulations for smoke-free schools

Implementation activities

Being guided by rules and obedience
  Obeying HPS rules
Holding a start-up meeting
  Holding mobilization meeting for the HPS project
Prioritizing "Health is first"
  Putting priority on health
Popularizing the HPS concept
  Communicating the HPS concept widely among teachers, students, and communities
Cooperating with governmental departments
  Cooperating collaboratively with various governmental departments
Ensuring community cooperation and participation
  Viewing health promotion as a coresponsibility of school, family, community, and government
Obtaining input from students, parents, and teachers
  Giving students, parents, and teachers opportunities for input and suggestions
Being a role model
  Having headmasters, teachers, and parents as role models for healthy behaviors
Choosing interventions
  Choosing interventions according to plan, requirements, or students' characteristics

                                                                                          (Continued)

Table 1 (Continued)

Providing training

    Participating in initial orientation workshop on HPS concept and plan

    Arranging school-based trainings by CDC, health department, hospital staff, and other experts

    Engaging in self-study, especially for psychological certification

Conducting study visits

    Visiting other Health-Promoting Schools to learn from their experiences

Utilizing the Internet

Utilizing the Internet as a source of information and for sharing

    Choosing class topics

    Choosing topics for a variety of reasons, including conditions in their city, students' input, students' development, and "practical condition"

Using new teaching and learning methods

    Starting to use participatory, interactive, democratic teaching methods

Teaching social skills and life skills

    Teaching social skills, including skills for career development and housework

New textbooks and materials

    Utilizing or creating new textbooks and materials or making modifications to existing ones

---

Monitoring and evaluation

Carrying out process evaluation

    Carrying out various assessments for record-keeping of activities, teacher appraisal, students' activities and behavior, and school management

Conducting baseline, mid-term and final evaluation

    Conducting pre and postassessment

    Documenting the many aspects in which the HPS project can make a difference

Changing standards of evaluation

    Making health and holistic development of students part of the goals and evaluation standards

---

On the other hand, teachers, parents, and students repeatedly noted that because parents have only one child, children wield tremendous influence in their families. They indicated that parents and grandparents are likely to follow the suggestions and advice from their child and grandchild. They consider the child "the little emperor." Indeed, parents seemed to make behavior changes, especially reducing or quitting smoking (mostly fathers or grandfathers) and changing dietary habits (mostly mothers) after the child shared new knowledge and expectations. Grandparents seemed to be especially responsive to their grandchild, whom they reportedly "spoiled." For example, grandfathers told us that they stopped smoking after their grandchildren convinced them to do so.

These observations indicate that the one-child policy contributes the risk factor of academic pressure that resulted in stress and affected mental health, but also contributes the success factor of effective outreach to family members and convincing them to change unhealthy behaviors.

Educational system. During multiple interviews, participants mentioned the fierce academic pressure in Chinese schools. In this type of scholastic environment, it is understandable that students do not want to help each other or tell each other the solution, and the atmosphere traditionally has been very individualistic. There is no focus on teamwork because school administrators traditionally believed that the best way for teachers to convey large amounts of information efficiently is for students to be passive, rote learners and to obey directions.

Education in China traditionally serves foremost as a tool to strengthen the country. Standardized textbooks are common, and teachers have a high level of authority. Students are not encouraged to challenge knowledge from teachers and textbooks. Learning traditionally involves passive methods such as listening, thinking, and silent practice (Marlow-Ferguson & Lopez, 2002). However, the government recognized some of the shortcomings of this system (Wang, 2003). Since 1999, the Chinese government had advocated a policy of "quality education" that calls for holistic development of students. Particularly parents told us that the HPS concept fits exactly with the government-mandated quality education.

Viewed in the context of this transitional state of education in China, it seems that the HPS project has come to China at an opportune time. During the project, teachers implemented more participatory activities. Students reportedly started working together and supporting each other. Teachers started to evaluate students not only according to their academic achievements but also according to physical, emotional, and social health and development.

Thus, the participants' reported ability to engage in new methods of teaching and learning indicates that the proposed changes in the educational system are likely to contribute to the successful implementation of the HPS project in China.

Gaining Leadership Support

Implementing HPS started with strong support from the leadership – in the province, municipality, and school. This included "paying attention" – or giving priority – to the HPS project as well as obtaining financial support. As one teacher said, "everything can be done if the leadership pays attention to the issues."

Principals received programmatic and financial support from the education bureau, as well as support from WHO, CDC, and experts at the national and provincial levels. Some school administrators communicated with the government to win their support. A vice headmaster reported that since the school became a Health-Promoting School, they got "much attention from the leaders," and one of the teachers responded that they receive "help from everywhere."

In a rural school, administrators reported that leaders at higher levels offered supportive help and paid attention. Teachers told us that officials at all levels "tried their hardest to make all resources they could find available to support the implementation of this project." In an urban school, administrators said that it was helpful to get "support from leaders at different levels of the municipal public health departments." Helpful also was "the concern from WHO."

In addition to the support from the municipal government, and especially in cases where strong support from the municipal government was lacking, the strong leadership of the school principal and administrators was crucial. Some principals became role models for healthy behavior by stopping smoking or by walking to school. Teachers often followed suit. School principals or designated teachers led the special HPS committees. Some schools had a team of administrators who considered themselves "coworkers" on this project.

These reports show that governmental agencies gave support and principals provided the inspiration and ability to motivate people to pursue the vision.

Administrative and Management Support

A further factor in implementation is administrative and management support. Schools set up special *HPS planning committees*. Principals and/or vice-principals led or co-led these committees. Committee members included administrators and teachers with authority from various areas throughout the school (e.g., morality education, physical education, logistics, teaching, student works, school health service, counseling), selected according to the positions and roles they already held, so as to attach the project to their regular work systematically throughout the school. In some cases, students, parents, and/or community members also served on this committee. The committees discussed the policy to carry out, made a plan, and discussed details and assignments of tasks and strategies to carry out the plan. They set up and perfected various systems in the school, made modifications to the school policy, and took responsibility for project implementation. They developed a work plan, based on their regular work, integrating HPS interventions and making them part of the overall school responsibility.

Popularizing the HPS concept through various means of communication also played an important role in the administrative and management support of this project. Schools used wallboards and bulletins for propaganda, students passed on materials to parents and community members, and schools held parents' meetings and sent letters to parents. One school reported using news media and the Internet for publicity.

This combination of special HPS committees with frequent and various communication to popularize the HPS concept and interventions seemed to ensure that the HPS concept and interventions could be spread efficiently throughout the school and to the community.

Adaptation to Local Concerns

A further factor in implementation is adaptation to local concerns. while interventions were needed to ensure fidelity of the overall HPS concept, they also had to be adapted to local situations. Each school developed a *work plan* according to the

HPS project and related it to the school's condition. The basic principle was to adapt this project by taking the "practical situation" of each school into consideration. For example, vocational school students previously experienced failure, so they needed to develop confidence. In rural schools, students and families had lower basic educational levels, so they needed to learn about basic safety and injury prevention. In urban schools, students experienced a lot of pressure to achieve high academic scores, so they benefited from psychological consultation. Some schools were concerned about *balancing health and academics*, especially when parents were worried that the HPS project might have a negative impact on their child's academic education.

Developing a work plan tailored to each individual school helped to adapt the HPS project to local needs and concerns.

Training

Another important factor in implementation is training. Training is a crucial part of capacity building. Participants needed initial training to support them in *learning the HPS concept*. Delegates from each school went to an initial workshop with CDC, national, and international experts. Part of the training also included *visits to other HPSs* in the province. Then each school organized meetings in which those who had participated in the trainings passed on their knowledge. Administrators and teachers studied the WHO-issued HPS documents, and, in some cases, schools offered additional *trainings by CDC staff and/or other experts*. We saw pictures in which the whole schoolyard was filled with participants for trainings by CDC staff; these were sometimes truly team trainings. Some teachers engaged in *self-study*, for example, to gain psychological certifications. Parents were "trained" through information passed on to them by their children and through parents' meetings.

Despite these training efforts, many interviewees mentioned a lack of knowledge, skills, methods, theoretical guidance, and experience in health promotion; a lack of technical support; and a lack of qualified staff. For instance, in one school, teachers first thought that their nutrition knowledge was enough, but when the project gained in intensity, they felt a need for more professional instruction and hoped for more expert talks, though they also acknowledged that "knowledge is not enough" and that some students knew better than teachers. In another school, teachers reported a "lack of health promotion theory" and of the "health" concept. In several schools, administrators hoped that WHO would provide more guidance and good examples of international HPS achievements, to help them define specific goals for themselves. School administrators also expressed a desire to visit other places with experience with health promotion. In one school, the school nurse was the only one who had psychological training. Since many students had psychological issues, they needed more teachers with this knowledge. Parents suggested

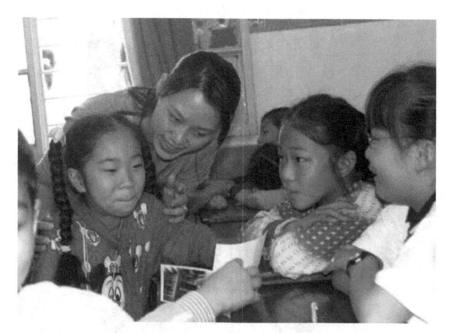

Picture 26

offering more good training for teachers to improve the quality of the staff and introducing more advanced ideas and theories to help them toward good achievements.

Thus, while various means of training initially enabled schools to establish Health-Promoting Schools, participants requested more training, guidance, and sharing of experiences. Study results indicate that training plays an important role in effective HPS implementation.

Conclusions, Insights, and Recommendations

Several factors contributed to the successful implementation of this project:

- Government officials, administrators, teachers, school staff, students, and parents were sincerely committed to improving the health status and all-around development of their communities. They felt ownership in valuing their schools as a community and were committed to working together to improve it.
- Schools put top priority on health, and it was seen as a coresponsibility. Schools viewed the HPS concept as part of the overall responsibility of the school rather than an extra task to be carried out, and parents recognized that they shared responsibility with the school to promote health.

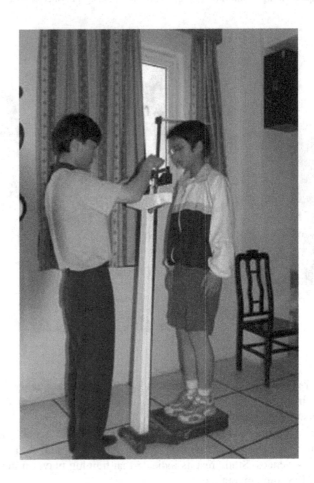

Picture 27

- The schools participating in this project had vast differences in health-related issues and resources among communities. As a consequence, each school needed to focus on different issues and tailor to its specific situation, in order to achieve necessary site-specific changes. The HPS model could be adapted for each school.

Several of the success factors were related to the macroenvironment, such as the one-child policy and the mandate for quality education.

- The one-child policy, while placing great pressure on the one child to perform well academically, also gave the single child a special role as a change agent in his or her family, convincing parents and grandparents of health-conducive behaviors, such as the need to stop smoking. This was supported by the fact that many parents had low levels of education and were eager to learn.

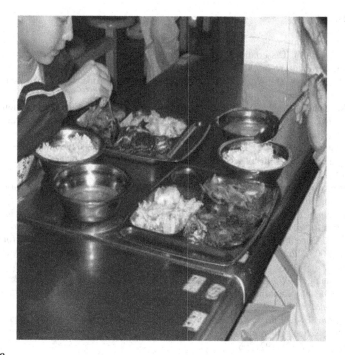

Picture 28

- The recent mandate from the Chinese government for quality education calls for a holistic approach to child development and education. The WHO HPS model provided a useful structure for implementing these changes. Parents and teachers came to value the whole child's development and its implications for learning.

One factor could be strengthened: There was a definite need for more training and professional development in health promotion concepts, knowledge, skills, and experiences about Health-Promoting Schools and related issues.

Overall, this study showed that implementing HPS in Zhejiang Province was successful and provided a comprehensive model for HPS implementation, though some aspects were definitely specific to China.

Acknowledgments The project has been implemented by the Health Education Institute of the Centers for Disease Control and Prevention (CDC) in Zhejiang Province, China, under the leadership of Dr. Zhang Xin-Wei and Dr. Liu Li-Qun. The data collection and analysis for this case study have been assisted and guided by Dr. Yu Sen-Hai, Mr. Jack Jones, Dr. Jared Kass, Ms. Cheryl Vince Whitman, and Dr. Gene Diaz.

References

Aldinger, C. (2007). Dissertation: *The process of implementing health-promoting schools in Zhejiang Province, China*. Cambridge, MA: Lesley University.

Hesketh, T., Li, L., & Zhu, W. X. (2005). The effect of China's one-child family policy after 25 years. *New England Journal of Medicine, 353*(11), 1171–1176.

Lynagh, M., Schofield, M. J., & Sanson-Fisher, R. W. (1997). School health promotion programs over the past decade: A review of the smoking, alcohol and solar protection literature. *Health Promotion International, 12*(1), 43–60.

Ma, H. L., Geng, L., Xia, S. C., Hou, J. X., Xu, S. Y., & Yu, W. P. (2002). Development of Health-Promoting Schools with tobacco use prevention as entry point. *Chinese Journal of Health Education, 18*(7), 414–417.

Marlow-Ferguson, R., & Lopez, C. (Eds.). (2002). *World education encyclopedia* (2nd ed., Vol. 1). Farmington Hills, MI: Gale Group.

Stewart-Brown, S. (2006). *What is the evidence on school health promotion in improving health or preventing disease and, specifically, what is the effectiveness of the health promoting schools approach?* Copenhagen, Denmark: World Health Organization Regional Office for Europe.

Wang, X. (2003). *Education in China since 1976*. Jefferson, North Carolina: McFarland & Company.

Xia, S.-C., Zhang, X.-W., Xu, S.-Y., Tang, S.-M., Yu, S.-H., Aldinger, C., & Glasauer, P. (2004). Creating health-promoting schools in China with a focus on nutrition. *Health Promotion International, 19*(4), 409–418.

Xu, L.-S., Pan, B.-J., Lin, J.-X., Chen, L.-P., Yu, S.-H., & Jones, J. (2000). Creating health-promoting schools in rural China: A project started from deworming. *Health Promotion International, 15*(3), 197–206.

Chapter 22
Hong Kong: Health-Promoting Schools

Albert Lee

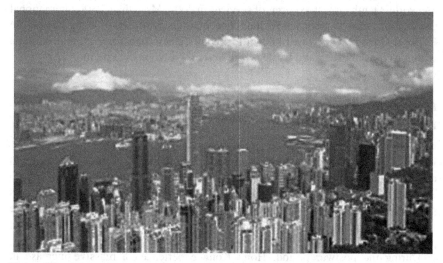

Picture 29

Contextual Introduction

Hong Kong Special Administrative Region

Hong Kong, described over 150 years ago as a "barren rock," has become a world-class financial, trading, and business center and, indeed, a great world city. Hong Kong became a Special Administrative Region (SAR) of the People's Republic of China on July 1, 1997, after a century and a half of British administration. Under Hong Kong's constitutional document, the Basic Law, the SAR enjoys a high degree of autonomy. Hong Kong's population was about 6.88 million in mid-2004, with a population density of 6,380 people per square kilometer. Hong Kong had a large foreign population of about 524,200. Chinese and English are the official languages. English is widely used in the Government and by the legal, professional, and business sectors.

A. Lee
Department of Community and Family Medicine, and Centre for Health Education and Health Promotion of School of Public Health, The Chinese University of Hong Kong (CUHK), Shatin, N.T., Hong Kong, China

C. Vince Whitman and C.E. Aldinger (eds.),
Case Studies in Global School Health Promotion: From Research to Practice,
DOI: 10.1007/978-0-387-92269-0_22, © Springer Science + Business Media, LLC 2009

Social and Economic Status of Hong Kong SAR

Hong Kong is the world's eleventh largest trading economy, sixth largest foreign exchange market, thirteenth largest banking center, and Asia's second biggest stock market. Hong Kong is one of the world's top exporters of garments, watches and clocks, toys, games, electronic products, and certain light industrial products; it was the world's tenth largest exporter of services in 2004. More than 3,800 international corporations have established regional headquarters or offices in Hong Kong. The HKSAR Government is well known for its efficiency, transparency, and fairness, with a well-established and trusted legal system based on the common law.

Hong Kong Health Education Environment and Health-Promoting Schools

During the early colonial period, from the late nineteenth to the early twentieth century, education policy was for the Colonial Government to provide assistance to enlighten the upper classes of Chinese rather than to force new ideas on the mass population. It was believed that civilized ideas among the leaders of thought were the best and perhaps the only means at that time for permeating the general population (Sweeting, 1990).

During the postwar period, Hong Kong experienced a massive increase in population and emerged as one of the world's largest financial centers. As the economy grew, the schools focused more on the forms of high-status knowledge (particularly English, Chinese, mathematics, science, and information technology) that were most directly linked to certification and admission to higher education institutions; that is, priority shifted to academic subjects.

Two main factors were perceived by parents as the key determinants of a school's status: its banding, determined by the pupils' performance in selective academic examinations, and its policy on the language of instruction (Morris & Chan, 1997). Schools claiming to use English have generally been accorded a higher status. With the change of sovereignty and growing economy of Mainland China, it is expected that the teaching of Putonghua (Mandarin) will also be accorded high priority for high-status schools.

Another critical point in schooling is the internal school examination system. Over 65% of the aggregate mark is derived from students' performance in languages, mathematics, and science (Morris, 1996). "Soft" subjects such as physical education, art, music, humanities, and home economics are assigned grades rather than marks. Health education is supposed to be integrated into the curriculum of those subjects. As the schools have allocated more time to high-status subjects, fewer periods are allocated to the *soft* subjects that would provide opportunity for health education to be integrated. Those soft subjects do not constitute a discrete and specialized field of study with clear linkage to further study at University. Time allocated to health education becomes thinner and thinner.

Level of Development of Health-Promoting Schools

In 1999 the Centre for Health Education and Health Promotion of the Faculty of Medicine of the Chinese University of Hong Kong (CUHK) conducted a large-scale survey of 26,111 students aged 10–19. Results showed that about 14% of students felt that their physical health and emotional health had interfered with their normal daily activities most of the time, about 15% of students had consulted doctors more than three times over the last 6 months, and about 15% admitted that they had been regular smokers (Lee & Tsang, 2004). Students in higher grades had more health problems in physical and psychological aspects, and a lower proportion of students in higher grades adopted healthy lifestyles. This is due to the heavier workload of their study and also to less emphasis on health education in their formal curriculum.

The research findings have provided evidence of the need to develop Health-Promoting Schools (HPS) in Hong Kong. The main provision of student health services in Hong Kong has been by the Department of Health. It operates a center-based health screening service rather than school-based student health services. There is a need to change the long-established traditional approach to school health education. The better approach should focus on the interaction of the informal and formal school curricula, and on the involvement of new partners in health promotion at schools, such as teachers, school education administrators, parents, community leaders, and students themselves, in addition to health professionals. The HPS concept is an effective approach to promote health in schools (Young, 1986) as it embodies a whole-school approach going beyond the school curriculum to include components – such as the physical environment, school ethos, school-based health policies, linkage with health services, and partnerships with community – that would have strong impact on the health of students (McDonald & Ziglio, 1994; Nutbeam, 1987; Parsons, Stears, & Thomas, 1996; World Health Organization, 1996; Young & Williams, 1989). In 1998 CUHK aimed to develop HPS, shifting the paradigm of school health into a more dynamic and political domain (St Leger, 2001).

Overview of the School Health Program

Date Boundaries

Figure 1 depicts the development and growth of the school health program.

Key Players Putting HPS in Practice

In 1998, CUHK decided to promote and implement the concept of HPS. It worked in collaboration with several groups:

Embryonic stage 1998 – 2002

Professional Diploma in Health Education and Health Promotion for school educators
1998 –
Hong Kong Healthy Schools Award Scheme starting 2001 –
Master program in Health Education 2001 –
Certificate program in Health Education for early childhood educators (preschool)
2002–
Development of Practical Manual for Health-Promoting Schools
Youth Risk Behavioral Survey 1999–
⇓
Growing stage 2002–2005

Hong Kong Healthy Schools Award for Kindergartens (early childhood education)
2005–
Health - Promoting Schools Mentorship Scheme 2005–07
Color and Bright Fruit and Vegetable program 2005–07
School Resiliency program 2005–06
School against SARS 2003
Training workshops for Health - Promoting Schools for educators and health
professionals in Hong Kong, Macao, Taiwan, and Mainland China 2003–05
Preparing schools for outbreaks of influenza 2004
Establishment of Health - Promoting Schools Network in different districts
International publications on evaluation framework of Health - Promoting Schools
⇓
Consolidation stage from 2005

Development of Self - Evaluation Scheme for Health - Promoting Schools
International Training Workshops for Health - Promoting Schools
Development of new Senior Secondary School Curriculum in Health and Social Care
(starts 2009)
CHILD (Children Harmonious Innovative Lifelong Development: mental health
promotion)
Building on the concept of Health Promoting Schools to develop an effective and
sustainable model of 'Healthy Campus (Starts 2009)
International publications on outcomes of Health - Promoting School Effectiveness

Fig. 1 Development of HPS in Hong Kong

- The Hong Kong Subsidized Secondary Schools Councils
- The Subsidized Primary Schools Councils
- The Hong Kong Special Schools Councils

(These groups thereafter were known as the *School Councils*).

Fullan and Stieggelbauer (1991) have asserted that "all major research on innovation and school effectiveness shows that the school principals strongly influence the likelihood of change." The three School Councils comprise the majority of the schools in Hong Kong with the principals serving as members representing the schools. As active partners, the three Councils have the power to influence policy and support the development of HPS.

Although there was no earmarked funding for HPS at that moment, the Hong Kong SAR Government had established a US $640 million (HK $5 billion) Quality Education Fund (QEF) to fund worthwhile projects to raise the quality of school education. CUHK and the School Councils successfully convinced the QEF that both health and education are linked to the economic performance and social cohesion of modern industrialized society. Therefore, funding of US $1.9 million in 1998 and US $1.1 million in 2000 was awarded to launch the initial HPS program.

The objectives of the initial HPS program were to overcome the barriers experienced by other countries. Teacher development in health education, including training and ongoing support, has been shown to increase teachers' feeling of preparedness to teach specific health topics (Hausman & Ruzek, 1995). A training course was launched at the CUHK in 1999, in the format of a Professional Diploma in Health Promotion and Health Education (Lee, Tsnag, Lee & To, 2000).

In addition to acquiring essential knowledge and skills of health education, the participating teachers conducted school-based health promotion projects in groups, to gain practical experience in implementing the concept of HPS and to accept the challenge of moving away from didactic health education to a settings approach to health promotion (Rowling & Ritchie, 1996–1997). Those projects provided good opportunities for involvement of school staff, parents, students, and community. Most of their projects had gained the support and participation of Parent-Teachers Associations of their schools, community leaders, nongovernment organizations, government departments, and business companies; so a strong community partnership was established for future action. By the end of September 2004, 513 participants (from around 500 schools) had graduated from a diploma course.

Reaching Out to Schools

Many schools are adopting school-based management to enhance productivity and learning (Cohen, 1988; David, 1989). It requires the involvement of all six segments of a school's community: the headmaster, teachers, supporting staff, parents, students, and other community members. The concept of HPS as a new initiative in school-based management would move beyond individual behavioral change, to consider organizational structure changes, such as improving the school's physical and social environment, its curricula, teaching, and learning methods. This would enable school effectiveness efforts to focus on social/affective outcomes, such as attitudes and behaviors of students, rather than just on academic achievement (Mortimore, Sammons, Stoll, Lewis, & Ecob, 1988). The gap between practice and "what ought to be" is greater for school health promotion than for most other areas (Seffrin, 1990). The CUHK launched the Hong Kong Healthy Schools Award

Scheme (HKHSA) to facilitate the development of school-based management and HPS practices (Lee, 2002). QEF funding of US $2.75 million in 2001 and US $0.5 million in 2005 was awarded for Hong Kong Healthy Schools Award and Health Promoting Kindergarten (early childhood education), respectively.

The Healthy Schools Award scheme provides a structured framework for implementation as well as a system to monitor and recognize achievement (Rogers, Moon, Mullee, Speller, & Roderick, 1998). Positive award-related changes have been demonstrated (Moon, 1999) in children's health behaviors and in the culture and organization of the school. However, the core business of schools is more concerned with educational outcomes than with health outcomes. The concept of HPS has an interesting parallel in models of school improvement developed in the education sector, for example, by the School Improvement Research Group at Cambridge University (Hopkins, 1994).

Scope of Implementation

Development of an Evaluation Framework

The Award Scheme in Hong Kong covers six key areas (health policy, physical environments, social environments, community relationships, personal health skills, and health services) based on World Health Organization (WHO) guidelines (WHO Regional Office for the Western Pacific [WPRO], 1996). Each country was encouraged to develop indicators to meet the local needs. The indicators and guidelines developed were evidence-based and have a broad range of objectives. They were designed to be relevant, adaptable, and achievable, so they can be used to develop good practices (Centers for Disease Control and Prevention, 2002; Pattenden, 1998; Piette et al., 2002; St Leger, 1999). Each key area has a number of components with targets for the school to achieve. The components cover school-based changes/initiatives as well as the involvement of parents, school management committees, the community, and teacher training. Evaluation of success would mean measuring the success of a complex of initiatives.

The process for the development of the indicators for the HKHSA and the process of audit/accreditation for schools have incorporated advice and guidelines and validation from a number of international experts in the field (Lee et al., 2004). CUHK then developed a practical manual with detailed guidelines and indicators for each component to achieve the standard for the six key areas documented by WHO/WPRO (Centre for Health Education and Health Promotion [CHEP], 2003a). The report of the process of accreditation was submitted to WHO/WPRO, and the awards were endorsed by WHO/WPRO as meeting the WHO standards in 2002 and 2003 (CHEP, 2003b, 2004). Evidence from the comprehensive mapping of the status of Health Promoting Schools and from student surveys does show encouraging outcomes as well as identify priority issues to be addressed in the next 5 years (Lee, Cheng, St Leger, & Hong Kong Healthy School Team, 2007).

Instruments Used to Measure Outcomes

The indicators measure outcomes at different stages. CUHK had already developed a system for monitoring progress and assessing schools' performance on the HPS. Questionnaires covering the items of the six key areas were produced and issued to each school. They were designed in template format to allow much of the information to be entered as quantifiable data. The template also facilitated the collection of qualitative information. A team of health promotion coordinators from CUHK visited the school and supplemented the information by reviewing school documents (e.g., policies), analyzing the school curriculum, observing the school environment, and interviewing school teachers and head teachers. Table 1 describes how different outcomes were measured by different instruments (Lee, Cheng, & St Leger, 2005). The details of development of rating systems and evaluation framework for HKHSA have been published in detail (Lee et al., 2004; Lee, Cheng, et al., 2005; Lee, Cheng, Yuen, et al., 2007).

Table 1 School health outcomes

Types of outcomes	Indicators to be measured	Measuring instrument
Health and social outcomes	Depressive symptoms, life satisfaction, perceived health status, and perceived academic achievement	Validated questionnaires: LIFE, DSRS, and YRBS
Intermediate outcomes	Attitudes, lifestyles, and risk behaviors	Questionnaires to students and schools, school observation, documentary review, interviews, and ethnography
	School environment and school ethos	
	School health services	
Health promotion outcomes	Health skills and knowledge, self-efficacy	Questionnaires to students and schools, curriculum review, documentary review, interviews, focus groups, and participant observation
	School health policies	
	Networking with parents, community, and other schools to launch health programs	
Health promotion action	School timetable for health education activities (formal and extracurricular)	Documentary review
	PTA and community involvement	

This summary shows the indicators and measuring instruments used for the different types of outcomes for school health promotion

Scaling of HPS Movement

When the Healthy Schools Award was first implemented in 2001, only 42 schools were involved. As of June 2007, there are 210 schools involved in the Healthy Schools Award Scheme, including 63 primary schools, 36 secondary schools, 11 special schools, and 100 kindergartens (preschools). As of June 2006, there were three schools with Gold Awards, 21 schools with Silver Awards, and 21 schools with Bronze Awards. In regard to training of schoolteachers, more than 500 school-teachers have graduated with a Professional Diploma, and 20 schoolteachers have obtained a Master's degree in Health Education and Health Promotion.

After SARS appeared in 2003, the Team Clean Report of Hong Kong SAR Government recommended HPS as a strategy for the education sector to promote better health and hygiene in order to prevent possible outbreaks of infectious diseases. The Education and Manpower Bureau commissioned CUHK to conduct workshops for schoolteachers to promote the concept of HPS to all schools in Hong Kong; 1,232 school principals and teachers attended. It has now been modified as a short course suitable for both local and overseas participants. CUHK has conducted two international HPS workshops commissioned by WHO WPRO for health and educational professionals from Asian and Pacific Island countries. CUHK has visited Laos as consultants to help them develop HPS. CUHK has conducted several workshops for Macao SAR and Mainland China. The Centre director has also been invited as keynote speaker in Australia, Britain, Canada, Japan, Korea, Macao, Mainland China, and Malaysia. CUHK also presented many papers related to HPS during the 2004 and 2007 World Conferences in Health Promotion.

Local and Overseas Seminars and Workshops

From 2001 to 2004, the Centre has conducted more than 50 seminars and work-shops for school coordinators, teachers, and school heads. A total of 64 school representatives have taken part in 5-day training and exchange trips to Taiwan in 2001 and 2002. Forty-four school principals, teachers, school nurses, and school social workers have participated in a 4-day exchange and training program in Melbourne during the World Conference in Health Promotion in 2004. Seminars sharing the inspiration of the training after each trip were organized for other schoolteachers.

Supporting Schools in Crisis Management

During the SARS period, the concept and implementation of HPS contributed to preventing the spread of SARS in Hong Kong. The framework of the HKHSA prepared the schools with the following:

- A structuralized crisis management system
- Proper documentation and follow-up with students' sick leave records
- A policy on prevention of infectious disease
- A supportive and harmonized school environment to encourage sharing and mutual support

The crisis, then, became an opportunity for the whole community, including the schools, to overcome what then seemed an insurmountable challenge (Lee, Cheng, Yuen, Ho, & Healthy Schools Support Group, 2003). In 2005, the teaching material for prevention of Avian Flu was produced in CD format for the schoolteachers. Several seminars were conducted to teach students how to step up measures at schools and to educate the students, staff, and parents on prevention of Avian Flu.

Health Promotion Activities for Families, Staff, and Communities

From 2002 to 2004, the HKHSA participating schools organized health promotion activities for the families and the networking communities. A total of 119 and 46 health topics were delivered to the families and communities, respectively, by the 32 participating schools. After joining the HKHSA, the participating schools improved their ability to involve and mobilize parents in health promotion activities. Various kinds of health-related workshops and seminars have been conducted for the participating schools for staff health. Topics include back care, foot care, and crisis management.

Development of Ten Health Content Areas for Different Grades

CUHK has devised a booklet of 10 Health Content Areas with reference to the contents of health education implemented in other countries. They are Personal Health; Food and Nutrition; Mental and Emotional Health; Family Relationship and Sex Education; Prevention and Management of Disease; Smoking, Alcoholism, Drug Use and Abuse; Consumer Health; Safety and First Aid; Environmental Health and Conservation; and Life, Aging, and Death. By acquiring the knowledge and skills from the ten Health Content Areas, students are enabled to resist various temptations of unhealthy elements in the environment by building up their capabilities in problem-solving, stress management, wise decision-making, acquisition of health information and services, risk-identification and analytical thinking, effective communication, life-long learning, goal setting, self-management of health, refusal techniques, and coordination and cooperation. The booklets of 10 Health Content Areas have been sent to the participating schools joining the HKHSA as the recommended footprint for planning health education in different school grades. All of the 32 schools that underwent the audit process have integrated the 10 Health Content Areas into their school curriculum or extracurricular activities. The mean coverage of the health topics was up to 95%. A guideline booklet has also been produced for kindergartens to help preschool educators develop a health curriculum (Lee, Ho, et al., 2007). The personal health skills development laid down the foundation for developing the new Senior Secondary School Curriculum in Health and Social Care.

Specific Aspects of Implementation

Table 2 summarizes specific aspects of implementation.

Summary of Achievements and Impact

Improvement in School Management and Student Health

The participating schools have achieved remarkable results in the key areas, as indicated by the comparison of the baseline assessment with the audit result (Lee, St

Table 2 Specific aspects of implementation of HPS in Hong Kong

Vision	Innovative approach to improve teaching and learning and also to strengthen school-based management
National guidelines	Practical guidelines for HKHSA, including preschool (early childhood education)
Administrative support	University Centre for Health Promotion
Data-driven planning	Periodic youth risk behaviors surveys, school assessment data. HPS Registry for Western Pacific Region
Training	Professional Diploma/Master in Health Promotion, short courses for HPS training
	International Training Workshops
Critical mass	Engaging key schools with leadership roles, engagement of parents and community. Also started HPS movement for preschool setting
Resources	Quality Education Fund, Health Care Promotion Fund, private donations
Attention to external forces	Education reform for board-based learning and health care reform shifting toward community care and prevention
Local adaptation	For the new Senior Secondary School curriculum, public health and disease prevention will be taught as core modules under Liberal Study, a compulsory subject for all secondary school students. A new academic subject, Health Management and Social Care will be introduced
Champion and leaders at all levels	CUHK is aiming to become an education hub for HPS in the region, with development of a comprehensive evaluation framework with practical guidelines and a self-evaluation scheme, also with international publications of HPS effectiveness

Leger, & Moon, 2005). At follow-up evaluation, 98.2% of the participating schools had set up a working group or committee for school health promotion and education whereas only 53.4% of the participating schools had such kind of working group at the baseline assessment. For promoting healthy eating, all participating schools have laid down a healthy eating policy for their students, whereas only 57.1% of the participating schools had this policy in the baseline assessment. For the maintenance of student health, only 5.4% of the participating schools were analyzing and following up on students' body weight, and 19.6% of these schools informed the parents and students of students' body weight at baseline. At follow-up evaluation, 76.8% and 73.2%, respectively, analyzed and followed up students' body weight, and informed parents. In regard to infectious disease control and management, 91.1% of the participating schools kept a comprehensive record of students with special needs as shown in the audit result, whereas 32.1% kept the record in the baseline assessment. Please refer to Tables 3 and 4 for details of the results. The early results demonstrated significant improvements in various aspects of student health and well-being.

A recent study tested the hypothesis that students from schools that had comprehensively embraced the HPS concept as indicated by the Healthy School Award were better, in terms of health and education outcomes, than students from schools that only partially followed the HPS concept (Lee, Cheng, Fung, & St Leger, 2006). The results presented came from nine schools (four primary and five secondary) applying for accreditation of the Healthy Schools Award after adopting the HPS framework for 2 years. Students had completed pre and postsurveys to assess their health behaviors, self-reported health status, and academic standing, prior to the 2-year intervention and at its end. Data from the pre and postsurveys of the students attending schools that reached certain levels of HPS standard as indicated by the award were compared with that of students whose schools did not receive the award, and the results showed differences. Some differences were found to be more significant among the primary school students than among the secondary school students. This indicates that early intervention for lifestyle changes is more effective. Students' satisfaction with life also improved if their schools adopted the concept of HPS comprehensively. The results suggest that comprehensive implementation of HPS would contribute to differences in certain behaviors and self-reported health and academic status. Students in the HSA category were also found to be better than those in schools that did not achieve an award. Results reached statistical significance in personal hygiene practice, knowledge of health and hygiene, and access to health information. HSA schools were reported to have better school health policy, higher degrees of community participation, and better hygienic environments (Lee et al., 2008).

Conclusions and Recommendations

The HKHSA emphasizes the combined efforts of education and health professionals to enable the HPS program to be more comprehensive and related to school

Table 3 School improvements

Components	At baseline (%) $N = 56$ schools	At evaluation (%) $N = 56$ schools
School health promotion and health education		
School has a working group or committee for school health promotion and education	53.4	98.2
Student health promoting organizations or activity group	32.7	67.3
Cross-curriculum program includes health topics	26.8	83.9
At least one staff trained or under training to promote health education	57.1	94.6
Provides diversified and well-managed health education resources for staff	58.9	78.6
Healthy eating		
Has healthy eating policy	57.1	100
Committee to monitor school healthy eating policy	75.0	96.4
Student health maintenance		
Has student health maintenance policy	51.8	91.1
Statistics on attendance of body check	37.5	98.2
Follow-up of body check	25.0	80.1
Statistics on attendance of dental check	23.2	69.6
Follow-up of dental check	19.6	72.9
Student health data is kept	60.7	98.2
Analysis and follow-up of students' body weight	5.4	76.8
School informs parents and students of students' body weight	19.6	73.2
Measures the weight of school bags	3.6	50.0
Infectious disease control and management		
Has policy on prevention of infectious diseases	46.4	96.4
Comprehensive system for monitoring, control, and management of infectious diseases	8.9	94.6
Follow-up of students immunization status	23.2	78.6
Encourages students' participation in large-scale school cleaning activities	38.2	80.0
First aid and emergency management at school		
Has first aid and safety policy	78.6	98.2
Has at least 2 qualified providers of first aid service	42.9	69.6
Analysis and follow-up of student injury records	0	46.4
Crisis management		
Establishes committee to handle crisis	83.9	98.2
Measures to handle students' emotional instability	89.3	96.4
Measures to handle students' traumatic events	69.6	76.8
Measures to handle staff's emotional instability	28.6	60.7
Measures to handle staff's suicidal attempts	26.8	42.9
Measures to handle staff's traumatic events	25.0	42.9
Addressing the needs of students		
Has policy to prevent violence and bullying	64.3	96.4
To reward students who actively participate in community services and activities	83.9	94.6

(Continued)

Table 3 (Continued)

Components	At baseline (%) N = 56 schools	At evaluation (%) N = 56 schools
To reward students who have behavioral improvement	75.0	80.4
Students' involvement in policy making	28.6	55.1
Has a student mentor system	75.0	84.9
Keeps a comprehensive record of students with special needs	32.1	91.1
Promoting occupational health and safety		
Has policy on staff health promotion	26.8	96.4
Formulated a committee or group for occupational health	25.0	76.4
Formally encourages staff to have OSH training	66.1	91.1
Form to record injury of staff	0	67.9
Analysis and follow-up of staff injury records	0	30.4
Encourages staff to have periodic checkups	21.4	75.0
Encouraging parent involvement in school life		
Parents participate in formulating and reviewing of annual health promotion plan and health policies	16.1	66.1
Parents involve as instructors of school activities	21.4	62.5
Parents serving as active volunteers	21.4	57.1
Proactive leakage with community		
Involves community members or organizations in formulating and reviewing of school health policies	12.5	82.1
Involves community members or organizations in development of school's annual health promotion plan and discussed school needs	10.7	89.3
Networks with other schools in health promotion activities	46.4	71.4
Participates in local health education exchange activities	21.4	75.0
Transport safety		
Closely monitor school bus services	33.3	100
Actions to ensure road safety	41.1	52.1

School improvements are shown here by comparison of the findings of the baseline assessment and the audit evaluation result

outcomes. This project shows some promising changes occurring among the students from award schools. The findings suggest that if the HPS framework is embraced comprehensively, there will be substantial gains in health and educational outcomes.

The results of the HPS movement in Hong Kong also highlight the importance of health policies, empowerment, capacity building, and creation of supportive environments and partnerships to implement HPS successfully. The findings suggest that HPS would provide a framework and strategic focus to enhance the health and well-being outcomes of students.

The Director of Audit's 2005 report of Hong Kong SAR Government includes a full review of the Government's efforts to involve the community in keeping Hong

Table 4 Improvement in students' health and well-being

Mental health	Baseline (%)	1-Year (%)
Primary schools (7 schools; 820 students)		
Students with depressive symptoms[a]	25.95	21.92
Students feeling hopeless[a]	24.49	15.49
Students with mild self-harm[a]	11.64	5.94
Students considered suicidal	10.08	8.06
Secondary schools (8 schools; 2,661 students)		
Students feeling hopeless	25.22	22.88
Students with mild self-harm	14.82	14.03
Students ever planned suicide[a]	9.97	8.28
Bullying		
Primary schools (7 schools; 820 students)		
Students threatened by someone[a]	5.94	2.59
Students feeling unsafe	3.49	1.38
Students with property stolen or damaged by someone[a]	29.40	20.75
Secondary schools (8 schools; 2,661 students)		
Students carrying a weapon to school	7.60	6.53
Students injured because of fighting	15.08	13.84
Students with property stolen or damaged by someone[a]	24.23	20.16
Eating habits		
Primary schools (7 schools; 820 students)		
Students with crisps $\geq$ 4 times/week[a]	18.60	11.76
Students with sweets $\geq$ 4 times/week[a]	27.09	19.80
Secondary schools (4 schools; 599 students)		
Students with crisps $\geq$ 4 times/week	18.72	13.75
Students with sweets $\geq$ 4 times/week	29.66	24.20

Improvements are shown here for three categories
[a]P value < 0.05

Kong clean. In the section on Civic and Health Education, it compliments CUHK's effort in initiating the HKHSA and launching the Professional Diploma Program in Health Education. The Audit observation indicates that "the evaluation results of these projects are very positive. The overall assessment of the Diploma Program is excellent and that of the Award Scheme is very favorable. In view of the encouraging results, the Audit considered that the Education and Manpower Bureau (EMB) needs to decide on the best way forward to make full use of the benefits derived from the Diploma Program and the Award Scheme." It also recommends that "the Secretary of Education and Manpower should evaluate the need for providing a trained health educator in each school, as initiated by the CHEP and the desirability of encouraging all schools to achieve the status of a health promoting school."

It is hoped that more schools in Hong Kong will develop along the concept of HPS and also that the existing HPSs will further their development on health initiatives. The concept of HPS should be embedded as one of the important missions of education for the young generation, and all students should have the right to be nurtured in a HPS.

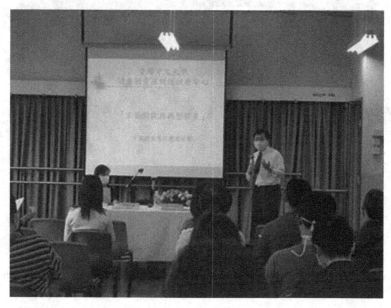

Picture 30 Using the concept of Health Promoting School as crisis management against SARS in Hong Kong, 2003

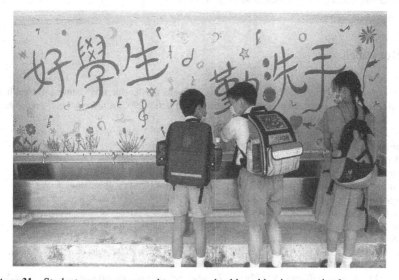

Picture 31 Students were empowered to promote health and hygiene at school

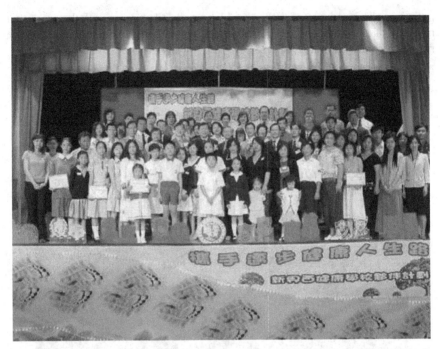

Picture 32 Health Promoting School mentorship Scheme linking Preschool, Primary Schools, and Secondary Schools

Acknowledgments The author had support from Health School coordinators of the Centre for Health Education and Health Promotion and grants from the Quality Education Fund of Hong Kong Government of Special Administrative Region.

References

Centers for Disease Control and Prevention, National Center for Environmental Health and Division of Environmental Hazards and Health Effects. (2002). *Environmental public health indicators project*. Atlanta: Author.

Centre for Health Education and Health Promotion. (2003a). *Practical guide to the health promoting schools: The Hong Kong healthy schools award scheme*. Hong Kong: The Chinese University of Hong Kong.

Centre for Health Education and Health Promotion. (2003b). *The Hong Kong healthy schools award scheme special issue 2003*. Hong Kong: Chinese University of Hong Kong.

Centre for Health Education and Health Promotion. (2004). *The Hong Kong healthy schools award scheme special issue 2004*. Hong Kong: The Chinese University of Hong Kong.

Cohen, M. (1988). *Restructuring the education system: Agenda for the 1990s*. Washington, DC: National Governors' Association.

David, J. L. (1989). *Restructuring in progress: Lessons from pioneering districts*. Washington, DC: National Governors' Association.

Fullan, M., & Stieggelbauer, S. (1991). *The new meaning of educational change*. New York: Teachers College Press.

Hausman, A. J., & Ruzek, S. B. (1995). Implementation of comprehensive school health education in elementary schools: focus on teacher concerns. *Journal of School Health*, 65(3), 81–86.

Hopkins, D. (1994). School improvement in an era of change. In P. Ribbins & E. Burridge (Eds.), *Improving education: Promoting quality in schools* (chap. 6). London: Cassell.

Lee, A., Tsang, K.K., Lee, S.H., To, C.Y. (2000). 'Healthy Schools Program' in Hong Kong: Enhancing Positive Health Behavior for School Children and Teachers. *Special joint issue of Education for Health, and Annals of Behavior Science and Medical Education, 13(3)*, 399–403.

Lee, A. (2002). Helping schools to promote healthy educational environments as new initiatives for school based management: The Hong Kong Healthy Schools Award Scheme. *Promotion and Education, Suppl 1*, 29–32.

Lee, A., Cheng, F., Yuen, H., Ho, M., & Healthy Schools Support Group. (2003). How would schools step up public health measure to control spread of SARS? *Journal of Epidemiology and Community Health, 57*, 945–949.

Lee, A., & Tsang, K. K. (2004). Youth risk behaviour in a Chinese population: A territory-wide youth risk behavioural surveillance in Hong Kong. *Public Health, 118*(2), 88–95.

Lee, A., Ho, M., Leung, T. C. Y., Cheng, F. F. K., Tsang. K. K., Suen, Y. P., & Yuen, S. K. (2004). Development of indicators and guidelines for the Hong Kong Healthy Schools Award Scheme. *Journal of Primary Care and Health Promotion, 1*(1), 4–9.

Lee, A., Cheng, F., & St Leger, L. (2005). Evaluating health promoting schools in Hong Kong: The development of a framework. *Health Promotion International, 20*(2), 178–186.

Lee, A., St Leger, L., & Moon A. S. (2005). Evaluating health promotion in schools meeting the needs for education and health professionals: A case study of developing appropriate indictors and data collection methods in Hong Kong. *Promotion and Education, XII (3–4)*, 123–130.

Lee, A., Cheng, F., Fung, Y., & St Leger, L. (2006). Can health promoting schools contribute to the better health and well being of young people: Hong Kong experience? *Journal of Epidemiology and Community Health, 60*, 530–536.

Lee, A., Cheng, F., St Leger, L., & Hong Kong Healthy School Team. (2007). The status of health promoting schools in Hong Kong and implications for further development. *Health Promotion International, 22*(4), 316–326.

Lee, A., Cheng, F., Yuen, H., Ho, M., Lo, A., Leung, T., & Fung, Y. (2007). Achieving good standard of health promoting schools: Preliminary analysis after one year implementation of Hong Kong healthy schools award scheme. *Public Health, 121*, 752–760.

Lee, A., Ho, M., Leung, C. Y., Suen, Y. P., Chan, G., Wu, Y. S., Chan, L., Chan, M. S., Ma, S. W., Leung, Y. L., Lo, Y. Y., & So, S. L. (2007). *Guidelines for Developing Health Education Curriculum for Kindergartens (Chinese)*. Hong Kong: Centre for Health Education and Health Promotion of the Chinese University of Hong Kong and Department of Early Childhood Education of Hong Kong Institute of Education.

Lee, A., Wong, M. C. S., Cheng, F., Yuen, H. S. K., Keung, V. M. W., & Mok, J. S. Y. (2008). Can the concept of Health Promoting Schools help to improve students' health knowledge and practices to combat the challenge of communicable diseases: Case study in Hong Kong? *BMC Public Health, 8*, 42. Retrieved 30 January 2008 from http://www.biomedcentral.com/1471-2458/8/42

McDonald, H., & Ziglio, E. (1994). European schools in a changing environment: Health promotion opportunities not to be lost. In C. M. Chu & R. Simpson (Eds.), *Ecological public health: From vision to practice*. Brisbane: Griffiths University.

Moon, A. (1999). *Does a healthy school award scheme make a difference? The evaluation of the Wessex Healthy Schools Award*. Unpublished PhD thesis, Department of Public Health Medicine, University of Southampton, UK.

Morris, P. (1996). *The Hong Kong school curriculum: Development, issues and politics* (2nd ed.). Hong Kong: Hong Kong University Press.

Morris, P., & Chan, K. K. (1997). The Hong Kong School Curriculum and the politicization, contextualisation and symbolic action. *Comparative Education, 33*(2), 247–64.

Mortimore P, Sammons P, Stoll L, Lewis D, Ecob, R. (1988) *School matters: The junior years.* Wells: Open Books.

Nutbeam, D. (1987). The health promoting school: Organisation and policy development in Welsh secondary schools. *Health Education, 46*, 109–115.

Parsons, C., Stears, D., & Thomas, C. (1996). The health promoting school in Europe: Conceptualising and evaluating the change. *Health Education Journal, 55*, 311–321.

Pattenden, J. (1998). *First workshop on practice of evaluation of the Health Promoting School - models, experiences and perspectives, 19–22 November 1998* (Executive Summary. 39–41). Bern/Thun, Switzerland: ENHPS.

Piette, D., Roberts, C., Prevost, M., Tudor-Smith, C., Tort, I., & Bardolet, J. (2002). *The final report of the EVA2 Project - Tracking down ENHPS successes for sustainable development and dissemination.* Brussels, Belgium: ENHPS.

Rogers, E., Moon, A. V., Mullee, M. A., Speller, V. M., & Roderick, P. J. (1998). Developing the "health-promoting school" – A national survey of healthy school awards. *Public Health, 112*, 37–40.

Rowling L., & Ritchie, R. (1996–1997). Health Promoting Schools: Issues and future directions for Australia and the Asia Pacific region. *Asia-Pacific Journal of Public Health, 9*, 33–37.

Seffrin, J. R. (1990). The comprehensive school health education curriculum: Closing the gap between state-of-the-art and state-of-the-practice. *Journal of School Health, 60*, 4.

Shek, D. T. L. (1992). "Actual-ideal" discrepancies in the representation of self and significant-others and psychological well-being in Chinese adolescents. *International Journal of Psychology, 27*(3 & 4), 229.

St Leger, L. H. (1999). The opportunities and effectiveness of the health promoting primary school in improving child health: A review of the claims and evidence. *Health Education Res, 14*(1), 51–69.

St Leger, L. H. (2001). Schools, health literacy and public health: Possibilities and challenges. *Health Promotion International, 16*(2), 197–205.

Sweeting, A. E. (1990). Education in Hong Kong, Pre-1841–1941: Fact and opinion. Hong Kong: The Hong Kong University Press.

WHO Regional Office for the Western Pacific. (1996). *Health-Promoting Schools Series 5: Regional guidelines. Development of health-promoting schools – A framework for action.* Manila, Philippines: Author.

Young I. (1986). *The Health Promoting School, report of a WHO (Euro) conference, at Peebles, Scotland.* Edinburgh: SHEG.

Young, I., & Williams, T. (1989). *The healthy school.* Edinburgh: SHEG.

Chapter 23
India: Implementing Health-Promoting Schools: HOPE Initiative

Gourdas Choudhuri, Uday Chand Ghoshal, and Elton D'Souza

Contextual Introduction

Brief Introduction to the Country

India is a country of 3.3 million km^2, comprising 28 states and 7 union territories, with a population of 1.13 billion making it the second most populous country in the world. One-third of India's households are in urban areas and two-thirds in rural areas. Sixty-eight percent of households (56% of rural and 93% of urban) have access to electricity, and 45% have access to toilet facilities. Eighty-eight percent of households use an improved source of drinking water (95% urban, 85% rural), but only 25% have water piped into their dwelling, yard, or plot. One-third of households treat their drinking water to make it potable (National Family Health Survey, 2005–2006).

India is a country with gross disparity in wealth and opportunities: While four Indians are listed among the top ten richest men in Forbes list, a third of the world's poor reside in this country (The World Bank, n.d.).

The State of Uttar Pradesh

The state of Uttar Pradesh has an area of 240,928 km^2 and a population of 166.20 million. With its capital at Lucknow City, it has 70 districts, 813 blocks, and 96,383

G. Choudhuri(✉)
Sanjay Gandhi Postgraduate Institute of Medical Sciences, Lucknow, India

C. Vince Whitman and C.E. Aldinger (eds.),
Case Studies in Global School Health Promotion: From Research to Practice,
DOI: 10.1007/978-0-387-92269-0_23, © Springer Science + Business Media, LLC 2009

villages. The state has a population density of 690/km^2 (compared to the national average of 324). The decadal growth rate of the state is 25.85% (compared with 21.54% for the country), and the population of the state continues to grow at a much faster rate than the national rate.

Thirty-one percent of the population of Uttar Pradesh is living below the poverty line (compared with 26% of the national population). The female literacy rate for the state is 43% (as of Census 2001), which is 11% below the national rate. The infant mortality rate is 71 per 1,000 live births, and the maternal mortality rate is 517 per 100,000 live births (Ministry of Health and Family Welfare, 2001–2003), both higher than the national average (National Family Health Survey, 2005–2006).

Social and Economic Indicators of India

Health Indicators

Health care. The overall annual expenditure on health care in India in recent years is less than 2% of the GDP. There are wide variations in health statistics across India, from the populous northern state of Uttar Pradesh (with an infant mortality rate of 71/1,000) to the southern state of Kerala (15/1,000), whose health indicators rank among those of developed countries (Registrar General India, 2007). Table 1 shows the rural-urban contrasts.

Child health. Less than half (44%) of children aged 12–23 months are fully vaccinated against the six major childhood illnesses – tuberculosis, diphtheria, pertussis, tetanus, polio, and measles.

Table 1 Vital statistics for India: rural and urban

Infant mortality rate	*Per thousand live births*
Rural	62
Urban	39
Total	57
Birth rate (2006)	*Per thousand*
Rural	25.2
Urban	18.8
Total	23.5
Death rate (2006)	*Per thousand*
Rural	8.1
Urban	6.0
Total	7.5
Natural growth (2006)	*Per thousand*
Rural	17.2
Urban	12.8
Total	16.0

Vital Statistics (Registrar General India, 2007)

Adult health. In a recent survey by World Health Organization (WHO), the major cause (60%) of death in India was attributed to incommunicable diseases. India is emerging as the diabetic capital of the world, with about 7% of adults from urban India suffering from diabetes mellitus (National Family Health Survey, 2005–2006). About 2% suffer from asthma, and about 57% of men and 11% of women use some form of tobacco, which is more common in rural areas and among those with less education. About one-third of men consume alcohol. About 418 persons per 100,000 are estimated to have medically treated tuberculosis.

Education Indicators

Only 83% of primary-school age children attend school (88% in urban areas and 81% in rural areas). School attendance drops to 75% for children of age 11–14 years and is only 41% for children of age 15–17 years. Among children of age 6–10, there is no gender disparity in school attendance in urban areas, but school attendance in rural areas is higher for boys (84%) than for girls (74%). At older ages (11–17), too, gender disparity in school attendance remains small in urban areas, but is pronounced and increases with age in rural areas. About 41% of women and 18% of men of age 15–49 have never been to school, while 35% of men and 22% of women have completed 10 or more years of education.

The Indian education system has primary, secondary, and tertiary education, including technical education, and is run by government as well as nongovernment organizations. Its good aspects include low cost, as it is highly subsidized, and wide availability. Technical education offered by most Indian universities is of fairly high quality. The system's major shortcomings are the lack of adequate attention to primary education, particularly in rural and semiurban areas; wide variations in quality; low literacy rates in many parts of the country; and lack of adequate attention to women and health education. Failure to adopt modern technology more uniformly in all sectors is also a limitation of the country's current education system. The Health Oriented Program and Education (HOPE) Initiative is a step toward health education in India.

Impetus, Origin, and Leadership of the School Health Program

It all began with the lead author's visit to the Department of Public Health, University of Sydney, in April 2004 on a WHO fellowship on IEC in Health Promotion. During the 1-month visit to observe implementation of health promotion strategies in Australia, especially the Health-Promoting School (HPS) program, the authors decided to implement a similar model in India. The WHO India office supported a project on Health Promotion in 2004 with the author as the principal investigator. A staff member of the WHO Regional Office provided encouragement, guidance, and technical support. Apart from promoting health in the hospital, the project extended its reach to the campus school (Health Promotion In, n.d.). The HOPE Initiative was conceptualized when a team visited the Kendriya Vidyalaya branch within the campus of Sanjay Gandhi Postgraduate Institute of Medical Sciences (SGPGI), with its health promotion programs for the students. Also, the Principal of La Martiniere College, the most prestigious and popular school in Lucknow, lent his support to this venture by becoming one of the founders of HOPE Initiative and joined in the launching of the first phase of activities in his school. The tremendous response received from this school, and the positive publicity that the initiative received through the local media, gave birth to the idea of promoting health awareness in schools throughout the city. As a result, an organization by the name of HOPE Initiative was established in November 2004 (HOPE Initiative, n.d.).

Levels of Schools

HOPE Initiative began as a pilot project in the city of Lucknow, initially targeting English medium city schools. After establishing its credibility, HOPE expanded operations to Hindi medium schools within the city and then to rural schools in three districts of the state of Uttar Pradesh under a UNICEF project. With the help of a recently obtained grant, HOPE is targeting 1,000 schools in 10 districts of Uttar Pradesh by 2010.

It targets all strata of school students – senior, middle, and junior – with programs tailored to each. For instance, debates are popular in the senior sections while poster-making competitions and quizzes are popular in the junior sections. Because of immense demand, HOPE Initiative expanded its reach to target college students as well.

Overview of the School Health Program

The idea of a health program for schools was new to all the principals of schools and colleges in this region. Although most school principals agreed to its need, they did not consider it important enough for allocation of time, resources, and policy. With academic performance of students as assessed by examination results being the yardstick of a school's performance, administrators and teachers allocated low priority to health and left the onus for "homes" to fulfill. The initial attitude of students was not very different; they were apprehensive that health sessions would be boring sermons on eating veggies and apples and would, at best, provide a temporary respite from studies.

The challenges for HOPE Initiative, therefore, were to make programs exciting and attractive to students and teachers, avoid didactic style, and encourage partici-pation. We thought that after thoroughly sounding out and motivating students and teachers on health issues, administrators would become more receptive to change and would implement policy (Choudhuri, Umar, Chopra, et al., 2006; Choudhuri, Umar, Jain, & Kacker, 2006).

Date Boundaries

The school health program started in 2004 as an offshoot of a WHO-sponsored project, "Making SGPGI a Health Promoting Hospital," with our targeting the Kendriya Vidyalaya school, located in the institute's campus and catering to the children of the institute's employees. In late 2004, it was an ordained HOPE Initiative, acquired an agenda and constitution, and was registered under the Society's Act of the Government of Uttar Pradesh, with eight founding members. It continued to receive technical guidance from WHO India, as it started generating its own financial resources and reaching out to increasing number of students and institutions.

Key Cast of Players/Agencies

HOPE Initiative shaped itself on the lines of HPSs, with the technical support and guidance of WHO India. It was registered as a separate body with the lead author, who is a professor and head of the Department of Gastroenterology, SGPGI, as its founder and Secretary; the other founders included a retired judge of the high court; an Associate Professor of Gastroenterology and a junior colleague of the founder; the principal of La Martiniere College, the best-reputed school in Lucknow; three female philanthropists; and an educator with special experience in dealing with handicapped children. The first school coordinator contributed her immense enthu-siasm and energy to give the organization a head start.

In 2007, UNICEF partnered with HOPE Initiative to reach out to nine rural schools in three districts of Uttar Pradesh. In 2008, HOPE Initiative received a grant from BMS Foundation to reach out to 1,000 schools in 10 districts of the state, and is expanding its scope rapidly.

Selection of Schools

As the concept of HPS was rather new in this region, HOPE Initiative adopted a top-down marketing approach. It sought the permission of a few principals of the best-reputed schools in Lucknow to provide a time slot for orientation of their teachers. A high-impact event, centered on a health issue, was then organized for the students of the school, and the press media were invited to give it wide coverage. With this approach, HOPE Initiative became immensely popular in Lucknow very quickly, and we started receiving requests from other schools to conduct our programs in their institutions. Requests from colleges also followed.

Reach

In a short period of time the number and reach of the activities of HOPE Initiative grew exponentially, as shown in Figs. 1 and 2.

Scope of Implementation

The broad health issues addressed by HOPE Initiative were as follows:

- Lifestyle: fast food, cola drinks, exercise, and obesity
- Road safety and prevention of road traffic accidents
- Sanitation and hygiene
- Stress, especially during examinations
- Tobacco, alcohol, and drugs
- Hepatitis B

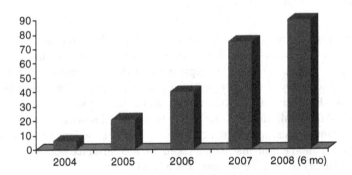

Fig. 1 Number of events (cumulative) conducted by HOPE Initiative

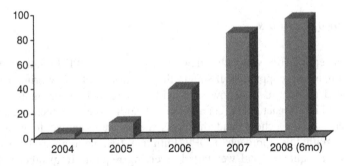

Fig. 2 Number of schools (cumulative) reached by HOPE Initiative

- Safe celebrations of festivals: Healthy Holi and Safe Diwali
- Environment: global weather change, water, pollution, deforestation
- Mosquito-related health hazards: malaria, encephalitis, dengue; preventing the mosquito menace
- Special issues: sex education, HIV, violence, bullying

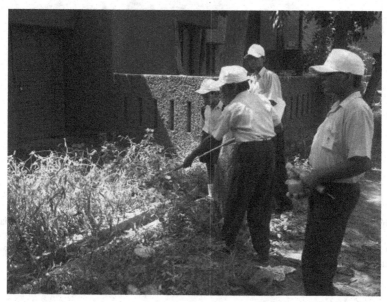

Picture 33 Children of Kendriya Vidyalay school taking part in the mosquito control community project. Mosquito-borne disease (malaria, Dengue, and Japanese Encopholity) are common in Uttra Pradesh after the rains in July, and take a heavy toll each year. Getting children as agents of school acting and change made a major difference in the community

These health issues are of contemporary and local importance. Recent surveys indicate that about 10% of Indian urban school children are obese, due to increasing consumption of fast food, decreasing physical activity (lack of time, place, and incentive for outdoor games and increased TV viewing), while lack of sanitation and hygiene continue to be major health hazards among rural children (Mohan et al., 2008).

Road accidents are emerging as a major killer on congested Indian roads, due to increasing numbers of vehicles, bad roads, alcohol, and the use of mobile phones while driving. Examination stress continues to take a heavy toll, as several young lives are lost to suicides each year when the results of the school final examinations are announced.

While the prevalence of hepatitis B continues to be about 4% in India, the government has not yet been able to include hepatitis B vaccination in the expanded program of immunization. Tobacco, alcohol, and drug addictions are on the rise in India among children, and education about sex and HIV remains rudimentary, especially among rural children.

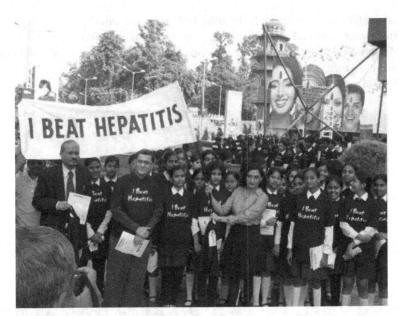

Picture 34 School children at a rally near a shopping mall to create awareness about Hepatitis. They distributed pamphlets to shoppers on Do's and Don't's of Hepatitis. In the process, they learn about Hepatitis and the need for vaccination to protect aginst Hepatitis B. In the foreground are Director of the hospital, Dr. G. Choudhuri, and Asma Hussain – a local celebrity

Mode of Action

Care was taken to ensure that each session was interesting, innovative, and participatory in nature. The health issues were addressed through one or more of the following methods: interactive sessions, quiz programs, elocution and poster contests, audiovisual films, antitobacco oath-taking ceremonies, intra and interschool debates, articles in school newsletters, teacher orientation programs, creation of a Web site for the initiative, magic shows, rallies, printing and distribution of pamphlets with health tips and figures, and nutritional counseling of parents during parent–teacher meetings. Table 2 gives an overview of activities to date.

Analysis of Specific Aspects of Implementations

Health promotion in schools was unknown in schools in Uttar Pradesh. The concept was introduced successfully to schools in the state across the recent 3 years. Since health is regarded as a boring and unimportant subject by students and teachers, the approach had to be innovative, interesting, and motivational. We have avoided didactics and use of the word "should" when talking with students. Most issues have been discussed with facts and figures, collected and presented in an interesting

Table 2 Activities of HOPE Initiative through May 2008

Activity	Number
Schools included for activities (urban/rural)	84/12
Distribution of health pamphlets	25 schools (>10,000 students)
Teachers' orientation program	6
Quizzes	21
Hospital visits by students from school	3
Intraschool and interschool debates	30
Poster-making competition	4
Awareness program about diseases, which were reported frequently at that particular time	8
Interactive sessions with students on health issues	9
Lectures by experts in the field	2
Fete	1
Stress-management sessions to reduce stress of the examination	6
Health camp	1
Rally	1
Major conference on health promotion	1
Magic shows giving health message	3
Workshop (5 days)	1

manner. The administration has been sensitized on issues and encouraged to act in "healthy directions." We have, however, tried not to enforce or pressurize through the government machinery in the formative years of the venture.

The approach taken by HOPE Initiative to date has been creating awareness, through authentic facts and figures, and encouraging youngsters to adopt healthy habits by shaping their attitudes. In fact, the approach has been largely promotive and student-centric, with methods designed to send messages home to parents.

The programs were considered successful on the basis of popularity and strong demand for them by students and schools; by a significant decrease in consumption of cola drinks and fast food by students (their own reports in subsequent sessions as well as changing sales pattern in school canteens); by their increasing awareness of the harmful effects of addictive agents; by their increasing use of helmets while driving two-wheelers; and by the recent willingness of school administrators and district inspectors of schools to collaborate with HOPE Initiative to discuss healthy policies for schools.

Having gained wide and public acceptance and appreciation, HOPE Initiative now contemplates working through the government as well. The approach will still remain stimulatory and motivational, with screening of interesting documentary films specially prepared, stimulating and encouraging leadership roles amongstudents through recognition by awards, bringing in new information through quizzes (very popular in India), and opening minds to new ideas through debates.

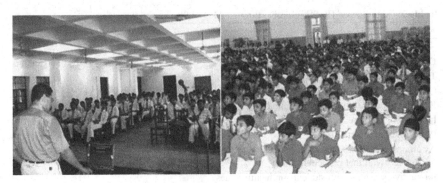

Picture 35 Students taking part in a health quiz competition conducted by HOPE Initiative

What Worked and Was Successful?

The biggest challenge was to create and sustain interest in health promotion programs, create awareness of contemporary health issues, make the sessions interactive, encourage children to choose and adopt healthy life styles, and create an environment for administrators and students to agree to "healthy policies." Generating participation and motivation among individual students was challenging (Choudhuri, Umar, Chopra, et al., 2006; Choudhuri, Umar, Jain, et al., 2006). We tried to popularize a health promoting Web site (www.hope.org.in) for creating health awareness among students by coupling it with names and pictures of students and schools. This recognition of individuals and institutions led to a 316% increase in hit counts to the HOPE Initiative Web site.

Another strategy that worked well was to provide material on the Web site on a topic prior to a debate and encourage participants to research the topic well using this resource.

What Did Not Work or Was Challenging?

While students were easy to enthuse and stimulate, teachers often proved difficult. Many lacked enthusiasm and energy to experiment with anything new and often viewed HOPE activities as wasting time (meant for formal lessons) on a low-priority topic of health.

Leadership proved to be very vital; the enthusiasm of the principal was reflected in the behavior of the teachers.

The other major limitation was the lack of trained manpower to coordinate and conduct these programs. HOPE Initiative initially started as a small philanthropic venture. As funds were small and came initially from voluntary donations from philanthropists, engaging and retaining high-quality people with zeal and creativity proved difficult.

What Barriers Needed to Be Overcome?

Health should be included in the curriculum of students in schools and colleges. Achieving it through governmental action and policy is bound to increase its reach, but whatever is brought about through education policy in India tends to become theoretical and boring. A partnership of the education department with an enthusiastic health promoting society might be more effective in shaping attitudes and changing behavior of students. The feasibility of this kind of venture has not yet been fully explored.

Conclusions, Insights, and Recommendations

Our attempts at promoting health among students in schools and colleges have been challenging. In this venture, "The ends are ape-chosen, only the means are man's." (Aldous Huxley). Hence creativity, innovation, and constant change are what make all the difference between an inspiring event and a dull one. Talented, motivated manpower to create these programs and a dedicated large field force to take them to schools are prerequisites for a successful outcome. As most attitudes and habits are formed in childhood and youth, adequate investment of resources for promoting health in schools could pay large dividends in terms of good health of our future generations.

A Web site, www.hope.org.in, has been posted on the Internet. The site is dedicated to students, providing them with interesting health-related facts and figures. It also details the efforts taken by HOPE Initiative toward school health promotion.

Acknowledgments The authors and HOPE Initiative gratefully acknowledge technical support and guidance from Dr. Cherian Varghese, WHO India Country Office. The project is supported under the WHO Government of India Collaborative Program. The founder members of HOPE Initiative are Justice D.K. Trivedi, Mrs. Sandhya Singh, Mrs. Manju Tayal, Mrs. Surabhi Kapoor, Mr. Kiron Chopra, Dr. U.C. Ghoshal, Mr. Elton D'Souza, and Dr. G. Choudhuri.

References

Choudhuri, G., Umar, S., Chopra, K., D'Souza, E., Ghoshal, U.C., Trivedi, D.K., et al. (2006). *Strategies of popularizing health promoting Web sites among young students: Proceedings of Global Convention & Expo on Telemedicine & e-Health, P-06.* Lucknow: School of Telemedicine and Biomedical Informatics, Sanjay Gandhi Postgraduate Institute of Medical Sciences.

Choudhuri, G., Umar, S., Jain, N., & Kacker, A. (2006). *Use of Internet to increase the level of participation in health promotion campaigns: Proceedings of Global Convention & Expo on Telemedicine & e-Health, P-07.* Lucknow: School of Telemedicine and Biomedical Informatics, Sanjay Gandhi Postgraduate Institute of Medical Sciences.

Health Promotion In. (n.d.) *Developing SGPGIMS as health promoting hospital*. Retrieved August 29, 2008, from www.healthpromotion.in

HOPE Initiative. (n.d.) *Health oriented programmes and education*. Retrieved August 29, 2008, from www.hope.org.in

Mohan, V., Mathur, P., Deepa, R., Deepa, M., Shukla, D.K., Menon, G.R., et al. (2008). Urban rural differences in prevalence of self-reported diabetes in India – The WHO-ICMR Indian NCD risk factor surveillance. *Diabetes Res Clin Pract*, *80*(1), 159–168.

Ministry of Health and Family Welfare (2001–2003). Sample Registration System (SRS), 2001–2003. New Delhi, India: Government of India

National Family Health Survey [NFHS-3]. (2005–2006). *India: Key findings*. Mumbai, India: International Institute for Population Sciences. Retrieved August 29, 2008, from www.nfhsindia.org

Registrar General India, Vital Statistics Division. (2007). *SRS Bulletin* (Sample Registration System), *42*(1). Retrieved August 29, 2008, from www.cesusindia.gov.in

The World Bank. (n.d.) *India: Data, projects and research*. Retrieved August 29, 2008, from www.worldbank.org.in

Chapter 24
Lao PDR: Strengthening the School Health Initiative

S. Phoungkham, Ly Foung, and P. Khatthanaphone

Contextual Introduction

Geography and Population

Lao People's Democratic Republic (PDR) is a landlocked Southeast Asian nation of approximately 5.6 million population with a population growth rate of 2%. The population is ethnically varied, with 47 distinct ethnic groups identified in the 1995 census; the ethnic, or lowland, Lao make up 52.5% of the total (Lao PDR – National Statistical Center, 2003). The ethnic Lao tend to predominate in the lowlands; the ethnic minorities, in the highlands, although there is some mixing through migration and resettlement. The ethnic minority areas in the highlands have higher rates of poverty, worse health indicators, and fewer services available for a variety of reasons, including remoteness, lower levels of educational achievement, and increasing land pressure that limits their ability to achieve food self-sufficiency (Lao PDR, 2003). Ethnic diversity also presents communication challenges, as many of the ethnic minority people do not speak Lao.

Governance and Political System

The Lao PDR is a one-party state under the lead of the Lao People's Revolutionary Party. The levels of government include 1 central, 16 provincial, 1 municipal, 1 special zone, 142 districts, and 10,868 villages (Lao PDR – National Statistical

S. Phoungkham(✉)
Research Institute for Education and Sciences, Ministry of Education, Vientiane Capital, Lao PDR, e-mail: phouangkham@yahoo.com

C. Vince Whitman and C.E. Aldinger (eds.),
Case Studies in Global School Health Promotion: From Research to Practice,
DOI: 10.1007/978-0-387-92269-0_24, © Springer Science + Business Media, LLC 2009

327

Centre, 2003). The government is promoting decentralization with the center responsible for policy, the province for strategy, the district for planning and budgeting, and the village for implementation. The details of implementation of decentralization are being worked out, and certain functions such as tax collection are being recentralized.

Social Economic Indicators

The Lao PDR is politically stable; it has undergone substantial change on development. Economic growth was 6% annually in the 1990s but fell to 4% with 110% inflation during the Asian financial crisis. Stabilization measures were implemented; growth and inflation in 2000/2002 were at about 6% and 15%, respectively. Inflation was estimated at 11% and economic growth at 5.8% in 2003. Revenue collection was 13.5% of GDP in 2002/2003 (World Bank, 2003). There are wide urban-rural disparities, with a poverty rate of 12% in Vientiane and 53% in northern Laos (Lao PDR, 2003).

Health and Education Status

Malaria is a leading cause of morbidity and mortality across the Lao population (all ages) and has become a major health concern. Children are the most vulnerable once infected. Dengue fever, another mosquito-borne disease, is prevalent in cities and increasing in rural areas. Other issues such as poor nutrition contribute to half of all child mortality. Poor sanitation and personal hygiene practices also contribute to a high incidence of soil-transmitted helminths and other oral health issues.

According to Ministry of Education (MOE) Statistics, the number of primary schools reached 8,600 in 2006 with almost 800,000 children. It is important to note that a large proportion of children enter primary school at greater than 10 years of age and that the average age for primary school completion is around 14 years. Generally, schools run about 8 h per day. Not every school has a school food shop to provide lunch service for children who stay in school. It is estimated that about 20% of schools have latrines. Lack of sanitation in schools is always a difficulty for boys and girls; it is recognized as a particular difficulty for girls. It is not yet mandatory that latrines accompany any school that is built; this remains a critical lack to address.

A national curriculum exists for both primary and secondary schools. It includes a section called *The World Around Us*, which covers some aspects of health education.

Start of the School Health Program

Schools are recognized as effective vehicles for the delivery of health education and the promotion of health-related behavior change. Participatory, interactive education on health issues is used to influence children's current and future health practices. Also, children, if properly motivated and empowered, have proven to be effective vehicles themselves for the spread of health education messages to their families, to other children, and to other community members. Children who learn proper preventive practices or health-seeking behaviors during the educational periods are likely to remember and apply such practices during their adulthood.

It is recognized that improved hygienic conditions are the best long-term, sustainable measures to prevent infectious disease, but achievement of universal high hygienic standards is expensive and difficult. Waiting for improved hygienic standards means that another generation of children is exposed to the risk of impaired intellectual and physical development. Therefore, supporting health promotion in the education system is the most important element to prepare children in both education and health. Good health supports successful learning as much as successful learning supports health. Healthy children have higher daily school attendance, learn better, take full advantage of every opportunity to learn, and thus achieve higher academic excellence.

Using the basic concepts and principles of modern health promotion from the Ottawa Charter (World Health Organization, 1986), Lao PDR has focused on four areas of actions that can be used for initiating the concepts: (1) school health instruction/healthful school environment (building, rooms, and fences in condition, school canteen, latrine, waste incinerator), (2) school health education (including *The World Around Us* and first-aid training for teachers and school children), (3) school health services (first-aid service in schools, including the essential drugs and some equipment for very simple injury management), and (4) school-community partnerships (establishing parent associations).

Overview of the School Health Program

Although Lao PDR has several agencies involved in implementing health activities in schools, they are not large and systematic. So far, the school health program has been initiated to strengthen cooperation between the MOE and the Ministry of Health (MOH) to introduce or expand health subjects in the school curricula, using effective, participatory, and interactive teaching methods.

During 1993–2000, the MOH was implementing a pilot project, funded by the World Health Organization (WHO), to establish Health-Promoting Schools in 30 schools. The MOH had difficulty in meeting the high level successfully on its own. During the same period, the MOH had some cooperation from the Centre for

Information and Education in Health (CIEH), and the MOE. The project has begun to provide a safe school environment, including hygiene and sanitation, skills-based education, and access to health services.

A discussion among education and health ministries was held to improve the project. In 2002, the discussion yielded a promising Memorandum of Understanding (MOU) between the Ministries of Education and Health. They agreed to form a National School Health Project that covers all health-promotion activities in the school setting. It was agreed that MOH should play a facilitating role to the MOE to institutionalize, expand, and improve health promotion in schools and to ensure high-quality and appropriate health promotion topics, through adoption of modern teaching methods and interactive participatory learning. This became an initial collaboration between the key ministries to enhance gradual improvement of primary schoolchildren's health effectively.

The signed MOU reflected a significant achievement that creates a basis for collaborative activity in the future. It also presents an opportunity for coordination of donor activities around school health issues in the provinces. The concepts and vision of school health that support educational outcomes had been reintroduced to provincial and district education and health administrators in the annual meeting. At present, almost 450 primary schools in 17 provinces throughout the country have joined the project. (Some of them were among the 30 schools in the pilot project.)

The Joint National School Health Taskforce, which consists of staff from related departments of the MOE and MOH, was established at central and lower levels to oversee the school health implementation in certain schools. Duties and responsibilities had been assigned and endorsed by the two ministries. The task force plays multiple roles in a cycle of school health implementation; for instance, it supports assessment and research, develops guidelines and tools, and assists provinces to plan and implement school activities. In addition, it is responsible for monitoring and evaluation.

Both vertical and horizontal coordination mechanisms are used to encourage collaboration and coordination between education and health sectors. The central task force is divided into four small groups; each group consists of two to three members who respond directly to coordination, monitoring, and supervision in the assigned provinces. This coordination framework encourages all task force members to participate fully in carrying out the activities with better leadership and commitment. Regular meetings among central task force members are held once in a month to share and exchange experiences and information.

Since 2005, the school health task force at each level has been performing the school deworming campaign for all primary school-aged children under the framework of school health. This demonstrates good progress on coordination and collaboration of education and health sectors at all levels.

With support of a grant from Luxembourg through the WHO during 2003–2005, coordination and collaboration have been strengthened and progressively highlighted between the education and health sectors at all levels. Their commitment has been shown by facilitating some of the achievements listed in the next section.

Specific Aspects of Implementation

Development of the School Health Policy and Strategic Guidelines

In 2005, the first Lao's School Health Policy (SHP) paper was formulated by the school health task force with strong support from the WHO, Japan International Cooperation Agency (JICA), and UNESCO. It responds to Education Vision 2020, Health Vision 2020, Millennium Development Goals, Health for All, and Education for All for Lao PDR in its commitment to provide quality education for all children (Lao PDR, 2005). The targets of this policy are pregrade 1 and primary school students. The goals are to improve the health status of school children, to increase enrollment, to reduce absenteeism and dropouts, and to give equal opportunities for girls and the disadvantaged groups in this multiethnic society. All key components and items included in the policy have been considered carefully; they are not too difficult and not too expensive to change in a very initial step.

The policy prioritized five components:

1. Personal health and life skills: Improve the current health education curriculum to emphasize prevention skills, develop educational materials, and build teachers' capacity for a student-centered learning approach.
2. Healthy school environment: Promote improvement for both physical and psychosocial environments.
3. Health and nutrition services: Focus on basic regular health checks, conduct school deworming campaigns, promote good practice on oral health, and address basic hygiene in school canteens.
4. Common diseases control and prevention: Conduct extra-educational activities that link to prevention of common diseases of school children.
5. School and community partnership: Encourage the community to participate in school development by joining the school health team, identifying problems, planning, implementing, and assessing progress.

In addition, the strategic implementation guidelines contain the General Strategy for Coordination, Implementation, Monitoring, Evaluation, and Reporting as well as Indicators and a Checklist for Accreditation based on the National SHP (Lao PDR – National School Health Taskforce, 2005).

The accreditation system has been created as an incentive for the schools to improve their health and sanitation standards. The basis of the accreditation system is a checklist covering all five SHP components. This checklist is not only a tool for checking whether the school can get awarded; it also functions as a guideline of standards, giving a practical example of what aspects schools should address in order to improve their health and sanitation norms and conditions.

The accreditation system has three levels (gold, silver, and bronze), which schools are encouraged to achieve. Achieving a gold medal means that the school will be recognized as an outstanding Health-Promoting School. Although reaching this level should be the ideal for all schools, many schools are still too far away from this goal. Most schools' first goal will be to reach the silver or even the bronze, only after that pursuing the highest standards and a gold medal.

Improvement of Existing Health Education Curriculum

The primary school curriculum already included several health topics under the subject of *The World Around Us*. The topics mostly gave general information about diseases, such as malaria, diarrhea, cholera, and intestinal parasites. The curriculum also covered the topics of food, nutrition, road traffic, and personal hygiene. To help children develop prevention skills against diseases and knowledge of how to maintain good health, the topics have been revised with support from the WHO. The revised curriculum was taught in six selected schools in two provinces. School-teachers accepted the revised curriculum; however, it needs more improvement to apply child-to-child approach techniques.

Educational Material Development

First, a review of the existing health education materials was completed. Almost 400 materials had been collected and considered, but agreement was made for improvement of the existing *Blue Box* materials, originally promoted by UNICEF. Revisions were made to modify the materials in the box, not only focusing on the issues of hygiene and sanitation, but also concentrating on malaria, diarrhea, parasite control, dengue, nutrition, dental health, and waste management. The materials in the box were revised, and some new materials were created to match the health education part of *The World Around Us*.

The number of materials in the box has increased from 13 to 20 items. Production of the boxes was supported by WHO, UNICEF, and a nongovernmental organization. Dissemination mechanisms are key to help teachers familiarize themselves with the tools and enable them to use them effectively. A training course was conducted for province and district trainers, who then conducted a course to train teachers in targeted schools. The Blue Box was distributed to all 450 schools targeted by the school health project. UNICEF and another nongovernmental organization also distributed the box to additional schools. A first, rapid assessment found the materials very useful to teachers delivering health information about behavior change for students. The materials are both entertaining and educational; they create both fun and relaxation during the class.

Integration of School Health into Teacher-Training Institution

It is recognized that health skills development for schoolchildren may not be sufficient when teachers lack certain skills and knowledge on disease control and maintaining health. Therefore, an advocacy workshop to introduce the SHP and related documents has been conducted for the directors of eight Teacher Training Colleges (TTCs) together with the representatives of the Provincial School Health Task Forces and Provincial Trainers from eight provinces where the TTCs are located. It is important to ensure that teachers understand the national project well and are competent to implement school health activities in their colleges.

The TTCs include Health Education in the subject called Demographic and Environmental Studies. It takes up 40% of the subject, which is about 64 study hours of the preservice primary schoolteacher training. Topics taught include reproductive health, human body, personal hygiene, environmental health, and common infectious diseases. People from related health and education sectors jointly developed the subject. In the TTCs, Health Education is also part of the two subjects of Demography and Science, which comprise 5 study hours per week.

These are the government efforts to integrate the school health activities into an existing educational system. Through these efforts, both teachers and students can learn pedagogy as well as other school health issues. The *Blue Box* and checklist tools are being utilized to support health information delivery to teacher students, for use during their last 3 months of intensive practice in schools before graduation. Thus, teacher students are well-prepared with the SHP and assessment tools that will enable them to assist principals in their future schools to carry out the Health-Promoting School activities.

This government initiative implements SHP at the national level. Several schools, especially in the capital city, Vientiane, have developed their own policies that relate to the components of the national policy. The formerly weak relationships between school and community are now improving. Many schools are reaching out to the community to help on dengue surveillance (check larvae in water containers of household), cleanliness for the surrounding villages (collect rubbish and recycle), and promotion of personal hygiene (arrange for hand-washing facilities). In addition, issuing of the national SHP helps to strengthen the implementation of MOE's *Green School* policy. It directly encourages schools to keep a safe school physical environment and to beautify by gardening, planting shade trees for shade, etc.

Conclusions and Recommendations

In recent years Lao PDR has witnessed substantial progress in addressing Health-Promoting Schools and integrating the national deworming program for primary school-aged children into the school health framework. Through the introduction and dissemination of the SHP/accreditation scheme and the Blue Box to schools and teacher training institutions, the country is now gradually moving toward the national goal on health promotion in schools. Under the leadership of MOE and MOH, a coordination framework among partners has been established. This initial progress marks a significant achievement for the government, donors, and development partners in school health in Lao PDR.

Although the implementation of Health-Promoting School activities in Lao PDR has been initiated, there is a critical need for strong leadership and ownership by task forces at every level, to move the initiative forward and to strengthen the implementation of the newborn SHP in primary schools. Each school principal needs to perform a self-assessment to recognize the health problems in his or her school, and then develop a plan of action for further school development. Some recommendations can help to move the initiative forward:

- Political support is needed to move the initiative forward and integrate it as a part of a government *Model Cultural Village* project, in order to mobilize participation from communities and other key sectors.
- Currently – as several partners are carrying out the health promotion activities in schools – the task force needs strong leadership to identify a coordination and collaboration mechanism, planning and implementation, and information flow management. Good leadership can ensure effective sector-wide collaboration and avoid duplication.
- To translate the national SHP into effective action to improve the health of school children, we need a powerful leadership; a strong support system from the central, province, and district levels; and financial resources.
- We need to intensify the development of a framework between schools and teacher training institutions that will support Health-Promoting School activities. The limited support of school health activities for preservice teacher students in TTCs allows some students to become teachers who are not familiar with the issue of health promotion in primary school; thus, it may harm the sustainability of health promotion in schools. At the same time, TTCs need to improve their own physical environments to become part of the reinforcing factors for health behavior change in students.
- Appropriate monitoring and supervision frameworks should be set up at every level.

Acknowledgment   The authors had support from Ms. Chitsavang Chanthavisouk, World Health Organization, Lao PDR.

References

Lao People's Democratic Republic (Lao PDR). (2003). *The National poverty eradication programme background document*. Vientiane, Lao PDR: Author.

Lao People's Democratic Republic (Lao PDR). (2005). *National school health policy*. Vientiane, Lao PDR: Author.

Lao People's Democratic Republic (Lao PDR) – National School Health Taskforce. (2005). *Strategic implementation guideline*. Vientiane, Lao PDR: Author.

Lao People's Democratic Republic (Lao PDR) – National Statistical Centre. (2003). *Basic Statistics 2002*. Vientiane, Lao PDR: Author.

Lao People's Democratic Republic (Lao PDR) – State Planning Committee/National Statistics Centre. (1997). *Results from the population census 1995*. Vientiane, Lao PDR: Author.

World Bank. (2003). *Lao PDR economic monitor*. Vientiane, Lao PDR: Author.

World Health Organization. (1986). *Ottawa charter for health promotion*. Geneva: Author.

Chapter 25
Philippines: Supporting Health Promotion in Schools Through the Urbani School Health Kit

Sheila R. Bonito, Lurenda S. Westergaard, and Raman Velayudhan

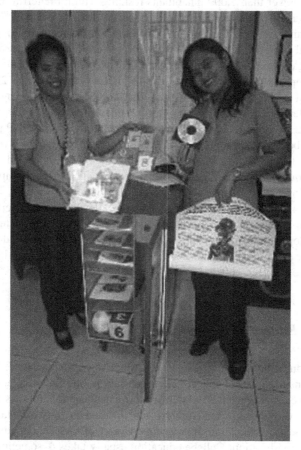

Picture 36 Teachers receiving the Urbani School Health Kit

S.R. Bonito(✉)
University of the Philippines Open University, Los Baños, Laguna, Philippines

C. Vince Whitman and C.E. Aldinger (eds.),
Case Studies in Global School Health Promotion: From Research to Practice,
DOI: 10.1007/978-0-387-92269-0_25, © Springer Science + Business Media, LLC 2009

Introduction

Country Profile

The Philippines is an archipelago made up of more than 7,000 islands. The country is divided into three geographical areas: Luzon, Visayas, and Mindanao. It has 17 regions, 81 provinces, 118 cities, 1,510 municipalities, and 41,995 barangays (villages). The barangay is the basic unit of the Philippine political system. It consists of fewer than 1,000 inhabitants residing within the territorial limit of a city or municipality and administered by a set of elective officials, headed by a barangay chairman. It is the primary planning and action unit for government programs and projects. It is a forum for the collective opinion of a community. Every barangay is required to have a health center and a school.

The Philippines has a population of 88.5 million as of August 2007, with a growth rate of 2.04% (National Statistics Office, 2008a). It has a young population: 37% are under 14; 59% are between 15 and 64; and only 4% are over 64. The median age is 21 years (National Statistics Office, 2008b). The GDP per capita is estimated to be US $5,000 in 2006, with a real growth rate of 5.4% reflecting the continued resilience of the service sector, together with improved exports and agricultural output (World Bank, 2006). However, given the Philippines' high annual population growth rate and unequal distribution of income, it remains a challenge to make appreciable progress in the alleviation of poverty. The life expectancy at birth is 65 years for males and 72 years for females. Child mortality is 40/1,000 population among males and 28/1,000 among females. Adult mortality is also higher among males, with 269/1,000 population, compared with 149/1,000 among females (WHO, 2007).

The Basic Education System

Philippine education is patterned after the American system, with English as the medium of instruction. Schools are classified into public (government) or private (nongovernment). The general pattern of formal education follows four stages: preprimary level (nursery and kindergarten) offered in most private schools; 6 years of elementary education, followed by 4 years of high school education, plus optional higher education. College education usually takes 4, sometimes 5, and in some cases – like medical and law schools – as long as 8 years. Graduate schooling is an additional 2 or more years. Classes in Philippine schools start in June and end in March.

The goal of basic education is to provide the school-age population and young adults with the skills, knowledge, and values they need to become caring, self-reliant, productive, and patriotic citizens. The country has a high literacy rate: 92.6% of ages 15 and over can read and write. A system of free and compulsory elementary education has been in place since the beginning of 1900. In 2006, the Department of Education listed 42,152 elementary schools, 89% of which are public schools and 11% private schools. At high school level, 8,455 schools were listed, 60% public and 40% private. Available data (SY 2003–2004) show the gross enrollment ratio (the total enrollment in a given level of education as a percentage of the population based on 2000 Census of Population and Households, National Statistics Office) at 99.87% for ages 6–11 and 79.50% for ages 12–15. The functional literacy rate among ages 10–64 in 2003 is 84.10% (Department of Education, 2007).

Public schools (and most private schools) follow a standard curriculum and learning competencies. At the elementary level, health is taught together with science (in the Science and Health subject). The average student at elementary level is exposed to 40–60 h of health education. The learning competencies on health focus on body systems and growth and developmental changes, but rarely on health behaviors. The teachers are not adequately trained on effective teaching of health concepts. There is room to enrich the teaching and learning of health concepts.

The Department of Education is mandated to promote, protect, and maintain the health and nutritional status of students and school personnel through the provision of various health and nutrition services and education. The Department of Health and other public and private institutions help schools to be child-friendly and conducive to learning, growth, and development.

Promoting Health in Schools

Research shows that targeting just a handful of risk factors can significantly reduce major causes of death, disease, and disability. These risk factors can be addressed by developing healthy behaviors early in life. Children must develop healthy habits while they are young. When children are healthy, they have a greater capacity to learn and achieve their full potentials. And with good education, they can aim for a better quality of life, and better health, overall.

The school is one of the best places where health education and health promotion among children can take place. Children spend a great deal of time in this setting. They enter the school open to learning new things. They should have teachers who serve as guides and role models. They should be in a caring and supportive environment, where each child is encouraged to develop vital life skills. They should be in Health-Promoting Schools. A Health-Promoting School is one that constantly strengthens its capacity as a healthy setting for living, learning, and working. An effective school health program is one of the most cost-effective investments a country can make to improve education and health simultaneously. A Health-Promoting School is a place where all members of the school community work together to provide students with integrated and positive experiences and structures that promote and protect their health.

The Philippines, through different initiatives of government and private sectors, aims to uphold the principles of Health-Promoting Schools. It supports projects such as Universal Medical and Dental Check-up, Food for School Program, Deworming, Vision Testing, National Drug Education, and other collaborative programs through the Department of Health, UNFPA, UNICEF, and others. However, teachers are given few opportunities to train on what to teach about health, how to teach health, and how to support health promotion in schools.

The project described in this case study addresses the question of how to promote health in schools by providing elementary schools with teaching resources and training teachers on how to use them. The project targets schools far from the cities in Palawan, a province in the southwestern part of Luzon, and in the Davao region in Mindanao. These schools are known to have endemic cases of malaria and dengue. Malaria is a public health concern in these endemic areas, and dengue epidemics are not uncommon in some schools. Malaria is predominantly a rural disease affecting mostly poor indigenous population groups while dengue is an urban disease that is spreading to semiurban and rural areas of the country. By using schools as entry points, it is hoped that health behaviors needed in the prevention and control of malaria and dengue will be learned by students and, eventually, by their families and communities.

Overview of the School Health Program

About the Urbani School Health Kit

The Urbani School Health Kit is *an integrated package* containing materials that can support health education and health promotion activities in schools. The integrated package concept has been developed at the WHO Regional Office for the Western Pacific to cover a number of health issues for Health-Promoting Schools. The kit was named after the late Dr. Carlo Urbani, an expert in the control of parasitic diseases including helminths and malaria. He developed the concept that schools could be provided with a kit that would help teachers to educate children about prevention of health problems and to implement appropriate interventions. He was the first person to discover severe acute respiratory disease syndrome (SARS) in Viet Nam. His efforts prevented many cases from spreading, especially among hospital staff. However, during this work he himself contracted SARS and died.

The kit *exemplifies the principles of the Health-Promoting School*. It fosters health and learning. It engages health and education officials, teachers, students, parents, health providers, and community leaders in making the school a healthy place. It strives to provide a healthy environment, health education, and health services in schools, along with community projects. It implements policies and practices that respect an individual's well-being and dignity, while it provides multiple opportunities for success and recreation. It strives to improve health of students, school personnel, families, and communities.

The kit *emphasizes the role of teachers in promoting health* among children. It encourages teachers to be champions of health promotion, to start with a positive inquiring and caring attitude to (1) find out about the most important health problems in the community, (2) be a role model for health promotion, (3) advocate the creation of supportive environments in schools that will encourage children to make healthy choices, and (4) develop creative ways to help children understand the importance of healthy living and to take action to improve their own health. Teachers are also challenged to explore how health promotion can be linked to the topics covered in the basic education curriculum. For example, promoting healthy lifestyle such as balanced diet, regular physical activity, and the avoidance of harmful substances can be linked to the biological systems and chemical process in the Science subject. Counting calories in the diet or comparing daily intake with recommended dietary guidelines can be an example taken in the Math subject. Socioeconomic determinants of health can be a fascinating topic in Social Studies. Teachers are encouraged to have at least one health promotion lesson everyday.

The kit considers the *different health needs of children at different ages*. The kit targets two groups of children: ages 5–9 years and 10–12 years. Learning objectives specify the knowledge, skills, and attitudes that school children should attain by completing a lesson. Each age group is given learning objectives and strategies appropriate to the children's age and preference.

The kit *showcases important health issues, health activities, and resource materials* for a healthy school program. The kit focuses on seven key issues:

- Improving personal hygiene
- Improving oral health
- Improving diet and nutrition
- Keeping the environment clean and healthy
- Preventing worm infections (including Schistosomiasis)
- Saying no to tobacco
- Preventing malaria and dengue

A resource booklet for each key issue describes the knowledge areas, skills, and attitudes that the teacher could emphasize among students. Specific learning objectives, key messages, learning activities, material/resources, and relevant reading materials are described. A Teacher's Resource Book is also provided, which explains the concept of Health-Promoting Schools, the roles of teachers in promoting health, how the kit can be used, how to evaluate use of the kits, and how to share them with other teachers.

The kit encourages *innovative ways of teaching health*. The materials are contained in a wooden cabinet with wheels that are durable and easily transported within schools. Design considerations include visibility (not tucked away in an office or closet), usability (appropriate, answers needs of teachers and schools), and durability (able to withstand the elements and rough handling). The box with its flip top can also be used as a platform for teaching in class. A collection of flashcards can easily stand on the platform as visual aids in teaching. The sides of the cabinet can be used to hang tarpaulin posters (which are provided for each key issue). Other materials are provided for indoor and outdoor activities, such as models of human mouth with teeth, toothbrushes, toothpaste mimic, rubber mats, game cards, a soft ball, and soft dice. A booklet on games explains basic rules on how to play several games (for teaching and evaluation), using the materials provided. The learning activities are designed to allow easy implementation in a variety of contexts. Even with very limited access to resources, teachers and students should still be able to perform the activities.

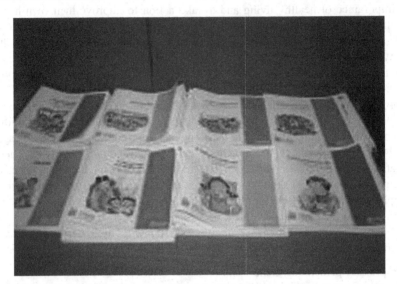

Picture 37 Sample booklets from the Urbani School Health Kit

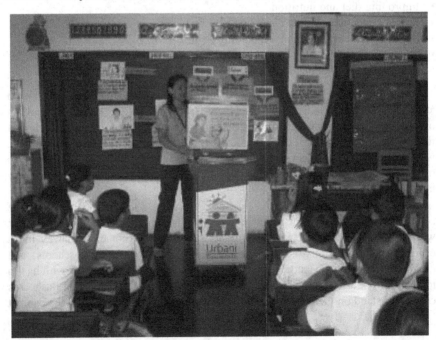

Picture 38 A teacher using the Urbani School Health Kit during a class session

Teachers' Workshop on Using the Urbani School Health Kit

One-hundred eighty eight teachers from 56 public elementary schools in Davao and Palawan participated in the training workshops on how to teach health concepts using the Urbani School Health Kit. The schools were selected by the Department of Education regional offices together with the Department of Health in Davao and the Pilipinas Shell Foundation in Palawan. The schools received two Urbani school health kits each. Observers from the provincial and local health offices, officials from the Department of Health Regional Office and from the Department of Education were also part of the workshop, as well as technical experts from the World Health Organization and the Department of Health.

During the workshops, the background of the project, the concept of Health-Promoting Schools, and the features and contents of the kit were explained to the participants. The orientation emphasized the key messages that teachers should communicate to students with the use of the different learning materials found in the kit. They were asked to design a short lesson plan and conduct a class demonstration using the kit. Issues of implementation were discussed, such as timing and integration with the present curriculum in Science and Health. Teachers showed confidence that they could easily integrate the key messages of the kit in their lessons. Monitoring and evaluation measures were agreed upon. Teachers were also encouraged to explore ways to integrate the use of the kit in teaching other subjects.

Implementation of the Urbani School Health Kit

The Urbani School Health Kit was implemented in 56 schools in Davao and Palawan during the school year 2007–2008. The project has reached about 23,460 students. Teachers who attended the workshop were asked to conduct class demonstrations on the use of the kit in their classes and were observed by external reviewers from the Department of Education and the Department of Health. They were asked to do a self-evaluation and were interviewed to get their views about the experience and on how to improve the content and use of the Kit.

Results of the Monitoring Activity

Class Demonstration on the Use of Urbani School Health Kit

Teachers were asked to demonstrate the use of the kit in at least one actual class session. Two to three observers were present to evaluate how the kit contributed to the effectiveness of teaching health concepts. The main focus of the observation was to review whether the goals (intended use) of the kit and its contents were achieved. The observation also considered the teachers' preparation and implementation of the classroom teaching demonstration to determine whether the contents were taught appropriately and effectively and to see how the schoolchildren responded to the key health messages and learning activities.

Class demonstrations showed that teachers prepared good lesson plans that integrated the use of the kit. They were able to use the key health messages and learning activities found in the kit, not only in the Science and Health subject, but also in Reading Comprehension in English, Character Education, and Social Studies. Teachers used the resource booklets to shape the lesson for the day, emphasized the key messages identified in the health topics, stimulated learning by using the activities in the kit, and encouraged full student participation. The greatest observed contributions of the Urbani School Health Kit include giving teachers a scaffold on which they can build lessons and providing clear health messages, creative learning activities, and the means for formative evaluation. The kit is flexible enough to be integrated with different topics in the curriculum, such as worm infections in human beings, waste segregation in the environment, and tobacco control in values formation. It offers visual appeal to students, which encourages them to participate more in the learning process. Some teachers need to check key health messages given to students to make sure that they are accurate and complete. Teachers need to encourage students to talk more about their experiences. Teachers need to help children develop good habits by being good role models and praising children who showed good behavior or actions.

Self-Evaluation of Teachers

The self-evaluation form is aimed at evaluating the teacher's experience after every use of the kit to (1) determine the importance and relevance of the key health messages, (2) identify the best parts of the experience, and (3) identify parts of the experience that need improvement. Teachers were asked to reflect on the activities done using the kit and to write what key messages were emphasized during the said activities. They were asked to note the best parts of the experience as well as the parts that need improvement. The cited best parts of the experience include having the students attentive, active, and responsive in answering questions; eager to demonstrate skills like brushing teeth, proper hand-washing, identifying mosquito breeding sites, telling stories about reminding parents not to smoke, meal planning, and more. Innovative learning strategies found in the kit – such as storytelling, role-playing, puppet shows and outdoor explorations – made teaching and learning fun and enriching. Parts that need improvement include time management, since students most often wanted to extend learning activities. Since classes usually have 40–50 students, there is also a need to make the pictures and letters of the visual aids bigger.

Teachers were asked to rate themselves on how they teach health topics. Most of the teachers rated well, but there is room for improvement, specifically in adopting higher order thinking skills in lesson preparation and in grounding the learning experience more thoroughly in everyday life.

Interviews of Teachers

Teachers who used the kit in the class demonstrations were interviewed to get their comments on the use of the kit and suggestions on how to improve it. They were also asked on how they envision their schools as Health-Promoting Schools. The teachers were mostly graduates of Bachelor in Elementary Education. Most were teachers of Science, some with specialization in Filipino, Math, or English. When asked about successes achieved through the use of the kit, they cited getting satisfaction in teaching by having students' attention the entire duration of class, having learning objectives that were easier to achieve, and seeing positive outcomes in students, such as interest in the lessons, demonstrations of healthy practices, and reports that they relayed some health lessons to parents.

Limitations that were cited in the use of the kit include difficulties in implementing some health messages, usually because of the limitations of families and communities where pupils live, such as lack of toothpaste, inability to afford slippers and shoes, and lack of available healthy food. There is also a need to unlock difficult words and even translate into the local dialect. Other topics were also suggested to be the focus of additional teaching materials, such as safety, first aid or emergency management, and reproductive health. Information materials for students to take home to parents should also be provided.

There is also a need for increased awareness on improving school environments and for policies to be more child-friendly. Another important issue is how to link better with parents and local community leaders to improve children's education.

Specific Aspects of Implementation

Vision and Concept

More than aiding classroom instruction, the Urbani School Health Kit introduces to teachers the concept of the Health-Promoting School, why they should promote health in schools, and their roles in making their schools become Health-Promoting Schools. The teacher's guide enjoins teachers to begin by finding out the most important health problems in the community, then advocating the creation of a supportive environment that will encourage children to make healthy choices, being a role model for health promotion, developing ways to help children understand the importance of healthy living and take action to improve their own health, and exploring how health promotion can be linked to the topics that they teach. The Urbani teacher's guide also encourages teachers to have at least one health promotion lesson every day and to share experiences with other teachers in their schools or other schools.

Champions, Leadership, and Advocacy

The support of the school principal is key to the successful implementation of the Urbani School Health Kit and its broader vision of helping schools become Health-Promoting Schools. The principals who were supportive of the teachers' efforts to find innovative ways of teaching and integrating healthy habits in their courses had the most energetic and creative teachers as well as students. Principals can be primarily concerned with academic achievement of the students. By emphasizing the significant role of health in the child's learning, it is not difficult to point out that the goals of education and health are the same: children who are healthy and able to reach their full academic potentials.

Team Training and Ongoing Coaching

Providing teachers with the framework and tools to teach health is an important mechanism for the successful implementation of the Urbani School Health Kit. The framework of Health-Promoting School and tools such as the teacher's guide and the resource booklets, visual aids, and learning activities found in the kit are all necessary to help teachers develop their capacity to teach health effectively. Training not just one teacher but a team composed of four teachers is part of the strategy of sustainability. The trained teams are tasked to "echo" what they have learned to other teachers in their schools and to be part of a network of potential trainers for successive implementation of the Urbani School Health Kit in other regions of the country.

Mechanism for Cross-Sector Collaboration

Collaboration between the health and education sectors is essential to the implementation of the Urbani School Health Kit. The Department of Health helped by identifying priority health issues, such as malaria and dengue, which were given emphasis in the Urbani School Health Kit. They also provided technical experts who became resource persons in schools to discuss with the teachers their role in preventing and controlling such diseases. The Department of Education's support is crucial in the participation of the schools and teachers. Without the directive from the Division Offices of the Department of Education in Davao and Palawan, teachers cannot attend the training workshops. The Department of Education also plays an important role in the sustainability of the project. An aspect of the monitoring activity of the Urbani School Health Kit is the class demonstration observed by division supervisors/coordinators or representatives from the School Health Office. This monitoring provides a point for gathering feedback from schools and teachers as well as motivation for teachers to continue using the School Health Kit.

Involvement of other sectors in the community such as the Kilusan Ligtas Malaria – a special private–public partnership program for malaria control involving of the Department of Health in Palawan for the prevention and control of malaria – as well as the Pilipinas Shell Foundation of Shell group of companies in the Philippines is also important in linking school health issues with their communities. Kilusan Ligtas Malaria and Pilipinas Shell Foundation were both tapped for technical experts to discuss the prevention and control of malaria. They also explained the ongoing efforts in the community to prevent and control malaria and engaged teachers to help by educating students and parents.

Conclusion and Recommendations

Evaluation showed that the Urbani School Health Kit helped teachers in conveying clear and accurate health messages in their lessons. They used the kit as the platform for the class session, and its contents helped to shape lessons for the day. They were able to emphasize the key messages and to stimulate learning using the activities included in the Kit.

Teachers mentioned that the kit is useful, helpful, and appropriate, since the materials are ready to use, encourage class participation, and motivate students with games and visual aids. They said that every class should be provided with the kit. They also said that schoolchildren were amazed, happy, curious, excited to use the materials, and very eager to perform the activities. They suggested, though, that the letters and pictures should be made bigger and the language simpler.

School children showed increased interests in the health topics because of the innovative learning activities. School children were seen actively participating in the learning activities, demonstrating healthy practices, and showing interest in an environment supportive of health.

The kit's presence in the school served as a reminder to have more discussions on health topics. The posters were kept posted in halls and boards in the schools. Teachers verbalized interest in joining other trainings or workshops related to teaching health and health promotion.

Future plans for the implementation of the Urbani School Health Kit include further distribution in rural areas where health services are a bit lacking than in other parts of the country. Teachers also suggested additional topics, such as safety in schools, mental health, and reproductive health. Good teaching aids from available resources at the local and international level can be incorporated to further enhance the kit and update the topics.

The Urbani School Health Kit is an innovative way of supporting health promotion in schools.

Acknowledgment The Urbani School Health Kit project was supported by AusAID, Department of Health, World Health Organization project to Roll Back Malaria in Mindanao.

References

Department of Education, Republic of the Philippines. (2007). *Factsheet on basic education statistics*. Retrieved August 19, 2008, from http://www.deped.gov.ph/factsandfigures/default. asp

National Statistics Office. (2008a). *2007 Census of population*. Retrieved August 19, 2008, from http://www.census.gov.ph/data/census2007/index.html

National Statistics Office. (2008b). *Quick statistics*. Retrieved August 19, 2008, from http://www. census.gov.ph/data/quickstat/index.html

World Bank. (2006). *Country brief*. Retrieved March 15, 2008, from http://www.worldbank.org. ph/

World Health Organization [WHO]. (2007). *Countries: Philippines*. Retrieved March 15, 2008, from http://www.who.int/countries/phl/en/

Chapter 26
Singapore: Health-Promoting Schools: The CHERISH Award

Rose Vaithinathan, Cheong-Lim Lee Yee, Wong Mun Loke, and Kelly Leow

Contextual Introduction

Singapore is a small island-country, about 700 sq km in area, with a total population of 4.5 million and a resident population of 3.6 million. Its rich ethnic mix comprises 76% Chinese, 13% Malays, 9% Indians, and 2% of other ethnic origins. Twenty percent of the population is under 15 years of age. The healthcare system is comprehensive and access is good, as reflected in the infant mortality rate of 2.6 per 1,000 live births and a life expectancy of 80 years. There are about 350 government primary, secondary, and preuniversity level schools attended by children from 6 to 18 years old. The first 6 years of education, starting at 6-years-old and covering primary one to primary six levels, are compulsory. There is opportunity for every child to have secondary school education (4 years). The mean number of years of schooling is 9.3 years, with 60% of the population currently holding a secondary or higher qualification. Postsecondary and tertiary education choices are offered by several polytechnics, institutions of technical education, three universities, and other specialty education institutions. The population literacy rate is 95.4%.

The origins of school health promotion can be traced to the 1970s and 1980s, when the Ministries of Health and Education worked together on the school health education syllabus and curriculum materials. Over those years, the Ministry of Health offered a wide range of programs in schools addressing smoking, nutrition, exercise, mental health, oral health, and sexually transmitted diseases (STDs) individually. These topics and activities were well accepted by schools and achieved a broad reach to students and teachers annually.

Recognizing the wider potential of health promotion and the benefits of a holistic approach embodying the principles of the Ottawa Charter over the traditional curriculum, the Health Promotion Board of the Ministry of Health sought to

R. Vaithinathan(✉)
Youth Health Division, Health Promotion Board, Singapore

C. Vince Whitman and C.E. Aldinger (eds.),
Case Studies in Global School Health Promotion: From Research to Practice,
DOI: 10.1007/978-0-387-92269-0_26, © Springer Science + Business Media, LLC 2009

establish a Health-Promoting School model that would fit well with the directions in which Singapore schools were developing. Program developers felt that an award scheme would be culturally appropriate and acceptable. A reward scheme would not be unfamiliar in the schools' context, particularly because the Ministry of Education already had an established system of school awards. Schools across Singapore were comparable as regards environmental, educational, and other characteristics, and they had already had many years' experience of health promotion activities in school.

The Health Promotion Board then established the Championing Efforts Resulting in Improved School Health (CHERISH) Award and began promoting it to schools in 2000. Modeled after the World Health Organization's Health-Promoting School initiative, the award offers a structured approach for schools to establish the Health-Promoting School framework for their staff and students. The CHERISH Award aims to encourage schools to develop comprehensive school health promotion programs and provides national recognition for their efforts in nurturing the physical, emotional, and social health of the school community.

Overview of the School Health Program: CHERISH Award

The CHERISH Award includes three main assessment criteria, consistent with the WHO model of the Health-Promoting School:

1. School organization, ethos, and environment: the structure, policies, procedures, and the physical and social environment in the school
2. Curriculum, teaching, and learning: formal curricular teaching and learning, cocurricular activities
3. Community links and partnership: collaboration between the school and the wider school community – parents, community members, government, and nongovernment agencies, service providers

Schools are urged to set up a proper organizational structure to plan and implement health promotion, such as a health promotion committee, with the principal or vice principal as advisor. They are encouraged to develop a charter or policy on health promotion and to incorporate it with their other school values. A comprehensive 70-item checklist for the three criteria is provided to schools, which also helps them to design their health promotion program, although they are assessed only on certain aspects. Guidance is given to schools for topic-specific interventions according to the needs of the school, such as smoking control, healthy eating, mental health, STD/AIDS. Recently, the Health Promotion Board has also guided schools to include more emphasis on evaluation, as well as on future plans and challenges.

Depending on the merit of their health promoting initiatives, schools may be awarded a Gold, Silver, or Bronze Award in recognition of their efforts. To reach a Silver Award, schools would have to show, among other programs and structures, evidence of a comprehensive school health promotion plan. For a Gold Award, self-evaluation is an essential component. In 2003, the Platinum Award was introduced to recognize schools that have demonstrated sustained achievements in health promotion. For a Platinum Award, schools must have achieved a Gold Award for two consecutive cycles, show positive outcomes for students and staff with trend data for 3 years, and show impact on the broader community, for example, parents and community members.

Although the Health Promotion Board champions the evaluation process, the Ministry of Education plays an important collaborative role, and they jointly assess all CHERISH Award applications. On-site visits and interviews are conducted for selected schools and all Gold and Platinum award contenders to validate their report submissions and give the schools feedback.

The Minister for Education has demonstrated his support by attending the award ceremonies and presenting the awards to schools.

Participation in the CHERISH Award

Since the Award was introduced in 2000, there has been a threefold increase in the number of schools vying for it (Fig. 1), and the number of schools achieving the award has risen from 84 in 2002 to 276 in 2006. This number comprises 145 primary schools and 131 secondary schools and preuniversities, reaching about 400,000 students. About 90% of all schools, covering 450,000 students, have now participated in the 2008 CHERISH Award. Apart from the increase in participation among schools, it has been encouraging to note that the number of schools achieving the Silver and Gold Awards (Fig. 2) has grown from 41 (49%) in 2002 to 230 (83%) in 2006. This increase suggests that the quality of health promotion efforts in the schools is also improving.

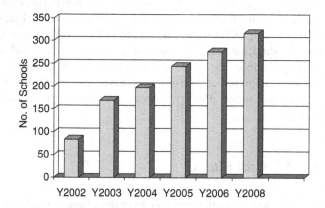

Fig. 1 Schools' participation in CHERISH Award 2002–2008

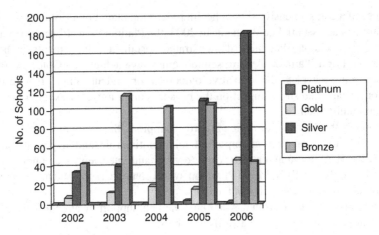

Fig. 2 Categories of CHERISH Award 2002–2006

Specific Aspects of Implementation

Health-Related Policies in Schools

Policies promoted by the Ministry of Education affect all schools. Many schools have added holistic school policies, which contribute toward their status as a Health-Promoting School.

Curriculum

All schools have health education in the curriculum. In the primary school years, health education is a separate subject that occupies a half-hour period each week. In the secondary school years, health education is featured in various subjects, such as general science (smoking, STD/AIDS), home economics (nutrition), and biology. The Ministry of Education has developed modules for social and emotional learning, including the teaching of life skills. In conjunction with other agencies (including the Health Promotion Board), they have also developed a sexuality education program for upper primary, lower secondary, upper secondary, and preuniversity levels.

Exercise and Physical Fitness

All schools have physical education classes two or three times a week, which, at the secondary level, are conducted by trained teachers. Schools also organize mass physical activities, such as sports day and game carnivals for their students. All these help students to become physically fit and to learn skills for sports. Many students also take up a sport as an extracurricular activity after school hours. Most schools have a playing field or playground, an outdoor fitness station, a health and fitness room, or a sports hall.

The School Tuckshop

Since the early 1990s schools have practiced a "green labeling" system, which places green indicators on the menu board of each stall in the tuckshop to help students identify healthy food. Principals and teachers are equipped with a set of school tuckshop guidelines, identifying healthier food (less fat, less salt and sugar, healthier ingredients, prohibited foods) and a list of drinks allowed to be sold in the tuckshop. All schools must have water-dispensing machines (sometimes called water fountains, dispensing water free-of-charge) in the ratio of 1:120 students.

The Model School Tuckshop

In 2003, the Health Promotion Board introduced the Model School Tuckshop Program (MSTP) to encourage and recognize schools that offer healthier food choices in their school tuckshops. Schools can choose to improve their tuckshop and attain Model School Tuckshop Status. The MSTP comprises seven food guidelines:

1. Sell drinks with no more than 8% sugar content.
2. Sell deep-fried food and preserved meat on only one day of the week.
3. Use low-fat milk to replace part of coconut milk in local dishes.
4. Use skinless poultry and lean meat when preparing food.
5. Provide the recommended amounts of vegetables in rice dishes and noodles.
6. Sell at least two varieties of fresh fruit daily.
7. Avoid serving gravy/sauce for rice dishes unless requested.

Starting in 2008, the guidelines were revised to:

- Replace the original drink guidelines and sell only drinks on the Health Promotion Board's Healthier Choice list. These drinks are easily identified by a "Healthier Choice" label on each drink can, bottle, or packet. This guideline will ensure that only drinks with 7 g/100 mL or less sugar content will be sold in schools.
- Have at least two water-dispensing machines inside the tuckshop. This change would encourage students to drink water, rather than other drinks, with their meals and not only when they are thirsty outside the mealtime.

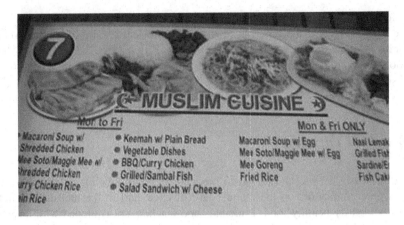

Picture 39 School menu "Muslim Cuisine"

The Health Promotion Board engages nutrition consultants to assist schools in implementing the MSTP by assessing the nutritional value of food and drinks sold in the tuckshop, recommending changes to ensure alignment with the guidelines, and conducting culinary training for tuckshop vendors to empower them to prepare healthier meals in schools. The participating school and the Health Promotion Board cofund the nutrition consultancy fee. Schools that achieve Model School Tuckshop (MST) status will be eligible for full reimbursement of these fees. The MSTP schools have a School Tuckshop Committee, which works with the tuckshop vendors to ensure their adherence to the MSTP guidelines through regular monitoring of the food and drinks sold.

In 2004, 16.6% of schools achieved MST status. This status rose to 46.5% in 2005. In 2006, about 90% of schools participated in the program and 75% of them achieved MST status. From 2008, only schools with a Model School Tuckshop are eligible for Gold and Platinum CHERISH awards.

Other Policies

All schools have a full-time, trained counselor for students. All schools are no-smoking or tobacco-free areas by law, so neither students nor teachers can smoke there at any time. There are school rules for safety and guidelines for emergency medical care. Health Promotion Board health teams visit all schools every year for a schedule of screening and booster immunizations. In-school and mobile dental clinics ensure that students in every primary and secondary school receive basic dental care. Regular fogging for mosquitoes is carried out. Following the SARS outbreak in 2003, many schools have also put in place comprehensive measures to be taken in the event of an outbreak of a serious communicable disease, to prevent its spread. These include daily monitoring of body temperatures of students and staff to identify infections early.

Policies of CHERISH Schools

In addition to these universal policies, individual schools have implemented health-related policies that contribute to becoming Health-Promoting Schools. Many schools have set up a health promotion committee and incorporated a "health charter" into their school values. Not forgetting staff, many schools ensure protected time for staff wellness, availability of sports facilities, courses, a staff social lounge, birthday celebrations. Realizing that students often come to school without breakfast, many schools have established a healthy breakfast program where students can have cereal and milk, sandwiches, or grilled potatoes for a token fee. In one school, every pupil has a chance to take responsibility as a student leader in class for at least one term, for example, as librarian, class monitor, classroom manager, or subject leader for subjects such as mathematics, science, or English language.

Specific Aspects of Implementation

The Health Promotion Board seeks to assist and support schools continuously in their efforts toward becoming a Health-Promoting School. Through the years, it has introduced several initiatives, described here.

Capacity Building

Capacity building in the area of health promotion is of paramount importance for the schools. The Health Promotion Board offers training courses free to school teachers. Courses such as, "Essential Updates on Current Health Issues and Concerns for Schools" and "Your First Steps Towards Planning a Health Promoting School" are organized annually and are well-attended. Such courses also provide feedback to the Health Promotion Board on schools' needs. Other courses are more issue-specific and train teachers in particular skills or in the use of health promotion modules prepared by the Health Promotion Board: The "Peer Assisted Learning (PAL) Smoking Prevention Program" course trains teachers to use peer leaders for classroom-based smoking prevention; the "School-Based Break Free Smoking Cessation Program" offers teachers a step-by-step guide to conduct a school-based smoking cessation program.

Various modules and guides are produced for teachers' use; many do not require much formal training and are distributed to schools with a brief introduction. The Health Promotion Board also provides training for tuckshop vendors on culinary skills for healthy cooking, healthy recipes, and training for tuckshop committees on maintaining a healthier tuckshop. The Health Promotion Board works closely with the schools, providing customized consultation to help them address their weaknesses and foster a health promoting culture among their staff and students. A list of courses by other reliable agencies (such as nongovernmental organizations) and a list of providers for health education talks and programs are disseminated to schools for easy reference. The Health Promotion Board facilitates the sharing of best practices among schools by the conduct of regular sharing sessions, publication of good practice books with exemplary or interesting programs by schools, and an online e-newsletter for teachers, HealthVine. These have proven to be effective and efficient ways of disseminating good practices among schools.

In addition to training teachers, the Health Promotion Board organizes teachers' wellness programs in an effort to encourage teachers to lead a healthy lifestyle, thus influencing their students to do likewise. In 2007, the Ministry of Education introduced a new department, the Staff Well-Being Unit, to consolidate and spearhead wellness programs for staff. The Health Promotion Board has collaborated with the unit to enhance the health promotion efforts for teachers. Further partnership will continue to provide more support for the teachers' health. To reach out to more teachers, additional programs will be organized at school-based and school cluster-based levels.

Recognizing that peers and role modeling play an important part to influence the decisions of youth, the Health Promotion Board also taps youth leaders to promote health among school students through a new youth-led initiative launched in 2005, called the Youth Advolution for Health (YAH) Programme. (The word *advolution* stems from the words *advocate* and *revolution*.) The program seeks to encourage young people to be advocates for health and to revolutionize health promotion for young people in school and community settings. Youth can join as committee members to plan and implement programs. The board provides training programs as well as guidance and funding for identified health projects.

School Health Promotion Grants

Three years after the launch of the CHERISH Award, the School Health Promotion Grant was set up, making financial support from the Health Promotion Board available for schools to mount appropriate health promotion initiatives for both staff and students, enhance existing programs, or develop a more comprehensive program and improve their standing within the CHERISH Award scheme. Issued on an annual basis, the grant is used for reimbursement of up to 50% of the amount expended, up to a maximum of SG$5,000 per school per year. These funds can be used for programs or services that increase awareness or knowledge or promote behavior change. All grant recipients must take part in the CHERISH Award for that year. If a school has received the grant previously, it will be awarded it in a subsequent year only if it has shown improvement in its CHERISH Award status. The grant is publicized extensively through brochures sent to schools, training courses for teachers, HealthVine, and the Health Promotion Board's Web site. Applications should include a plan for needs assessment, evaluation, and follow-up activities to ensure sustainability. In the 5 years since its inception, a total of 166 schools have benefited from the grant, implementing activities such as yoga instruction or health-related training courses for teachers, fruit days or fruit breaks, health camps, treks or excursions for students, purchase of exercise equipment, conducting surveys, or relevant health screening.

In preparation for the development of the Health-Promoting School concept in both preschools (kindergartens and childcare centers) and tertiary institutions, the Health Promotion Board has introduced the Pre-School Health Promotion Grant and the Tertiary Institution Health Promotion Grant. Sixty preschools have received a total of about SG$50,000 to implement nutrition and exercise programs for their students, teachers, and parents. Various health projects have also been implemented in institutes of technical education and polytechnics, utilizing the grant.

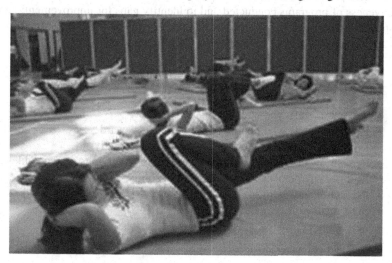

Picture 40   An exercise programme for staff funded by the school health promotion grant

Engaging Parents and the Community

Schools pursue parental involvement because they realize the benefits to the school community. Parents may be involved informally as helpers at events, but more often they participate within the structure of the school's parent support group. In many schools, parents help the school plan and implement activities for children. They take on duties – such as traffic warden, tuckshop facilitator to help younger students obtain their food, library helper, or arts and craft teacher – according to their individual talents and interests. In some schools, parents provide before- and after-school care for students. Many schools make available training or coaching for groups of parents so that they will feel confident to volunteer their time.

The Health Promotion Board is exploring more and better ways to work with parent support groups in schools. The aim is to provide health promotion initiatives and reach out to more parents via these groups.

For community involvement, students volunteer at nearby nongovernmental organizations, homes for the elderly, or facilities for the disabled. They learn to care for others and to be patient with the old or intellectually disabled. Some schools share their facilities with the neighborhood. One school with a swimming pool allows the neighboring community center to use its pool once a week.

Pre- and Post-evaluation

At the school level, pre and post data are often tracked at two levels: at the program level, where pre and post surveys are done with the stakeholders to ascertain the effectiveness of programs conducted and to identify gaps for improvement; and at the strategic planning level, where schools track health-related indicators for both staff and students. The data often include the following:

(a) For staff:

- Physical health

  • Percent of staff who undergo health screening
  • Percent of staff who obtain a physical fitness award
  • Percent of staff who engage in regular physical activity
  • Percent of staff who eat the correct number of servings of vegetables and fruit per day/percent of staff who eat healthily
  • Percent of staff who smoke
  • Staff medical leave rate
  • Staff turnover rate

- Social and emotional health

  • Staff morale and satisfaction
  • Staff stress level

(b) For students:

- Physical health

  • Percent of students who exercise the recommended number of times a week
  • Percent of students who have a balanced diet daily
  • Percent of students who have breakfast before going to school

- Social and emotional health:

  • Percent of students who feel safe in school
  • Percent of students who are happy in school
  • Indicators that track desired character traits identified by the school

- Others:

  • Percent of students who achieve at least a B grade in health education:

Many of these indicators are tracked using schools' annual health practice surveys. Such surveys are developed by the schools themselves, so as to better integrate their educational goals with health outcomes. In addition, the Ministry of Education requires schools to track other health-related indicators such as obesity rates and "healthy school climate." As these indicators are closely related to those the schools monitor for CHERISH, schools combine the two as overall health indicators.

Best Practices Among Health-Promoting Schools in Singapore

Tables 1–3, and 4 show examples of the best practices from the Health-Promoting Schools in Singapore. These examples have been sorted into broad categories, to demonstrate how schools have leveraged technology, school policies, and parent or community linkages to advance their health promotion efforts.

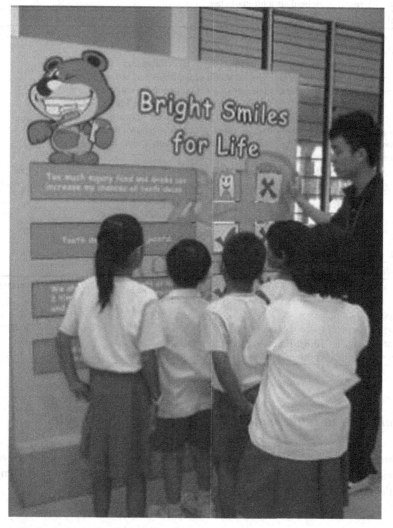

Picture 41   Students viewing health fair exhibits with a health fair facilitator

Table 1 Diffusion of innovation/technology

Health Promoting Initiative	School
Chowiz system	Canberra Secondary School
This system uses information technology to monitor calorie counts for the students as they have their meals in the school canteen. It also captures the nutritional value of food consumed by students in school	
AudioWaves 97.5	Whitley Secondary School
The students develop radio programs on a variety of issues and broadcast them weekly in school. Students also assume the role of broadcast journalists to provide "media" coverage for major school events. This program provides a platform for students to develop their confidence and boost their self-esteem	

Table 2 Leadership/school structure/policies

Health Promoting Initiative	School
Incorporation of the health charter into school values and CHERISH charter mural	Unity Primary School
The school's values are embodied in the acronym HEART, where H represents Healthy Lifestyle. The inclusion of health as part of the school's values demonstrates the school's commitment toward nurturing the health of the staff and students. A mural of the School's Health Promotion Charter is placed strategically in the canteen. Students, teachers, tuckshop vendors, and parents have shown their commitment to promoting health by planting their thumbprints in the border surrounding the mural	
Protected time for health	Catholic High Primary School
Staff have protected time to engage in regular physical activity	

Table 3 Parent support group

Health Promoting Initiative	School
Engaging parents in school activities	ACS Independent
Parents offer professional services, such as medical advice, sports coaching.	
Engaging parents in school activities	Hougang Primary School
Parents manage a CHERISH connect room for students waiting to participate in after-school activities	

Challenges in Implementing Health-Promoting Schools

Although Singapore has been relatively successful in establishing the Health-Promoting Schools initiative, several issues have commonly emerged as challenges for the future.

Table 4 Relationship with community

Health Promoting Initiative	School
School Health Fair	
The School Health Fair organized by the Health Promotion Board provides an opportunity for staff, students and parents to learn about health issues through interactive exhibits and activities. The host school invites neighboring schools and members of the community (including parents) to attend the fair. The fair thus encourages schools to foster links with their surrounding community	10–12 schools host the School Health Fair each year
Community Involvement Program	
Recognizing the importance of active citizenship and a sense of belonging to their community, the Ministry of Education introduced the Community Involvement Program in 1997, with the objective of building social cohesion and civic responsibility. Schools are given the autonomy to select appropriate activities for their pupils. Some examples of the activities are adoption of a park, visits to elderly homes and orphanages	Several schools

- Schools lack time to plan, develop, implement, and review health promotion initiatives.
- It is difficult to identify and address the "at-risk" and "unwell" groups in schools.
- Schools are reluctant to spend effort on evaluation, which is probably viewed as difficult to perform. The Health Promotion Board needs to spend more time increasing the capacity of teachers in this respect.
- The Health Promotion Board needs to spend more effort in performing systematic evaluation of groups of schools, if not all schools, to achieve collective gains of the CHERISH Award and to chart directions.

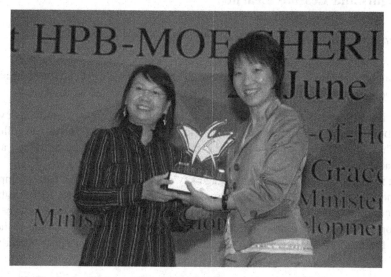

Picture 42 The Senior Minister of State for Education presenting the CHERISH Award plaque to a school recipient

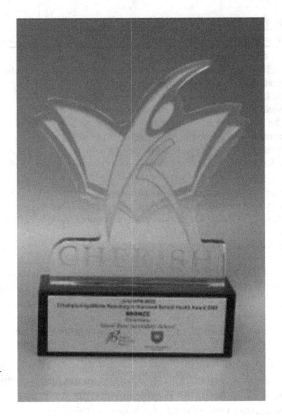

Picture 43 The Joint HPB –
MOE CHERISH Award
plaque

Insights and Lessons Learned

Recommendations

From our experience, we have found certain criteria that are essential to a Health-Promoting School initiative:

- It is necessary, when introducing a Health-Promoting School program, to develop and disseminate clear guidelines and strategic plans for schools to follow. These should be available from the outset and would best be presented as a package of handouts.
- It is important to identify and engage key stakeholders that can help to implement and propagate the Health-Promoting School. The Ministry of Education and interested individuals within it should be sought out early; and the benefits for education outcomes, shared with them. It would be appropriate to hold a formal presentation. Within the school, it would be important to identify a

Health-Promoting School coordinator. It would be ideal to make the coordinator a fixed position, for example, the physical education teacher of each school; however, this is not always possible.

- Teachers respond well to the program if they believe that it will improve the general well-being of the children and staff and make them happier. It may not always be necessary to show specific health outcomes that health personnel conventionally require. It is important to keep this in mind for marketing the Health-Promoting School.

- There is no substitute for building capacity to ensure that the teachers and other stakeholders have the knowledge and skills to implement the Health-Promoting School. Training sessions, workshops, dialogue sessions, focus group discussions are all important.

- It is important also to produce useful guides, anecdotes, and stories to motivate participants and to facilitate implementation.

- Many communication platforms must be made available. It is essential to be able to provide school-by-school customized consultation and feedback, looking into the strong and weak points of each school and, in many cases, making a trip to the school and communicating with the teacher in charge. It is also important to provide schools with direct access to the national coordinating agency in a personal way, giving names, telephone numbers, and e-mail addresses of persons dedicated to oversee the program for their school or group of schools. Platforms for networking among participating schools to share ideas and experiences are also useful.

- Incentive schemes and platforms for recognizing schools' efforts in implementing the Health-Promoting School are useful tools for encouraging participation, if it is deemed that the schools are fairly comparable.

Future Directions

In 2006, after 5 years of the CHERISH Award, the Ministry of Education, in a more inclusive approach, broadened its role from being a collaborator with the Health Promotion Board to becoming a joint owner and administrator. The award will henceforth be presented jointly by both organizations. This strategic move has strengthened the collaborative partnership between the health and education sectors, which is crucial for the advancement of the Health-Promoting School movement. The new joint CHERISH Award will also be included in the Ministry of Education's own master plan of awards and is thus poised to garner greater support among the schools. Already, we are seeing the participation of even more junior colleges in CHERISH as well as in the MSTP. Moving ahead, because so many schools have gained experience and are capable of implementing more comprehensive programs, the CHERISH Award will adopt a new 2-year cycle, in which schools will be given more time to address needs assessment, planning, evaluation, and review of their health promoting initiatives.

The board is currently developing, for the first time, a customized Health-Promoting School model to introduce the initiative to tertiary institutions (universities, polytechnics, and institutes of technical education); it is also studying the elements necessary for a Health-Promoting School approach in kindergartens and childcare centers. Besides the Health Promotion Grants, which have been set up as a first step over the past year, the Health Promotion Board has also started a certification program for Healthy Eating in Childcare Centers and Kindergartens, again as a critical preparation step for a Health-Promoting School scheme. Its assessment and certification span compliance with seven dietary guidelines (including an emphasis on provision of an adequate amount of milk daily for each child), healthy culinary skills training for cooks, and nutrition education in the classroom.

Conclusion

The award scheme has played a crucial role in providing a direction for schools toward holistic health promotion. While providing guidelines, the awards program has also left enough room for schools to design innovative activities that suit the particular needs and interests of the school community. The awards have encouraged the establishment of a school's health policies, an environmental focus, and community links. Noting its expanding acceptance by schools, the Ministry of Education evolved its support to the status of leading with the Health Promotion Board. Both organizations look forward to more schools aspiring toward and achieving Health-Promoting School status.

Chapter 27
Viet Nam

Bui Phuong Nga, Le Thi Kim Dung, Le Thi Thu Hien, Bernie Marshall, Nguyen Hung Lon, Nguyen Huy Nga, and Margaret Sheehan

Contextual Introduction

Viet Nam is a rapidly developing nation with a population of more than 84 million people, half of whom are under the age of 25. In recent years the socialist state has embraced far-reaching social and economic reforms and has come to be seen by many as an example of an effective development model. Viet Nam has lifted millions out of poverty and distributed the economic gains of its rapid growth fairly evenly across its society (International Development Association, 2007). According to the World Bank (2007), the country is "well positioned to achieve all the Millennium Development Goals by 2015."

Statistics:

Total population: 84,238,000
GDP per capita (Intl $, 2004): 3,298
Life expectancy at birth m/f (years): 69.0/74.0
Healthy life expectancy at birth m/f (years, 2002): 59.8/62.9
Child mortality m/f (per 1,000): 24/22
Adult mortality m/f (per 1,000): 197/122
Total health expenditure per capita (Intl $, 2003): 164
Total health expenditure as % of GDP (2003): 5.4

(WHO, n.d.)

M. Sheehan(✉)
World Health Organization, Hanoi, Viet Nam

C. Vince Whitman and C.E. Aldinger (eds.),
Case Studies in Global School Health Promotion: From Research to Practice,
DOI: 10.1007/978-0-387-92269-0_27, © Springer Science + Business Media, LLC 2009

Health Situation

Child nutrition has improved dramatically in recent years; both the underweight and the stunting rates among children under 5 show rapid annual reductions of around 2% between 1993 and 2004. However, the rates are still high, at about 26.6% and 30.7%, respectively, and micronutrient deficiencies are a significant problem.

Large disparities in health status exist between different geographical regions and population groups. Health indicators in the Central Highlands, the Northern Uplands, and the Northern Central Coast are considerably worse than in the rest of the country. Health status in rural areas is poorer than in urban areas, with ethnic minorities and people in mountainous areas lowest on the scale. Maternal and infant mortality among ethnic minority groups can be as much as four times higher than the national average. In remote and mountainous areas, maternal and infant mortality rates are increasing among the poorest 20% of the population.

The ten leading causes of mortality remained the same in 2004 as in the previous year, with acute respiratory infection, diarrhea, and parasitic infections being the most common childhood diseases.

New or reemerging diseases, such as tuberculosis, HIV/AIDS, dengue fever, and Japanese encephalitis, are increasing. On an average, there are more than 58,389 new tuberculosis patients every year. The proportion of HIV infections among persons under 30 years of age has been increasing in recent years. In 2004, HIV/AIDS, with a 44.2% increase in mortality over 2003, became the second most common cause of hospital deaths.

While the country has made great strides in improving the health and welfare of its population over recent years, it still suffers from a poor understanding of disease and illness and from a lack of basic health promoting infrastructure. For example, about half of all diseases in Viet Nam relate to unsafe water and poor sanitation.

Schools

School communities can be breeding grounds for communicable diseases – such as parasites, flu, measles, conjunctivitis, diphtheria, and whooping cough – which can spread quickly in schools and also from schools to families and communities.

Statistics:

Official primary school starting age: 6
Duration of primary cycle (years): 5
Official secondary school starting age: 11
Duration of secondary cycle (years): 7
Primary school-age population (2010)p: 7,773,484
Secondary school-age population (2010)p: 9,472,815
Lower secondary (age 11–14, 2005): 6,670,714
Upper secondary (age 15–17, 2005): 2,802,101
Number of teachers (all levels, 2005): 762,266
Primary level teachers: 360,624

However, schools are also an ideal forum for health interventions, since children account for a quarter of the population, and primary school attendance in Viet Nam is very high (98%). Studies both inside and outside Viet Nam indicate that the school environment influences children's physical health, self-esteem, and health behaviors, as well as their learning ability and development of life-skills. In addition to homes and families, school is also where children's moral behaviors and personalities take shape.

Impetus and Origin of the School Health Program

Viet Nam's interest and participation in school health promotion can be traced back to its participation in a Health-Promoting Schools (HPS) workshop in Singapore in January 1995. It also joined the working group for the development of HPS held in Shanghai in December 1995. The Ministry of Health (MoH), the Centre for Health Education in Hanoi, and the Health Information and Education Centre in Ho Chi Minh City all expressed interest in developing HPS in collaboration with the Ministry of Education and Training (MoET). The MoH, through its Preventive Medicine Department, was also interested in HPS as part of the Healthy Cities project, with a focus largely on water and sanitation.

Health education became an "official subject" in primary and secondary schools, crèches, and kindergartens in 1996, after its pilot implementation between 1990 and 1995 under a UNICEF grant. The MoET edited two manuals on health education for teachers and students. It also set up a subcommittee to edit all school manuals, including those on health education, by the year 2000.

In December 2000, the MoET and the MoH signed a joint declaration that HPS should be a priority area for action.

WHO advocates that health programs designed for schools both reduce common health problems and enhance the effectiveness of the educational system, thereby improving both public health and education and social development. School health programs should aim to address all facets of health, including physical, social, emotional, and – particularly – mental health. Being healthy allows children to do their best at school, protects them from specific illnesses, and gives them a positive start in life.

In keeping with this, WHO supported another HPS partnership with the MoH Preventive Medicine Department and the MoET Student Welfare Department, to initiate a specific Health-Promoting School project in 2001. In the early days of HPS, WHO both supported and drove the project and was one of many partners investing in the health of school children in Viet Nam. At the time of the HPS project's inception, others were also investing in school-based health in some provinces of Viet Nam, including UNICEF through its Child Friendly Schools project.

According to legislation and policy frameworks, the Education and Health sector share responsibility for school health in Viet Nam. Previously WHO had largely focused its schools work through the health sector. WHO determined that, in order to effectively integrate key health messages into the Vietnamese school curriculum, HPS would need to be an interministerial project, in partnership with the health and education ministries, something that is very unusual in Viet Nam and was a first for WHO in Viet Nam.

Overview of the School Health Program

During the years 2001–2006, WHO worked to support the MoH and MoET to develop, test, and disseminate a Vietnamese model for HPS. Over that period, HPS was implemented to varying degrees in 18 provinces, and when workshops planned for 2007 were complete, regional staff from both the education and health sectors of all 64 provinces received the HPS kit and the train-the-trainer manuals. Around 100 schools received small grants (ranging from $200 to $1,000) based on plans they submitted.

Guidelines and Training

In 2001 a steering committee drawn from WHO, MoH, and MoET was established to guide the project's implementation. The steering committee, working with a technical advisor from WHO, decided to adapt a model and guidelines for HPS developed in Australia to the Vietnamese context, drawing on the most appropriate elements. An important component borrowed from the Australian materials was the audit tool, which was used to help schools assess how "health promoting" they were. This tool was originally based on WHO global and WPRO guidelines (World Health Organization, 1996).

The initial objectives of the HPS project were to develop and document National Guidelines for implementing a HPS, to write support materials for classroom teachers (around the themes of a clean and safe school), to establish a group of demonstration HPS schools that could pilot the guidelines and classroom materials, and to build the capacity of selected individuals within provincial MoH and MoET departments to become trainers and experts in the area of HPS.

The Vietnamese Health-Promoting School model, as a settings approach, encouraged both individual behavior change and change in the environment of the school (to create a safe and secure environment to have the best impact on the health of school children). Four key elements, which form the four petals of the lotus flower used as the symbol in the project's logo, were selected by the steering committee to form the four pillars of the project (Fig. 1):

- *School facilities*: improving the physical environment of the school by having clean water and toilets available, decreasing rubbish, planting trees and garden beds, improving lighting, and ensuring the purchase of standard desks, chairs, and blackboards

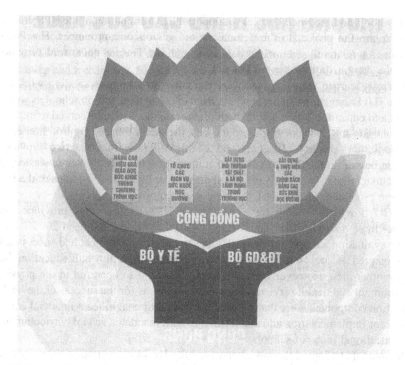

Fig. 1 The Viet Nam Health-Promoting School model

- *Health education*: encouraging certain health behaviors in children themselves, by integrating health education into the existing student curriculum
- *Health services*: engaging local health services and authorities to increase services provided on site, such as deworming, eye and dental checks, and vaccination sessions
- *Health policies*: implementing policies to promote school health, such as adopting a "no smoking and no drinking" policy within school grounds

The steering committee agreed on the broad guidelines for implementing HPS and employed two curriculum writers, one from the health and one from the education ministry, to develop materials that would complement the Vietnamese school curriculum.

The HPS guidelines and teaching materials were then included in a draft version of a Health-Promoting School kit. These kits included lesson plans for about eight to ten sample lessons, using an interactive teaching methodology, flip charts, picture sets, nutrition cards, a parasite control game, and a deworming poster, all designed to make health education for school children more active and engaging.

The WHO technical adviser, in collaboration with consultants, designed a draft 2-day train-the-trainer program. Training was delivered to small teams of people from schools and provincial offices to support the dissemination of the HPS draft kit and explain the project to the demonstration schools and provinces. Hai Phong province, a relatively well-off urban area, and Ha Tinh, a poor rural province, were the demonstration sites for Phase 1.

Lessons learned from the trial were presented to a large evaluation workshop held in Hai Phong, attended by teachers from every demonstration school as well as health and education officials from both provinces; the workshop served to improve the materials and add some topics to the kits, including tobacco control, household accidents, and puberty. Teachers and health officials from the two provinces provided input on the 2-day training of trainers program (ToT), which was developed into a more user-friendly, practical document. In 2005, 500 copies of the HPS kit were produced, and the ToT materials were completed.

WHO provided funding for expansion of HPS to three new provinces and another three districts in Ha Tinh, which took place during 2004 and 2005.

An evaluation, completed in April 2005, found that the project had successfully implemented its goals but that more activity had occurred in health education than in any other area. However, significant activity had also occurred in the physical environment and health services components. Reasons for the success of the health education component were that the area did not require significant financial contribution for implementation and that it fitted in with mandated school curriculum and the educational focus of schools.

Schools that adopted the model and used the HPS kit reported positive changes in the atmosphere of the classroom, related to the active teaching methods. Changes in children's behaviors have also been observed, including less littering in the school grounds and children paying more attention to their personal hygiene.

After these initial objectives were achieved, the project shifted its focus to training and engaging additional schools to adopt the HPS model, with local experts supporting and driving the process. The project funded an expansion in four more provinces and invited people from some provinces that were not funded.

A formal train-the-trainer manual was developed and printed as a training booklet in 2006, using a very clear and concise step-by-step approach to take teachers and health professionals through the guidelines and teaching materials.

In 2006 a train-the-trainer course was implemented for staff from 13 provinces previously not involved in HPS. Each province sent a team of three to four staff including Preventive Medicine, MoET, and one staff member from the People's Committee or Women's Union. Two large train-the-trainer sessions (for 30–40 people) were then held, one in the north of Viet Nam and one in the south.

The HPS kits were also disseminated by the MoH, which included a half-day training in one of its regular two-day training sessions for the Provincial Preventive Medicine Department.

Ten provinces received support for demonstration schools and province-specific training for teams of health workers and teachers from a range of schools.[1] This special support was mobilized especially in provinces that funded the local training event themselves, and the project then supported trainers' costs and the provision of kits and materials.

Small Grants

A small grants program operated as part of Phase 1 and Phase 2 was a key to gaining schools' buy-in to HPS.

WHO funded and/or helped mobilize small grants of around $500 to about 100 schools; many schools made remarkable progress with these funds, especially in the poorer areas. The audit tool helped many schools to identify and prioritize areas in need of improvement in their schools. The grants were then used to improve the physical environment of schools by planting trees, creating garden areas, cleaning up unused space to create play areas, installing large rubbish bins, paving paths, installing or repairing wells, building toilet blocks and modest kitchens, and purchasing drinking water containers for classrooms.

The grants were an important way of involving the whole community in the project. Schools were encouraged to work with local authorities, especially the local People's Committee and Women's Union, to secure additional funds to complete the work started from the small grants. Community involvement was high in many areas, with parents being asked to volunteer their time to implement the building projects. To secure a small grant, schools had to submit their plans to the MoH for funding and approval and agree to take action in all areas of the framework, based on the audit, and to identify priority areas and develop a plan accordingly.

Demand for grants outstripped WHO's capacity to supply funds; however, WHO was able to facilitate grants from several international organizations, including the Hanoi International Women's Club, the Australian Chamber of Commerce, and the United Nation's International School in Hanoi.

The revised HPS Guidelines Booklet, developed after the demonstration project in Ha Tinh and Hai Phong, included small case studies of how the schools had used their small grants and the steps they had followed, to help guide other schools through the process.

Impact

In early 2006, the Prime Minister requested that more be done to improve school health in Viet Nam. While not the only outcome, HPS added to the focus on school health and contributed to the call for national guidelines. Indeed many HPS report

---

[1]The ten provinces that received special support included Hai Phong, Ha Tinh, Ba Ria Vung Tau, Danang, Da Lat, Ha Noi, Ha Tay, Hai Duong, HCMC, and Ha Giang. The nature of the support varied, but all provinces had at least one designated training activity. Ha Tinh received the most significant resources.

that the model has helped them move toward meeting the national standards to become a recognized "national standard school."

The project also had a positive effect on the capacity of government ministries to work together, and the intersectoral model is now well understood.

The HPS kit proved a useful platform for rolling out new health messages in Viet Nam. The kit was refined with tobacco and injury prevention materials, added in 2006, and when the MoH received funding for glaucoma education, it added a glaucoma booklet to the Health-Promoting School kit.

The project took on a life of its own, with a number of provinces not directly involved in HPS seeking advice and access to training materials for their own schools. Critical to the success of the project was that eight to ten champions of the program sprang up, including key central figures in both MoET and MoH, two young enthusiastic teachers in the pilot province of Ha Tinh, and the Deputy Director of the provincial health centers in Ha Tinh and Hai Phong, whose enthusiasm for the program helped extend its reach and deepen its effectiveness.

Specific Aspects of Implementation

While Viet Nam is a country with a unique political system and a history that distinguishes it from many others, its establishment of HPS programs shares common factors for success with other countries. The Viet Nam experience places emphasis on a number of elements of Vince Whitman's model. Four significant factors are highlighted as integral in changing HPS policy and practice.

- *National and international guidelines.* The National Guidelines for HPS in Viet Nam drew on the original HPS principles developed in 1990 by WHO and were in line with WPRO HPS Guidelines. In addition the Viet Nam HPS model with its four components (Lotus flower) built on specific elements of the Victorian HPS Guidelines. One of the key elements of these guidelines was an audit tool that helps schools assess their current situation by allowing them to measure the level of health promotion being implemented in various areas, such as curriculum and facilities. This Vietnamese audit tool was adapted from the Victorian HPS Guidelines, 1996.
- *Team training and ongoing coaching.* Training was an integral part of the growth of this project; the training sessions were developed and refined to ensure success in building the capacity of those attending. A preliminary training session was provided, which involved teachers and other health professionals and served to detail the project as well as to present the HPS kit that would supplement all the work being done in the demonstration schools and provinces. Following the training session, those who attended gave input that later went into the development of a user-friendly document for the ToT program that would

provide future training sessions to more people, and eventually a formal manual was developed. More training sessions were then held, which extended to provinces not previously involved in the HPS project, and staff from a wide variety of sectors participated.

- *Adaptation to local concerns.* A steering committee that drew from expertise from the WHO and the local ministries of health and education was created to develop and refine a Vietnamese model for the HPS project. This model and accompanying guidelines for the implementation of this project drew from work done in Australia and was adapted to the Vietnamese context, taking care to use the most pertinent elements that would be most beneficial to Viet Nam. The Vietnamese model's approach targeted both behavior change and change in the physical environment in the schools. The key elements that the steering committee targeted included improving school facilities and increasing the breadth of health services provided, in addition to implementing health policies and improving health education within the schools.

- *Mechanism for cross-sector collaboration.* Because the Ministries of Education and Health recognized their shared responsibility for the well-being of schools in Viet Nam, both played active roles throughout the implementation of the project. The steering committee that was established to guide the project involved members from both ministries, as did the training sessions. In addition, to ensure widespread implementation for the project, staff from both ministries in their respective regions received the HPS kit and training manuals.

Conclusions and Recommendations

Drawing on a preexisting HPS model and adapting it to the Vietnamese context proved to be a very effective model for Viet Nam. While well-established health education principles were applied, the Viet Nam approach simplified and narrowed the focus of the Australian curriculum significantly before deploying it in the field.

The model was deliberately kept very simple and designed to complement the existing curriculum, but it gave teachers support to show them how to use it in a more interactive way.

While the project demonstrated the need for technical support to see it through the first phase, it must be written and driven from inside the local system in order to suit local needs. The project capitalized on already existing resources.

The project was labeled a "community project" rather than an "education project" from its inception. Community involvement was very strong and a key to success. Parents and local authorities committed time and money to the various small works projects that positively impacted the school environment. Training also went beyond the school gates, with a booklet on household safety made available to parents.

The model was successful in that it could be applied in different socioeconomic areas. However, significant differences in implementation, needs, and success were observed between urban and rural settings. The project had a very significant impact in the poorer provinces that were coming from a lower base of physical infrastructure and teaching capacity. In many poorer schools there had been virtually no teaching materials to support the curriculum. In the wealthier provinces, HPS helped to refine and elaborate the curriculum already in place and helped schools focus on what environmental improvements were needed. In Hai Phong, for example, additions of health rooms and nutrition programs were popular.

While policy setting at the school level was an aspiration of the project, there were only limited policy outcomes in the Vietnamese context, where the central authorities retain substantial control over policy. Some small policy gains were possible, however, such as in one school where a motorbike safety policy was initiated to regulate after school pickups.

The small grants were extremely successful in helping to mobilize additional community resources. The kudos of being involved in an external project (from WHO) was seen as a motivating factor. How to continue such enthusiasm for a project approach when HPS is integrated into a systems approach in such a large country remains an important question.

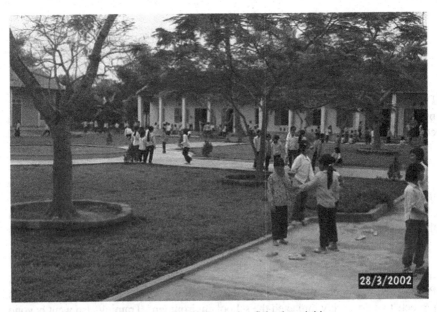

Picture 44 Students participating in Health-Promoting Schools activities

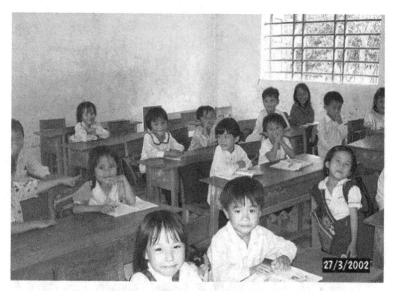

Picture 45 Students in Health-Promoting Schools

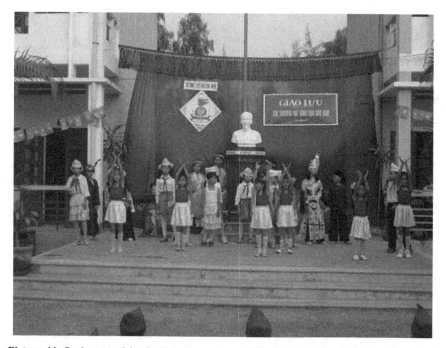

Picture 46 Students participating in a dance as part of Health-Promoting Schools

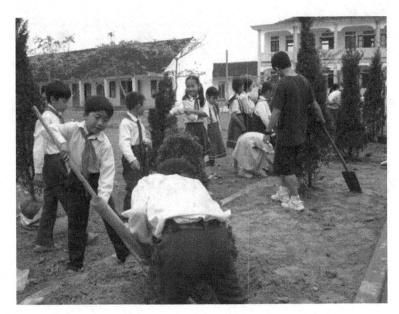

Picture 47 Students planting trees

References

International Development Association. (2007). *Vietnam: Laying the foundation for steady growth*. Retrieved from http://siteresources.worldbank.org/IDA/Resources/IDA-Vietnam.pdf

World Bank. (n.d.) *Vietnam country overview*. Retrieved February 2007, from http://web. worldbank.org/WBSITE/EXTERNAL/COUNTRIES/EASTASIAPACIFICEXT/VIETNA-MEXTN/0, menuPK:387573~pagePK:141132~piPK:141121~theSitePK:387565,00.html

World Health Organization (WHO), Regional Office for the Western Pacific (WPRO). (1996). *Regional guidelines. Development of health-promoting schools – A framework for action*. Manila, Philippines: WHO/WPRO.

World Health Organziation (WHO). (n.d.) *Viet Nam*. Retrieved from http://www.who.int/countries/vnm/en/

Chapter 28
Australia: The New South Wales School-Link Initiative

Danielle Maloney

Contextual Introduction

In 2008, the population of Australia was estimated at just over 21 million (Australian Bureau of Statistics, 2007). This creates particular challenges for Australia in delivering comprehensive programs across very large geographical areas with populations concentrating in towns around the coastline and small rural populations across the rest of the country. To put it into perspective, one of the rural Area Health Services (AHSs) of the State of New South Wales (NSW) is roughly the size of Germany and has a population of just over 305,000.

While most Australians enjoy a reasonable standard of living, there are pockets of disadvantage, with the Indigenous population experiencing health and education standards well below the average population. Australians, like populations from most other developed countries around the world, are showing increasing levels of obesity, diabetes, and mental health problems.

Australia has a three-tiered system of government. In relation to health and education, the Federal or Commonwealth government is responsible for setting a broad policy agenda and for distribution of money to the states for health and education initiatives and services. The state and territory health and education departments are responsible for the direct management of the state and territory health services and schools and for setting the curriculum in education. The management at the state level is further divided into regions or districts. The third tier, namely, the local governments do not have a direct responsibility but tend to link in with their local hospital and community health services or local schools. This creates a complex set of relationships for funding, policy development, and implementation of health and education initiatives.

In the late 1990s a national working party, brought together by the Commonwealth government, developed a National Mental Health Plan. Alongside it, a National

D. Maloney
Central Sydney Division of General Practice, Sydney, Australia

C. Vince Whitman and C.E. Aldinger (eds.),
Case Studies in Global School Health Promotion: From Research to Practice,
DOI: 10.1007/978-0-387-92269-0_28, © Springer Science + Business Media, LLC 2009

Action Plan for the Mental Health Promotion, Prevention, and Early Intervention was released in 2000. Along with this plan, States and Territories of Australia were given Mental Health Reform Incentive Funding to implement broad strategies outlined in the plan. While the Mental Health and Drug and Alcohol Office (formerly Centre for Mental Health), a division of the NSW Department of Health, has developed a number of key initiatives to address mental health at a state level, this case study will focus on their School-Link initiative as a comprehensive example of Health-Promoting Schools in practice.

School-Link, while being an initiative of the NSW Department of Health, was developed in collaboration with the NSW Department of Education and Training (Jones et al., 2002), based on a population approach to mental health problems. NSW at this stage already had a history of cooperation between the two departments on a number of health initiatives. The main purpose of School-Link is to systematically formalize partnerships between schools, Technical and Further Education (TAFE) Colleges, and mental health services and to work together to improve mental health outcomes for children and adolescents.

Not only was depression recognized for its increasing global burden at the time, but also we knew that mental disorders are at their most prevalent during adolescence and early adulthood (Commonwealth Department of Health and Ageing, 2004) and that their presence is commonly associated with serious risk factors and is linked with substance use and increased risk of suicide (NSW Department of Health, 2001). For this reason the original focus of the initiative, for the first 5 years, was secondary schools and TAFE Colleges. The second phase of the initiative has seen some forays into the primary school sector; however, without increased funding they have not progressed far at this stage.

Along with the funding to states and territories, a range of national programs was also being developed at the time, which would dovetail nicely with the School-Link initiative. One in particular is the MindMatters program, a mental health program for schools with a range of curriculum materials to address social and emotional learning. This resource was developed primarily by teachers for use by teachers. A number of prevention programs targeting either depression or anxiety were also developing an evidence base. What School-Link was able to do was lay the foundation and put in the infrastructure to support schools to implement whole of school, universal, and targeted programs.

Overview of the School Health Program

The NSW School-Link initiative was officially launched in late 1999. The initial round of funding was for 5 years. At that time, the state of NSW was divided into 17 AHSs. Funding was provided in the initial phase to each AHS to employ a School-Link Coordinator. The AHS was to provide the operating budget for the coordinator, demonstrating its commitment to the initiative. At the end of the first 5 years, another 3 years of funding was secured to distribute to the AHSs. A small number of

AHSs had absorbed these positions and made them permanent. They were able to use the extra funds provided to enhance their initiative. One AHS at this time used the extra position to pilot some work in the primary schools. Money was also invested in a formal training program for school and TAFE counselors and child and adolescent mental health workers. We are now close to the end of this funding cycle and awaiting further cabinet funding.

The focus for the initial development of School-Link was to build the relationship between schools, TAFE Colleges, and mental health services across NSW at all levels, including state, AHS/regional, and local. By first building the capacity of both health and education to work together in partnership, we have made a move from reactive to proactive mechanisms to address mental health issues.

School-Link provides a framework and structure to support child and adolescent mental health services (CAMHS) and schools in working collaboratively to promote mental health and to facilitate the early identification, management, and support of students with mental health issues. This follows closely the World Health Organization's model for school mental health. The implementation of School-Link has three main focus areas:

1. Support for the expansion of mental health promotion and prevention programs into schools and TAFE campuses
2. Improving pathways to care for children and adolescents with mental health problems through enhanced consultation, liaison, referral, and support between health and education staff
3. Professional development for school/TAFE counselors and CAMHS staff on mental health issues to improve early identification

The following diagram demonstrates the complex nature of the initiative with many tiers and levels of intervention. The top boxes indicate key partners and the bottom boxes indicate some of the strategies at each level. Only key partners are indicated here; however, flexibility allows for a number of other partners particularly at the local level (Fig. 1).

While the three focus areas of the initiative are consistent across the state, there is scope for flexibility in how each AHS implements School-Link. This flexibility is necessary as not all areas have the same services and structures. Geographical distances can also alter the way the School-Link Coordinator might be able to interact with schools. For example, an inner city coordinator may be able to have more direct contact with schools and provide more in-services, whereas due to large distances a rural coordinator might not be able to develop relationships in the same way and may not have access to the same services for young people. The flexibility also allows coordinators to address needs of specific communities in their local area; for example, some might have higher culturally and linguistically diverse populations, while others may have higher indigenous populations, highly affluent populations, and more socially disadvantaged populations.

While the initial thrust of the initiative was directed at school counselors, it was acknowledged that all staff in schools needed information and support with mental health issues. Apart from the statewide School-Link Training Program, School-Link

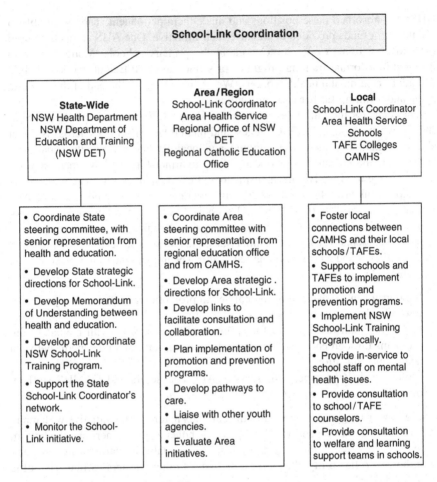

Fig. 1 School-Link Coordination Model

Coordinators have facilitated a range of professional development opportunities for both health and education staff including counseling and noncounseling staff.

A review of the initiative was conducted after the initial phase (Maloney, Jones, Walter, & Davenport, 2008). The School-Link review identified the crucial role the School-Link Coordinators play at the AHS level in achieving this aim. Both TAFE and school counselors identified negative impacts of communication between health and education with the loss of a School-Link Coordinator from an area. For instance, the loss of the School-Link coordinator was due to an AHS not putting in a position, which resulted in a loss of communication between health and education. Subsequently, increased communication between the sectors established better links to mental health services, resulting in better access for students and greater understanding, empathy, and awareness of mental health problems.

School-based programs, especially in the late primary and early high school years, offer opportunities for promotion and prevention targeting all children, at-risk groups, and/or for early intervention for children showing early symptoms of a mental health illness (Raphael, 2000). In each AHS, School-Link Coordinators work closely with schools to facilitate the implementation of evidence-based mental health promotion and prevention programs. From the School-Link review, we know that schools participating in School-Link reported an improvement in their knowledge and ability to manage mental health issues, improvement in their skills and confidence in delivering mental health programs, and structural changes within their schools, such as policy and curriculum changes.

Implementation of programs in the TAFE sector, however, has remained low. Work with the TAFE sector requires further investigation around barriers and suitability of programs for the TAFE environment. Most of the programs were developed for the school setting and the more independent and adult environment of TAFE does not suit the nature of many of these programs.

Specific Aspects of Implementation

Stage of Readiness

Mental health is an area in which schools have consistently asked the health sector for support, rather than the health sector trying to convince schools that they need to address a particular health issue. Commonly health issues that we are addressing in the school setting are about changing student's behaviors that will have an impact on their health into the future, but the impact in mental health is much more immediate. Schools globally are experiencing difficulties with students who are disengaged from schools, bullying and harassment, disruptive behavior, and suicide. In stepping into the School-Link role, some coordinators were inundated with requests for help from schools. This was quite different from having to knock on doors of schools and encourage them to participate.

Another factor that facilitated the rapid adoption by schools was the presence of a mental health staff member in the school (the school counselor), who quickly became a key facilitator of entry into the school. The other people in the schools who soon became allies were the welfare or pastoral care teams within the school. Support for them in their difficult role, for which many are undertrained and undersupported, facilitated the ability to move them from a reactive to a proactive position, where they could adopt a more holistic approach.

Vision and Concepts

The World Health Organization's model for mental health promotion in schools provided a very good framework from which to develop strategies under the

School-Link initiative. The four tiers of the model – whole of school, curriculum, targeted interventions, and treatment – are interrelated, and all must be addressed to have an effective impact on the mental health of students. For example, if we teach help-seeking behaviors in the curriculum as part of building resilience skills, but the school has no help available or the school is not supportive, it can lead to worse outcomes. On the other hand, if we provide the help for students with higher needs but do not create the supportive environment around them, they are likely to lose the gains they have made with the more intensive programs, rendering them ineffective in the long term. School-Link Coordinators provide school staff with in-service training to help them to unpack the model and understand their role.

At the time of inception of School-Link, there was a growing body of information on the protective and risk factors for mental health. Resilience became a buzz word, but what did that really mean? What was the role of the teacher? Assisting schools to understand the skills they could teach to develop resilience improved schools' ability to construct relevant classroom activities. Connection to school was also recognized to be one of the most important protective factors against mental health problems, particularly depression. But what does that mean? How do we achieve it? Schools have struggled with this for years, but with new insight into the factors involved they were assisted to explore new ways to address connection. The School-Link Coordinator's role as a "troubleshooter" or clarifier of concepts and referral pathways helped to raise the profile and improve connections and communication between health and education.

Dedicated Time and Resources

Often with large initiatives rather than a complete rollout, government departments tend to hedge their bets and pilot test the initiative in a small number of areas or – even worse – in one locality. The problem is that then only a small number of sites normally receive the benefit while more money than would be the typical case is poured into these pilot sites. This level of funding is unsustainable or cannot be replicated on a large scale, which makes the initiative look too costly to the funding body. This also tends to increase the disparity between sites and create competition for funds rather than cooperation. Government departments are run on short-term cycles, and it is often the case that pilots never go beyond that, even when they show very good results. This can create disillusionment in the workforce in areas that do not receive funding, as some areas typically attract all the funding.

The strength of the School-Link initiative is that each AHS across the state received the same amount of funding at the same time. This reduced the competitiveness and components such that the training could be rolled out across the state in a streamlined fashion. This consistent rollout also ensured a consistent message and helped to create a ground swell of support. Many School-Link Coordinators facilitated sessions where schools could share ideas and work through solutions to common problems they were facing.

Another strength of the initiative is the dedicated resources allocated to coordination. This includes the time and resources given to meetings at both the state and area/regional level. Both health and education were committed at each level to contribute to the development and ongoing management of the initiative. Having a dedicated coordinator to oversee the process meant that there was someone there who could provide the type of support that is required to assist teachers and clinicians to implement mental health promotion, prevention, and early intervention in a comprehensive way.

The coordinator needs to be of a sufficiently high position in the system to effect change. When the coordinators were not given sufficient power they lacked credibility and were not able to make decisions, thereby frustrating the process.

Team Training and Ongoing Coaching/Learning Community

The statewide training program recognized school and TAFE counselors as the primary mental health support for young people in the educational setting. They are employed by an educational institution whose professional development program is educational in nature. Health services are able to play a role in supporting these key players in mental health not only with professional development but also with a network of support, consultation, and collaboration. Many school counselors commented that it was the first time they really felt supported in their role.

The interdisciplinary nature of the training fostered an improved working relationship between the health and education sector. This training program is the first in Australia that has set out to systematically educate health and education professionals together. Coordinators are encouraged to organize the training around local CAMHS and their cluster of local schools and TAFE Colleges. Approximately 2,000 health and education professionals across the state are trained with the rollout of each module. To ensure that school counselors were able to attend from State schools, the Department of Education made it mandatory for them to attend. It prevented their principal vetoing them from attending. This demonstrates a high level of commitment from education.

Conclusions and Insights

Many mental health programs are currently available to schools. These programs tend to come and go and are usually short-term funded. To progress from improving knowledge and skills to changing practice requires structures in place to support this change. Rather than develop another program, School-Link put into place the infrastructure required to support schools to address mental health on multiple levels.

Often health services become involved in Health-Promoting School projects and are very good at advising schools on health promotion activities. What schools often want from health services is exactly that, health services. The Health-Promoting Schools model involves strengthening the partnerships of health services with schools. In the case of mental health this is particularly true; however, there will never be enough mental health services to meet the demand. Mental health services can support schools in delivering early intervention programs in schools and can play a role in supporting schools counselors to better assist students in the schools settings. This can ensure that more students get the help and support that they need, thereby reducing problems in the school and also reducing the burden on overstretched mental health services.

Long-term investment in coordination is a key feature of School-Link. Often sustainability is expected so that funding can be removed and reallocated to the next priority. The notion of sustainability is fraught with difficulty. The programs that are current today might not work in the future. If we go in and expect schools to continue doing the same thing from here on in, apart from being impractical, it might also be ineffective. Schools need continued support to address issues, someone with the time to keep up to date with the research and the time to research and address arising issues.

One of the successes of the School-Link program is that there is communication between health and education at all three levels of the system. This extended system of communication ensures support at all levels. School-Link Coordinators as drivers and supporters of change play a key role in maintaining communication channels.

It is much easier for principals to agree to become involved in a program if they know that it is supported by their department and they have a credible and trusted coordinator supporting their implementation.

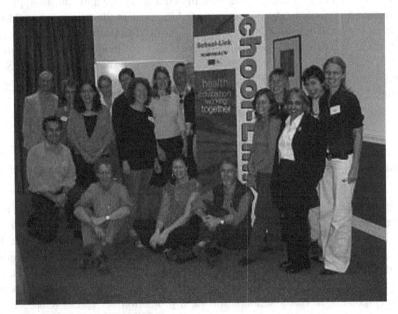

Picture 48 School link coordinators

Acknowledgment The author would like to thank Beverley Raphael, Former Director of the Centre for Mental Health, NSW Health, for having the vision to commence the initiative.

References

Australian Bureau of Statistics. (2007). *Population by age and sex, Australian states and territories, June 2007* (cat. no. 3201.0). Canberra, Australia: Author.

Commonwealth Department of Health and Ageing. (2004). *Responding to the mental health needs of young people in Australia.* Discussion paper: Principles and strategies, Mental Health Branch, National Mental Health Strategy. Canberra, Australia: Commonwealth Department of Health and Ageing.

Jones, J.E., Scanlon, K., Raphael, B., Hillin, A., McAlpine, R., Critchley, A., Stonehouse, R., McKie, D., Kerr-Roubicek, H., & Meerman, G. (2002). Health and education working together: The New South Wales School-Link initiative. *The International Journal of Mental Health Promotion, 4*(4), 36–43.

Maloney, D., Jones, J., Walter, G., & Davenport, R. (2008). Addressing mental health concerns in schools: Does School-Link achieve its aims? *Australasian Psychiatry, 16*(1), 48–53.

NSW Department of Health. (2001). *Getting in early: A framework for early intervention and prevention in mental health for young people in New South Wales.* Sydney, Australia: Author.

Raphael, B. (2000). *Promoting the mental health and wellbeing of children and young people.* Discussion paper: Key principles and directions, National Mental Health Working Group. Canberra, Australia: Commonwealth Department of Health and Aged Care.

Chapter 29
Cook Islands: The "Strengthening Project"

Debi Futter

Contextual Introduction

The Cook Islands is made up of 15 islands and atolls lying in the South Pacific Ocean, south of Hawaii and west of Tahiti. Spread across a zone of nearly 2 million km^2, they comprise a total land area of only 240 km^2. The Cook Islands is a self-governing nation with a population of approximately 15,000 people. Tourism is the major income source for the Cook Islands, with no major export or other income potential.

Spread across these 15 islands are 35 schools. Schooling starts with preschool at 3 years of age and is compulsory until the age of 16.

Overview of the School Health Program

With the health status of youth in the Cook Islands in an alarming position in 2002 (e.g., 32% of secondary school students overweight, mean age of first pregnancy 16 years and 3 months, and 48% of 14-year-olds smoking), the Ministry of Education realized that it needed to play a more central role in addressing these issues with its pupils. The first step began with the employment of a Health and Physical Well-Being Advisor to the curriculum advisory unit of the Cook Islands Ministry of Education. The Cook Islands Health and Physical Well-Being curriculum (CIHPWB) was then developed between 2003 and 2005.

Implementation of the curriculum document has taken the forms of the following:

- Professional development in content and pedagogical knowledge
- Resources to support the curriculum
- Support in the planning, implementation, and evaluation of programs

D. Futter
Ministry of Education, Rarotonga, Cook Islands

C. Vince Whitman and C.E. Aldinger (eds.),
Case Studies in Global School Health Promotion: From Research to Practice,
DOI: 10.1007/978-0-387-92269-0_29, © Springer Science + Business Media, LLC 2009

All schools have developed a plan on how they will implement the two essential learning areas of the curriculum and a 2-year health education long-term plan and an annual physical education long-term plan.

Specific Aspects of Implementation

Curriculum Adapted to the Local Situation

To begin the curriculum development process we required a *Cook Islands definition of health*; we also needed to know what Cook Islanders identified as the barriers to being healthy. Therefore, the curriculum development and consultation process focused on two questions presented to students and adults on different islands:

1. What does being healthy mean to you?
2. What makes it hard to be healthy in the Cook Islands?

Using the results from the consultation process, Cook Island health status statistics, and a multisectoral advisory committee, it was decided that five "key areas of learning" (KAL) would form the basis of the CIHPWB curriculum. These would be mental health, sexuality, food and nutrition, body care and physical safety, and physical activity.

The *Mental Health* KAL focuses on the following:

- Self-worth
- Examining how discrimination and stereotyping affect mental health
- Personal and interpersonal skills to enhance relationships
- Skills to support oneself and others during times of stress, disappointment, and loss
- Drug use and misuse
- Skills to recognize and respond to abuse and harassment
- Benefits of physical activity, relaxation, and recreation on mental health
- Values and attitudes that support the enhancement of mental health for oneself, other people, and society

The *Sexuality* KAL focuses on the following:

- Skills relating to sexual development
- Skills to enhance one's sexual and reproductive health
- Skills to enhance relationships
- Personal and interpersonal skills include the following:
    - The skills needed to examine people's attitudes, values and beliefs, and their rights and responsibilities
    - Attitudes of respect for oneself and other people
    - Attitudes of care and concern for oneself and other people

– Effective communication skills
– Problem solving and decision-making skills

The *Food and Nutrition* KAL focuses on the following:

- Healthy growth and development
- Understanding how nutrition, physical activity, and well-being are related
- Cultural significance of food
- Skills for selecting, preparing, and preserving food
- Meeting nutritional needs on a limited budget
- Preparing food successfully and safely
- Healthy eating patterns and the factors that influence food choices and food preparation methods

The *Body Care and Physical Safety* KAL focuses on the following:

- Personal body care
- Taking responsibility for one's own physical well-being and that of other people
- Knowledge and skills for the prevention of illness, injury, infection, disease, and common lifestyle disorders
- Practical ways of caring for oneself and other people during times of illness, injury or accident, and rehabilitation
- Identifying and managing environmental hazards
- Avoiding or minimizing harm to oneself and others
- Learning emergency procedures for managing risk situations

The *Physical Activity* KAL focuses on enjoying and encouraging participation in physical activity for life! It includes the following:

- Movement skills for physical competence, enjoyment, a sense of self-worth, and an active lifestyle
- Personal and interpersonal skills to strengthen one's awareness of personal identity and to enhance one's sense of self-worth and relationships with other people
- Knowledge and understanding of the importance of cultural practices in physical activities
- Knowledge and understanding of the significance of social influences on physical activity
- One's own values, attitudes, behaviors, and actions in physical activity settings

The curriculum has a health promotion philosophy (*Pito'enua*) that links it to Cook Islands culture, traditions, and values through the use of a *vaka* (Fig. 1) to represent the four dimensions of health in the Ottawa Charter – mental and emotional, physical, spiritual, and social. We have added a fifth dimension – environment.

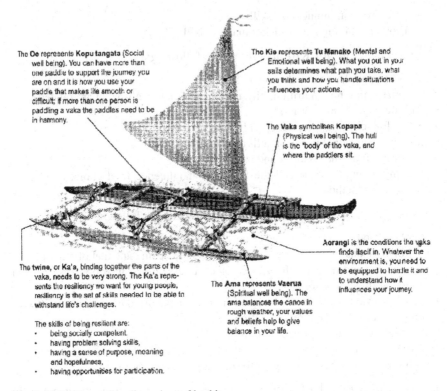

The **Oe** represents **Kopu tangata** (Social well being). You can have more than one paddle to support the journey you are on and it is how you use your paddle that makes life smooth or difficult; if more than one person is paddling a vaka the paddles need to be in harmony.

The **Kie** represents **Tu Manako** (Mental and Emotional well being). What you put in your sails determines what path you take, what you think and how you handle situations influences your actions.

The **Vaka** symbolises **Kopapa** (Physical well being). The hull is the "body" of the vaka, and where the paddlers sit.

Aorangi is the conditions the vaka finds itself in. Whatever the environment is, you need to be equipped to handle it and to understand how it influences your journey.

The twine, or **Ka'a**, binding together the parts of the vaka, needs to be very strong. The Ka'a represents the resiliency we want for young people, resiliency is the set of skills needed to be able to withstand life's challenges.

The skills of being resilient are:
- being socially competent.
- having problem solving skills,
- having a sense of purpose, meaning and hopefulness,
- having opportunities for participation.

The **Ama** represents **Vaerua** (Spiritual well being). The ama balances the canoe in rough weather, your values and beliefs help to give balance in your life.

Fig. 1 Vaka representing dimensions of health

Collaboration Between Ministry of Education and Ministry of Health

As part of the implementation of the curriculum document, the Ministry of Education and the Ministry of Health have been working closely together in many different ways. One example of this is a pilot project aiming to address obesity through physical activity in a school population of children aged 5–16 years in the Cook Islands. The pilot was initiated in 2004 as a collaborative effort of the Cook Islands Ministry of Education Health Education Advisor, the Ministry of Health Nutritionist, and the Papa'aroa School on the island of Rarotonga. The Papa'aroa School is a Seventh Day Adventist school, which begins at preschool and finishes at grade 11 or approximately 15 years of age.

During the development of the program, in what was a first for the Pacific, a memorandum of understanding was signed between the Ministry of Education and the Ministry of Health. This mutual agreement was fundamental in allowing the two ministries to collaborate on the project, fully utilizing the strengths of both organizations while also respecting the differences. Previously both ministries had tended to follow their own work plans without collaboration or consultation with each other. This often led to a double-up of work loads addressing similar issues, to programs unsupported (due to lack of consultation within the education), to unsuitable timing by the Ministry of Health in some of their work programs (due to the education sector having other priorities), and – at times – schools not fully supporting (due to lack of understanding) the work of the Ministry of Health.

The "Newstart" Program

Eighty schoolchildren participated in the program, which used the health promotion philosophy of the CIHPWB curriculum as a basis for all activities. The Papa'aroa School decided that it wanted to address not just the physical health of its students but the other four dimensions of well-being as well. Initially, the teaching staff, the Health and Physical Well-Being Advisor, and the Public Health Nutritionist worked together to develop a health education long-term plan and a physical education long-term plan for teachers to follow. These long-term plans became the basis for teacher planning, teaching, and learning programs. The long-term plans were based on the 2004 draft version of the CIHPWB Curriculum, which was gazetted as the official curriculum document for Health and Physical Education in the Cook Islands in 2007. The teachers named the pilot project the "Newstart" program, as it was attempting to change some behaviors for everyone in the school, not only the students, but also the teachers. The program was funded by the Secretariat of the Pacific Community (SPC) and was implemented over 10 months between February and December.

The focus for the Newstart Program was *enjoyment, confidence building, full participation, and skill development* in the areas of physical activity and health education.

Health education was taught during each school term for 3–4 weeks, with three to four 45-min lessons per week during that time. Topics covered were determined by the curriculum, including areas such as food and nutrition, mental health, making good choices, handling change, loss and grief, sexuality education, and self-worth.

Physical education sessions were conducted three times a week *all year*, including two lessons on skill development and one on school sports. The topics of these lessons, also determined by the curriculum, covered contexts such as large-and small-ball skills, aquatics, running, jumping, and throwing activities. Daily fitness sessions were conducted for 15 min immediately before lunch.

Teacher Resources and Professional Development

The Ministry of Health, the Ministry of Education, and the pilot school collaborated to facilitate program implementation, by developing a long-term plan of teaching programs/units of work to cover physical activity and health education topics. This included the creation of specialized teacher resources, such as a Health and Physical Education curriculum document and teacher planning resources, covering the many topics mentioned earlier. Professional development opportunities in physical activity were held for teachers of the pilot school, and teachers from other schools in the community were also invited. These opportunities comprised several after-school workshops to look at specific lessons that could be taken with students in different topics (e.g., fitness activities, ball skills, aquatics, athletics). The teachers who came to these workshops received a planning resource and a lecture, and then participated in the actual activities they would share with their own children. The Health and Physical Education Advisor also modeled teaching of health and physical education lessons to teachers who requested this support, and also observed and gave feedback to teachers when requested.

The purchase of physical education equipment was required to enable the teachers to have all children participate at all times during their physical education lessons. Previously the school had very limited balls, bats, ropes, etc. The teachers and Health and Physical Education Advisor went through the newly developed Physical Education long-term plan and created a list of equipment that would help the lessons to be implemented with maximum participation of all students. SPC funded the purchase of this equipment.

To enhance the types of food being offered to students and staff from the school canteen, some cooking equipment was purchased for preparation of healthy alternatives, such as a popcorn maker, a rice cooker, and a toasted-sandwich maker; this, too, was funded through the SPC. The Public Health Nutritionist worked with parents and staff to show them how to prepare such food as butter-free popcorn, juice ice blocks, a variety of sandwiches to appeal to children, and toasted sandwiches. Drinks available were limited to water, milk, flavored milk, and juices.

Adaptation and Awareness Raising

Special care was taken to tailor the program to schoolchildren; this included recognizing the pilot school's religious beliefs/foundation and the sensitivity needed when addressing the issue of overweight and obesity in the Cook Islands.

Information on the rationale and program goals was disseminated to the public via mass media. The principal of the school was interviewed for the television, as were teachers. They discussed what they were trying to do and why. Footage was shown of children participating in swimming lessons and using the new physical activity resources.

The parent community awareness of the program was raised through school newsletters, by a display board at parent/school events to show the statistics of the health checks of their children, by giving out information to parents about alternative school lunch ingredients, and through church announcements.

Physical activity levels increased in the pilot school as a result of this project; these increases were sustained following program completion, and they still continued in 2007. Formal evaluation examining changes in student's health status (height, weight, blood pressure, and waist circumference), activity levels, dietary intake, dietary preferences, and attitudes to healthy choices showed an improvement in attitudes, knowledge base, and ideas about making healthy choices; however, the health status stayed almost the same.

Conclusions and Insights

We learned the following lessons:

- The development of an in-country definition of health or well-being is *essential* to develop ownership by teachers, parents, and the community.
- A consultation process is imperative to providing the rationale in what should be included in a Health and Physical Education curriculum document, especially if there are some political agendas for exclusion (e.g., sexuality education).
- The use of traditional verses, analogies, or concepts creates a cultural anchor for the curriculum, which, in turn, enhances understanding for students, teachers, and the community.
- Partnerships are complex: A Memorandum of Understanding is important for defining roles and working to strengths, especially in a small nation where resources are limited. Success still depends on the right people being willing and able to work together. Leaders of organizations need to help this happen.
- The Newstart program taught us that ministries can work together successfully ☺!
- Creating understanding with teachers of *why* health education and physical education is important provides motivation for schools to adapt their timetables and practices.
- Teachers and schools need major, ongoing support to change if they have not had any preservice training in the areas of Health Education or Physical Education. (No Cook Islands teachers have had any comprehensive preservice teacher training in either of these two subjects.)
- Change of practice takes a long time, especially when both *content* and *pedagogical* strategies are new.
- Modeling and mentoring of best practices help Pacific teachers to feel confident to try new ways.
- If team teaching with Ministry of Health and Ministry of Education staff with classroom teachers is to be used, roles must be clearly defined. Otherwise, Ministry personnel are seen as "the experts" who can unintentionally intimidate teachers trying to implement new teaching strategies.
- From the Ministry of Health's perspective, having a focal point in the Ministry of Education curriculum unit was imperative.
- Cofacilitating professional development helped people from both Ministries appreciate and develop a respect for one another's roles.

Acknowledgments We acknowledge the support of the Papa'aroa School, the Ministry of Health, the Ministry of Education, and the Secretariat of the Pacific Community. This chapter was written with support from Karen Tairea.

Index